Lecture Notes in Computer Science   10347

Commenced Publication in 1973
Founding and Former Series Editors:
Gerhard Goos, Juris Hartmanis, and Jan van Leeuwen

More information about this series at http://www.springer.com/series/7409

Hsinchun Chen · Daniel Dajun Zeng
Elena Karahanna · Indranil Bardhan (Eds.)

Smart Health

International Conference, ICSH 2017
Hong Kong, China, June 26–27, 2017
Proceedings

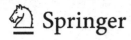 Springer

Editors

Hsinchun Chen
University of Arizona
Tucson, AZ
USA

Daniel Dajun Zeng
University of Arizona
Tucson, AZ
USA

Elena Karahanna
Department of Management Information
    System
University of Georgia
Athens, GA
USA

Indranil Bardhan
University of Texas
Richardson, TX
USA

ISSN 0302-9743   ISSN 1611-3349 (electronic)
Lecture Notes in Computer Science
ISBN 978-3-319-67963-1   ISBN 978-3-319-67964-8   (eBook)
https://doi.org/10.1007/978-3-319-67964-8

Library of Congress Control Number: 2017957536

LNCS Sublibrary: SL3 – Information Systems and Applications, incl. Internet/Web, and HCI

Printed on acid-free paper

This Springer imprint is published by Springer Nature
The registered company is Springer International Publishing AG
The registered company address is: Gewerbestrasse 11, 6330 Cham, Switzerland

Preface

Advancing informatics for health care and health-care applications has become an international research priority. There is increased effort to leverage information systems and data analytics to transform reactive care to proactive and preventive care, clinic-centric to patient-centered practice, training-based interventions to globally aggregated evidence, and episodic response to continuous well-being monitoring and maintenance. The annual International Conference for Smart Health (ICSH), which originated in 2013, intends to provide a forum for the growing international smart health research community to discuss the technical, practical, economic, behavioral, and social issues associated with smart health.

ICSH 2017 focused on studies on the principles, approaches, models, frameworks, new applications, and effects of using novel information technology to address health-care problems and improve social welfare. It successfully attracted scholars working on medical data/text mining and analytics, health community and social media, mobile health care, and economic impact and behaviors in health care. We are pleased that many high-quality papers were submitted, accompanied by evaluations with real-world data or application contexts. The work presented at the conference encompassed a healthy mix of different disciplines.

ICSH 2017 was held in Hong Kong SAR, China. The two-day event encompassed presentations of 31 papers. The organizers of ICSH 2017 would like to thank the conference sponsors for their support and sponsorship, including Hong Kong RGC Theme-based Research Project No. T32-102/14 N, City University of Hong Kong (the Information Systems Department as well as the Systems Engineering and Engineering Management Department) and the INFORMS College on Artificial Intelligence (CAI). We further wish to express our sincere gratitude to all Program Committee members of ICSH 2017, who provided valuable and constructive reviews. We further wish to express our sincere gratitude to all our sponsors.

December 2017

Hsinchun Chen
Elena Karahanna
Daniel Zeng

Organization

Conference Co-chairs

Hsinchun Chen   University of Arizona, USA
Elena Karahanna   University of Georgia, USA
Daniel Zeng   University of Arizona, and Chinese Academy
     of Sciences, China

Program Co-chairs

Indranil Bardhan   University of Texas at Dallas, USA
Jiexun Li   Western Washington University, USA
Xin Li   City University of Hong Kong SAR, China

Workshop Co-chairs

Hsin-Min Lu   National Taiwan University, Taiwan
Yu Tong   City University of Hong Kong SAR, China
Qingpeng Zhang   City University of Hong Kong SAR, China

Honorary Co-chairs

Youhua (Frank) Chen   City University of Hong Kong SAR, China
Choonling Sia   City University of Hong Kong SAR, China
Kwok Leung Tsui   City University of Hong Kong SAR, China
Weiguo (Patrick) Fan   Virginia Tech, USA
Ting-Peng Liang   National Sun Yat-Sen University, Taiwan

Publication Co-chairs

Hsin-Min Lu   National Taiwan University, Taiwan
Xiaolong Zheng   Chinese Academy of Sciences, China

Publicity Co-chair

Qingpeng Zhang   City University of Hong Kong SAR, China

Local Arrangements Chair

Yu Tong   City University of Hong Kong SAR, China

Program Committee

Muhammad Amith	Texas Medical Center, USA
Mohd Anwar	North Carolina A&T State University, USA
Ian Brooks	University of Illinois at Urbana-Champaign, USA
Zhidong Cao	Chinese Academy of Sciences, China
Xiaohui Chang	Oregon State University, USA
Michael Chau	University of Hong Kong SAR, China
Chien-Chin Chen	National Taiwan University, Taiwan
Guanling Chen	University of Massachusetts Lowell, USA
Xiaofeng Chen	Western Washington University, USA
Tingru Cui	University of Wollongong, Australia
Yimeng Deng	National University of Singapore, Singapore
Shaokun Fan	Oregon State University, USA
Qianjing Feng	Southern Medical University, China
Yuan Feng	Technische Universiteit, The Netherlands
Wai-Tat Fu	University of Illinois at Urbana-Champaign, USA
Xu Han	University of Connecticut, USA
Hung-Yu Kao	National Cheng Kung University, Taiwan
Kyoji Kawagoe	Ritsumeikan University, Japan
Dan Ke	Wuhan University, China
Erhun Kundakcioglu	Özyeğin University, Turkey
Juhee Kwon	City University of Hong Kong SAR, China
Jia Li	East China University of Science and Technology, China
Jiao Li	Chinese Academy of Medical Sciences, China
Mingyang Li	University of South Florida, USA
Yan Li	Harbin Institute of Technology, China
Yunji Liang	University of Arizona, USA
Yi-Ling Lin	National Chengchi University, Taiwan
Yu-Kai Lin	Florida State University, USA
Ben Liu	City University of Hong Kong SAR, China
Hongyan Liu	Tsinghua University, China
Na Liu	The University of Sydney, Australia
Xiao Liu	University of Utah, USA
Xuan Liu	East China University of Science and Technology, China
Yong Liu	Chinese Academy of Sciences, China
Zhong Lu	City University of Hong Kong SAR, China
James Ma	University of Colorado, Colorado Springs, USA
Deepti Mehrotra	Amity University, India
Mevludin Memedi	Dalarna University, Sweden
Riccardo Miotto	Icahn School of Medicine at Mount Sinai, USA
Jin-Cheon Na	Nanyang Technological University, Singapore
Radhakrishnan Nagarajan	University of Kentucky, USA
W. Nick Street	The University of Iowa, USA

Contents

Online Community

Predictive Diagnosis

Data/Text Mining in Healthcare

Poster Papers

Economic, Social, and Behavioral Concerns on Smart Health

Leveraging Social Norms and Implementation Intentions for Better Health

Che-Wei Liu[(⊠)], Weiguang Wang[(⊠)], Guodong (Gordon) Gao[(⊠)],
and Ritu Agarwal[(⊠)]

University of Maryland, College Park, USA
{cwliu, weiguangwang, ggao, ragarwal}@rhsmith.umd.edu

Abstract. One in eleven adults worldwide suffers from diabetes, and the disease accounts for 12% of global health expenditure(http://www.idf.org/about-diabetes/facts-figures). Although self-management and monitoring are critical for general control of the disease and for preventing diabetes-related complications, most patients fail to adhere to self-management regimens. We study what type of external intervention will amplify the self-monitoring frequency of Type-2 diabetes (T2d) patients. We conducted a randomized field experiment on a mobile health application with more than 500 T2d patients, and tested two well-known mechanisms for behavior change: social norms, and implementation intentions. Further, we combined social norms and implementation intentions and tested whether these two mechanisms can complement each other. Our results show that individuals who receive a message containing both social norms and implementation intentions perform the best in regard to self-monitoring. Our research paves the way to further investigate how different mechanisms may be combined to help users' form healthy habits.

Keywords: Social norms · Implementation intentions · Mobile health · Diabetes

1 Introduction

Self-management in diabetes is essential and especially useful in the prevention and detection of diabetes complications [1]. The process of self-monitoring of blood glucose (SMBG) is to collect blood sugar levels at different time points over a period of a time, so that a patient can identify high levels of blood sugar in a timely fashion and take corrective action [2]. In the past, typically patients would use a glucometer to measure blood sugar levels, and then manually record the values. Today, with the help of smart devices, patients can track their blood glucose with significantly lower effort. Forming a habit of SMBG has proven to be effective for both Type-1 diabetes (T1d) and Type-2 diabetes (T2d) patients because it enables more appropriate insulin dosage and a deeper understanding of the factors that affect their condition [3, 4]. However, despite the considerable effectiveness of self-monitoring, adherence to a consistent regimen has been found to be very challenging for many individuals. The barriers that impede regular self-monitoring range from insufficient knowledge to low self-efficacy [5, 6]. Karter et al. [3] show that patients' adherence to the recommended frequency of

© Springer International Publishing AG 2017
H. Chen et al. (Eds.): ICSH 2017, LNCS 10347, pp. 3–14, 2017.
https://doi.org/10.1007/978-3-319-67964-8_1

self-monitoring is roughly 34% for T1d patients, 54% for insulin-treated T2d, and 20% for oral agent only-treated T2d.

To the degree that SMBG is a key to controlling glycemic levels, it is imperative to improve patients' perceptions and actions related to adherence. The American Diabetes Association (ADA) recommends that measurements be taken 3 to 4 times a day for T1d and a minimum of once a day for T2d by [7]. Technologies such as mobile applications offer a unique opportunity for clinicians to increase patients' self-monitoring behaviors by providing a range of useful features. With the help of mobile applications, tedious procedures to manually record blood glucose can be eliminated. Additionally, most mobile health applications can set reminders, create spreadsheets, and generate graphs to help patients better understand their conditions. However, the biggest challenge for most mobile health applications is the sustainability of usage. According to a recent study[1], less than 15% of users of mobile health applications continued using the app beyond the first 7 days. Users who download the mobile health applications to record their blood glucose indicate that they do have intentions to monitor their blood glucose, but most people are unable to persist in using the apps. The gap between intentions and actual behaviors has been widely observed in the field, especially in health-related contexts [8]. Further, even when users continually use the mobile application, most T2d patients measure their blood glucose substantially less often than the recommended level of once a day.

In this study, we collaborated with one of leading diabetes monitoring mobile application providers in Taiwan to examine the effects of mobile messages on users' SMBG behaviors. Our goal was to motivate users who are underperforming relative to the recommended level of SMBG prior to treatment. We tested two mechanisms that have demonstrated efficacy in prior research for changing individual behaviors: social norms, and implementation intentions. The social norms approach is a well-studied mechanism whose aim is to motivate individuals by telling them what the majority of others do. Fundamentally, the social norms information is instrumental in initiating the psychological process of a desire for conformity, and individuals will seek to mimic what others within their referent group are doing. Implementation intentions, also known as an "if-then plan" [9], exert the power of environmental contexts. Once individuals develop an if-then plan, they are likely to do what they plan to do when they encounter similar contexts that have been articulated in advance. For instance, an individual might make the following plan: "If I finish work by 4:30 pm during a weekday, I will take a 30-minute walk." Once she finishes work at the time designated in the plan, she has a higher inclination and likelihood of going out for a walk.

We examine whether social norms and implementation intentions complement each other to help increase SMBG among T2d patients. Our expectation for such an effect is predicated on two reasons. First, a social norm constitutes an external motivation driving individuals to conform to the majority, but it might not always yield the desired outcomes. Often, social norms may succeed in correcting individuals' misperceptions about what others do, but fail to change their behaviors [10]. That is, social norms help

[1] Mobile benchmark Q3 2016 by "adjust" https://www.adjust.com/downloads/resources/mobile-benchmarks-q3-2016.pdf.

individuals realize what would be a feasible goal if they act like the majority of others, but do not necessarily specify a feasible *path* or guidance for accomplishing the goal (in our case, reaching the recommended number of self-measurements). Implementation intentions can play a role in overcoming this limitation and are especially beneficial when individuals have a strong goal commitment [9]. The implementation intentions provide users an "if-then" plan, which facilitates goal achievement. Therefore, the implementation intentions would complement social norms by providing situational cues that allow the individual to more easily conform to the average behavior of the reference group. Second, for implementation intentions to be realized effectively, it is imperative to select an effective goal-directed behavior. A measurement of blood glucose is a reasonable goal-directed behavior. Although it is possible to ask a user to set up when, where, and how to measure their blood glucose, the exact number of times one should measure in a week might not be clear enough for most patients. Therefore, social norms information can help individuals to set up a more realistic goal that fits the standard for the majority of others, thereby aiding individuals to adjust their "if-then" plans to achieve such goals.

To examine the theorized complementarity, we conducted a randomized field experiment using different push notifications. The control notification message is a standard message that reminds users how many measurements they took last week. The social norms message (SN) exerts the power of conformity by communicating the average number of measurements taken last week by T2d patients who use the application. The implementation intentions message (II) asks individuals to set up an if-then plan that specifies how many times they expect to measure in the following week, and when and where they will take the measurement. Finally, the combined social norms and implementation intentions message (SN+II) includes both social norms information and an if-then plan. As expected, we find that individuals in the control group barely improve the number of measurements taken after receiving the message. Both SN and II groups experience modest improvements as compared to the control group. By combining the SN and II message, we find a further increase in users' measurement frequency. Although the results are statistically only marginally significant, they are entirely consistent with the theoretical arguments. The findings offer useful insight on the potential gains from combining multiple mechanisms to improve users' SMBG behaviors. Our granular analysis paves the way to further examine the complex interaction between social norms and implementation intentions.

2 Literature Review

2.1 Social Norms

Social marketing approaches that harness the power of social norms have grown in popularity. Burchell et al. [11] define social marketing as an application of a program that aims to influence the behavior of target audiences in order to improve welfare. Individuals would conform to a norm because doing so might elicit the approval of the group and deviating from the norm might result in sanctions or punishment [12]. Substantial evidence has shown the effects of social norms on individuals' behaviors in diverse contexts. Allcott [13] conducted a randomized field experiment and demonstrated that a social norms treatment reduces energy consumption by 2%. Goldstein et al. [14] demonstrated that appeals incorporating descriptive norms can increase environmental protection for hotel guests more than the traditional appeals.

Social norms would be especially beneficial for T2d patients whose measurement frequency is lower than recommended because arguably they are the ones who need a proper guideline the most. It may be the case that individuals who under-measure their blood glucose simply do not have a correct understanding of appropriate measurement frequency. By exposing such low-intensity users to the social norm, we help them form a better understanding of the average measurement frequency for T2d patients in the online community.

2.2   Implementation Intentions

It is important to note that implementation intentions are distinct from goal intentions. While goal intentions indicate a desired future outcome that one wants to reach, implementation intentions have the following structure: if situation A occurs, then I will perform the goal-related response B. Formally, implementation intentions define when, where, and how one wants to act on one's goal intentions [9]. Implementation intentions exert the power of psychological mechanisms that create a mental link such that when individuals encounter an 'if' situation, they perform the subsequent 'then' action as planned before [17]. Such if-then plans have shown a moderate improvement of behaviors in various contexts such as influenza vaccination [18], voting rates [19], and weight loss [20]. Implementation intentions are especially useful when combined with a plan reminder because the reminder could increase the accessibility of the environmental cue [21]. Prestwich et al. [22] combined implementation intentions and SMS text messages to test their joint effect on exercise, and found that the effect of implementation intentions is enhanced when combined with plan reminders. Low-intensity T2d patients could plausibly benefit from implementation intentions because these individuals may lack a plan to properly measure their blood glucose.

2.3   Complementarity Between Social Norms and Implementation Intention

We propose the existence of a complementary between social norms and implementation intentions based on the theory of planned behavior (TPB) [23]. Attitude, subjective norm, and perceived behavioral control are postulated to determine an intention to perform a behavior. Despite decades of research using TPB for explaining health-related behaviors, a well-documented intention-behavior gap has persisted [24, 25]. Orbeil et al. [26] examined the integration of implementation intentions with TPB, and showed that implementation intentions do supplement intention to perform behaviors. Gollwitzer [27] specified that implementation intentions are volitional, which means that the effectiveness of implementation intentions builds on top of the presence of intention. Blanchard [28] found that intention significantly predicts implementation intentions, and underscored the importance of developing an action plan to translate intention into behavior. Trafimow [29] defined subjective norm as "opinion about what important others believe the individual should do", which has its roots in normative beliefs. The subjective norm is conceptually similar to social norms, which reflect the "beliefs about how one ought to act based on expectations of what other people would morally approve or disapprove [30, 31]". Therefore, sending a social norms message might change individuals' perception of what most others do, and in turn change individuals' intentions to increase their number of measurements, which would then be supplemented by implementation intentions to achieve the desired behavior.

3 Experimental Design

3.1 Research Context

To test the effect of different mechanisms on individuals' SMBG, we conducted a randomized field experiment. Following the recommendations of List and Rasul [32] in designing the experiment, we ensured that we were able to avoid the undesirable Hawthorne effect [33], also known as the observer effect, in which individuals may change their behaviors because they know they are under observation rather than as a response to the treatment. In our setting, the mobile application allows us to observe individuals' measurement behaviors before and after the treatments, and the participants are not aware that they are under observation.

Our research partner is one of the leading mobile healthcare providers in Taiwan. Its primary business focuses on providing a healthcare platform that incorporates mobile, digital health and cloud services for diabetes patients. The specific mobile application for our study offers a personalized care service to track individuals' blood glucose values and daily activities. Users who use the mobile application can input information such as blood glucose, blood pressure, weight, diet, medicine, and mood, accompanied by notes and photos to keep a complete record. The app also allows users to review their past blood glucose, blood pressure, and weight, and provides a trend tracking feature to visually detect any abnormal records. Beyond these basic functions, the mobile application also allows users to invite their family, friends, or even care providers to assist them in monitoring their status. The app comes with a smart cable which allows users to easily synchronize the records in the glucometer to the mobile application without tedious manual input.

3.2 Experiment Design

The two mechanisms included in our experiment are social norms and implementation intentions; we test their individual and joint effects on the SMBG behavior of T2d patients. For the social norms message, there is a well-known boomerang effect [16], where individuals who perform better than the norm tend to perform worse after receiving the treatment. To avoid this adverse outcome, we focus only on users whose SMBG is lower than the norm before the treatment. The norm on our mobile app for the week just prior to the experiment was 5.5. Therefore, we target users whose number of measurements in one week is below 5.5 before the treatment. To ensure that we avoid new users and those who are inactive, we select users who have been registered for at least one month, have had at least one measurement record in the past two weeks before treatment, and have read at least one message that the app provider sent in the two weeks prior to the treatment.

We randomly assigned users who qualified as specified above to one of four groups: (a) control group, (b) social norms (SN) group, (c) implementation intentions (II) group, and (d) social norms + implementation intentions (SN+II) group. All the individuals received push notifications, and needed to click the push notification to launch the mobile application to read the full message. Table 1 shows the messages sent to the individuals in each group. The control group received a customized reminder message, which mentioned the number of times the message recipient measured his/her blood glucose in the past 7 days. Individuals in the other three groups receive the same message, augmented with additional specific information based on the particular group the individual is in. For the SN group, the control message is augmented with information about the average number of measurements taken by T2d patients like them. For the implementation intentions group, individuals received a message encouraging them to set a plan to help them measure their blood glucose. Finally, for the social norms + implementation intentions group, individuals received both social norms related information and implementation intentions related information.

Table 1. Experimental messages

	N/A	Social norms
N/A	(Group 1: Control Group) Hi [first name], are you disappointed by your self-monitoring frequency? In the past 7days, you measured your blood glucose X times	(Group 2: Social Norms Group) Hi [first name], are you disappointed by your self-monitoring frequency? In the past 7 days, you measured your blood glucose X times. On average, Type II diabetes users who are like you in Health2Sync measure their blood glucose 5.5 times a week
Implementation intention	(Group 3: Implementation Intentions Group) Hi [first name], are you disappointed by your self-monitoring frequency? In the past 7 days, you measured your blood glucose X times. Many people find it helpful to make a plan. Click here to make your plan	(Group 4: Social Norms + Implementation Intentions Group) Hi [first name], are you disappointed by your self-monitoring frequency? In the past 7days, you measured your blood glucose X times. On average, Type II diabetes users who like you in Health2Sync measure their blood glucose 5.5 times a week. Many people find it helpful to make a plan. Click here to make your plan

Individuals in groups 3 and 4 who are willing to make a plan would click a link to the implementation intentions page. Table 2 shows the detailed information contained on that page. We asked individuals their measurement goal for the forthcoming week. We also asked individuals to construct a simple plan by indicating the dates, time, and locations they would perform the measurements. Finally, we asked about the extent of commitment to the plan they made.

Table 2. Implementation intentions page

An important goal for diabetes patients is to regularly measure their own blood glucose. The following questions will help you make a measurement plan for the following week to help you achieve the goal.

Please carefully think about the number of times you would like to measure your blood glucose next week. (total of 10 options)

1	2	3	4	5	6	7	8	9	>=10
o	o	o	o	o	o	o	o	o	o

In order to achieve your goal, we recommend you set up a simple plan. Please indicate which day you are able to measure your blood glucose (select all that apply).

Everyday	Mon.	Tue.	Wed.	Thu.	Fri.	Sat.	Sun.
□	□	□	□	□	□	□	□

Among the days you select, please contemplate when you feel it will be convenient to measure your blood glucose.

Get up	Before Breakfast	After Breakfast	Before Lunch	After Lunch	Before Dinner	After Dinner	At bed time	Midnight	Others
□	□	□	□	□	□	□	□	□	□

Among the days you select, please contemplate where you feel it will be convenient to measure your blood glucose.

Living room	Bed room	Study room	Kitchen	Restaurant	Restroom	Office	Others
□	□	□	□	□	□	□	□

Now you have made a feasible plan for the next week, please tell us how committed you are to this plan.

1 Not at all committed	2 Somewhat committed	3 Moderately committed	4 Very committed	5 Totally committed
o	o	o	o	o

We conducted our experiment at 16:40 pm on January 8th, 2017. Individuals who qualified for participation received the push notification for the group they were in. Since the process of assigning individuals to each group is purely random, individuals' performance should be orthogonal to the group, which means the assignment would be independent of users' preferences and capabilities.

3.3 Data

Since we are interested in estimating the effects of the push notifications for each message, we need to exclude users who do not read the message during the treatment period. Initially, we have 1,024 individuals in the experiment. Elimination of individuals who do not read the message during the treatment period results in a sample of 586 individuals across the four groups. The number of users in each group is spread relatively evenly, accounting for 25.2%, 22.7%, 26.6%, and 25.4% of the total sample.

All individuals receive the same push notifications before entering into the mobile application. This design avoids self-selection issue of clicking. As might be expected for T2d patients, the sample of users is middle-aged, with an average age of 51.9 years. Females constitute 35.7% of the sample, while average experience using the mobile application is 245.1 days.

Table 3 presents summary statistics for each group. We conducted a series of ANOVA tests on multiple characteristics as a randomization check. We checked for significant differences in the number of measurements in the pre-treatment period, age, gender (% of female), and tenure on this mobile application. The F-statistics in Table 3 confirms that randomization successfully produced balanced groups with no statistically significant differences among them.

Table 3. Summary statistics

	Control	Social norms	Implementation intention	SN+II	F-Stat
N	148	133	156	149	
# of measurement in pre-treatment	1.86 (1.37)	1.62 (1.27)	1.79 (1.26)	1.73 (1.48)	0.47
Age	53.02 (12.02)	51.34 (11.91)	52.14 (10.97)	51.13 (10.85)	0.49
Gender (female)	0.32 (0.47)	0.44 (0.50)	0.34 (0.48)	0.33 (0.47)	0.12
App tenure	239.18 (163.48)	235.33 (160.48)	247.08 (176.14)	257.81 (177.14)	0.69

Note: Standard deviation in parentheses

4 Results

4.1 Experimental Results

The key outcome of interest is the difference between the number of measurements taken in the pretreatment and posttreatment weeks. This difference is summarized for the four groups in Fig. 1. Individuals in the control group have the smallest improvement, which is roughly equal to 0.21 times per week. By contrast, all three treatment groups show higher improvement than the control group. Individuals in the social norms group improve 0.42 times, and individuals in the implementation intention group improve 0.29 times. As theorized, combining the social norms and implementation intentions message leads to the best outcome. Individuals in the social norms + implementation intentions group improve a striking 0.47 times after receiving the message.

Although the results in Fig. 1 are not statistically strong, they highlight the potential value of combining different mechanisms to change users' behaviors. Figure 2 shows a more granular analysis for SN, II, and SN+II groups. Since individuals in the SN group do not have an option to set a plan, all the individuals are regarded as having no plan. The SN group therefore serves as the baseline group for this analysis. As can be seen, individuals in the II group obviously experience a selection effect.

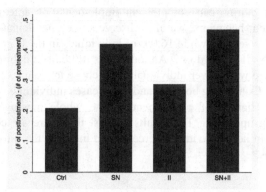

Fig. 1. Treatment effects

Those who set up a plan perform better than those do not set up a plan. If we compare those individuals to the individuals in the SN group, we can see that making a plan clearly polarizes individuals' performance. Individuals who are not affected by the implementation intentions message perform worse than the individuals in the social norm group, but individuals who are motivated by the implementation intentions message perform better.

If we combine the social norms and implementation message, we detect a strong complementary effect. Individuals in the SN+II group, regardless of whether they have a plan, perform at least equal to or even better than the individuals in the social norms group. This means that social norms can complement the effects of implementation intention. Individuals who set up a plan in the SN+II group perform well because they now have a guideline to follow. Interestingly, even individuals who do not set up a plan in the SN+II group perform well. Although they ignore the plan, it appears that they were still motivated by the social norms message. Therefore, when combining social norms messaging with forming an implementation intention, we observe the best way to improve individuals' measurement behaviors.

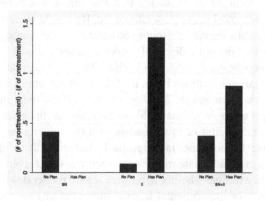

Fig. 2. The effects of Implementation Intentions

Although social norms can complement implementation intentions to improve patients' measurement behaviors, we also observe some unanticipated and somewhat surprising effects. We see that while 16.0% of individuals in the II group set up a plan, only 9.4% in the SN+II group do so. Although it is difficult to definitively answer the question of why there were fewer individuals who chose to set up a plan, we offer one possible conjecture. Combining both SN and II increases individuals' cognitive burden, which reduces the chances of comprehending the whole message and lowers the likelihood of setting up a plan. The results suggest that there are considerable complexity and nuance in how individuals perceive and interpret the information provided in push notifications.

5 Discussion

Mobile health applications offer a great opportunity for researchers and practitioners to orchestrate low-cost interventions to change users' behaviors. In this study, we examined the effects of two well-known mechanisms – social norms and implementation intentions – on motivating T2d patients' SMBG behavior. SMBG is vital to managing one of the world's most pervasive chronic diseases effectively. We combined both social norms and implementation intentions into one intervention and examined whether these two mechanisms complement each other. Our empirical study involved a randomized field experiment where different push notifications were sent to T2d patients in a mobile health application. As expected, both social norms and implementation intentions groups perform better than the control group. We find a complementarity between social norms and implementation intentions: individuals exposed to the combined message perform the best. Our granular analysis shows that individuals perform better than individuals in the pure social norms group when they set up an if-then plan. Even individuals who do not set up a plan have a roughly equal magnitude of improvement when compared to individuals in the pure social norms group.

Our study provides several insights and opportunities for future research. First, although the differences among groups in our randomized field experiment are not statistically strong enough to draw a firm conclusion, they are certainly suggestive of the power of combining multiple mechanisms to transform user's behaviors in domains such as SMBG that are notorious for low adherence. Researchers can also explore other combinations to test substitutive and complementary effects among different factors such as loss aversion or default rules [34]. Second, despite the lack of statistical significance in our experimental results, we hesitate to conclude that combining social norms and implementation intentions is not useful. We interpret our results with caution because our sample has, on average, 245 days of usage of the focal mobile application. For this length of app usage, it is reasonable to assume that these are committed users who have likely formed a habit of low measurement over a long period of time. Their behaviors might have become inertial, ingrained, and difficult to change, with push notifications alone being inadequate motivators. Future research could focus on a broad spectrum of users and examine whether app usage tenure moderates the effectiveness of the message. Finally, our experimental design allows us to observe only a one-time delivery of a push-notification. Future research might consider examining the effects of multiple interventions to determine whether the effects persist over time.

References

1. Haas, L., et al.: National standards for diabetes self-management education and support. Diabetes Care **36**(Supplement 1), S100–S108 (2013)
2. Welschen, L.M., et al.: Self-monitoring of blood glucose in patients with type 2 diabetes who are not using insulin a systematic review. Diabetes Care **28**(6), 1510–1517 (2005)
3. Karter, A.J., et al.: Self-monitoring of blood glucose levels and glycemic control: the Northern California Kaiser Permanente Diabetes registry∗. Am. J. Med. **111**(1), 1–9 (2001)
4. Evans, J.M., et al.: Frequency of blood glucose monitoring in relation to glycaemic control: observational study with diabetes database. BMJ **319**(7202), 83–86 (1999)
5. McCaul, K.D., Glasgow, R.E., Schafer, L.C.: Diabetes regimen behaviors: predicting adherence. Med. Care, 868–881 (1987)
6. Sigurðardóttir, Á.K.: Self-care in diabetes: model of factors affecting self-care. J. Clin. Nurs. **14**(3), 301–314 (2005)
7. McAndrew, L., et al.: Does patient blood glucose monitoring improve diabetes control? A systematic review of the literature. Diab. Educ. **33**(6), 991–1010 (2007)
8. Sutton, S.: How does the health action process approach (HAPA) bridge the intention–behavior gap? An examination of the model's causal structure. Appl. Psychol. **57**(1), 66–74 (2008)
9. Gollwitzer, P.M., Oettingen, G.: Implementation Intentions. Springer, New York (2013). doi:10.1007/978-1-4419-1005-9_1710
10. Clapp, J.D., et al.: A failed norms social marketing campaign. J. Stud. Alcohol **64**(3), 409–414 (2003)
11. Burchell, K., Rettie, R., Patel, K.: Marketing social norms: social marketing and the 'social norm approach'. J. Consum. Behav. **12**(1), 1–9 (2013)
12. Higgs, S.: Social norms and their influence on eating behaviours. Appetite **86**, 38–44 (2015)
13. Allcott, H.: Social norms and energy conservation. J. Public Econ. **95**(9), 1082–1095 (2011)
14. Goldstein, N.J., Cialdini, R.B., Griskevicius, V.: A room with a viewpoint: using social norms to motivate environmental conservation in hotels. J. Consum. Res. **35**(3), 472–482 (2008)
15. Neighbors, C., et al.: Are social norms the best predictor of outcomes among heavy-drinking college students? J. Stud. Alcohol Drugs **68**(4), 556 (2007)
16. Schultz, P.W., et al.: The constructive, destructive, and reconstructive power of social norms. Psychol. Sci. **18**(5), 429–434 (2007)
17. Gollwitzer, P.M., et al.: Planning promotes goal striving. In: Handbook of Self-regulation: Research, Theory, and Applications, vol. 2, pp. 162–185 (2011)
18. Milkman, K.L., et al.: Using implementation intentions prompts to enhance influenza vaccination rates. Proc. Natl. Acad. Sci. **108**(26), 10415–10420 (2011)
19. Nickerson, D.W., Rogers, T.: Do you have a voting plan? Implementation intentions, voter turnout, and organic plan making. Psychol. Sci. **21**(2), 194–199 (2010)
20. Luszczynska, A., Sobczyk, A., Abraham, C.: Planning to lose weight: randomized controlled trial of an implementation intention prompt to enhance weight reduction among overweight and obese women. Health Psychol. **26**(4), 507 (2007)
21. Prestwich, A., Perugini, M., Hurling, R.: Can implementation intentions and text messages promote brisk walking? A randomized trial. Health Psychol. **29**(1), 40 (2010)

22. Prestwich, A., Perugini, M., Hurling, R.: Can the effects of implementation intentions on exercise be enhanced using text messages? Psychol. Health **24**(6), 677–687 (2009)
23. Ajzen, I.: From intentions to actions: a theory of planned behavior. In: Kuhl, J., Beckmann, J. (eds.) Action Control. SSSP Springer Series in Social Psychology, pp. 11–39. Springer, Heidelberg (1985). doi:10.1007/978-3-642-69746-3_2
24. Hardeman, W., et al.: Application of the theory of planned behaviour in behaviour change interventions: a systematic review. Psychol. Health **17**(2), 123–158 (2002)
25. Norman, P.: Predicting health behaviour: a social cognition approach. Predicting Health Behav., 1 (2005)
26. Orbeil, S., Hodgldns, S., Sheeran, P.: Implementation intentions and the theory of planned behavior. Pers. Soc. Psychol. Bull. **23**(9), 945–954 (1997)
27. Gollwitzer, P.M.: Goal achievement: the role of intentions. Eur. Rev. Soc. Psychol. **4**(1), 141–185 (1993)
28. Blanchard, C.M.: Heart disease and physical activity: looking beyond patient characteristics. Exerc. Sport Sci. Rev. **40**(1), 30–36 (2012)
29. Trafimow, D., Fishbein, M.: The moderating effect of behavior type on the subjective norm-behavior relationship. J. Soc. Psychol. **134**(6), 755–763 (1994)
30. Doran, R., Larsen, S.: The relative importance of social and personal norms in explaining intentions to choose eco-friendly travel options. Int. J. Tourism Res. **18**(2), 159–166 (2016)
31. Lapinski, M.K., Rimal, R.N.: An explication of social norms. Comm. Theory **15**(2), 127–147 (2005)
32. List, J.A., Rasul, I.: Field experiments in labor economics. Handbook Labor Econ. **4**, 103–228 (2011)
33. Adair, J.G.: The Hawthorne effect: a reconsideration of the methodological artifact. J. Appl. Psychol. **69**(2), 334–345 (1984)
34. Sunstein, C.R.: Nudging: a very short guide. J. Consum. Policy **37**(4), 583–588 (2014)

Patient Satisfaction and Hospital Structure: How Are They Related?

Mingfei Li, Alina Chircu, Gang Li, Lan Xia, and Jennifer Xu[✉]

Bentley University, Waltham, MA, USA
{mli,achircu,gli,lxia,jxu}@bentley.edu

Abstract. This paper investigates the multiple dimensions of patient satisfaction measured by the HCAHPS (Hospital Consumer Assessment of Healthcare Providers and Systems) survey in the United States. The analysis reveals that even the highest rating hospitals do not excel on all dimensions of satisfaction. While satisfaction levels with nurse and doctor communication are high, satisfaction levels with discharge information and explanation of medications could be significantly improved. In addition, low rating hospitals seem to be doing better than the high rating hospitals on these critical dimensions for the quality of care. The paper also investigates how hospital structural characteristics captured in the American Hospital Association (AHA) survey affect different dimensions of patient satisfaction. The analysis reveals that these structural factors may have differential effects, i.e. the type of hospitals (e.g., teaching vs. non-teaching) has a relatively small effect on the hospital room environment than on communication and responsiveness. The results suggest that considering all patient satisfaction dimensions helps provide a more accurate picture of the care received by patients, makes it possible to pinpoint specific areas where hospitals are deficient that are not reflected in the overall satisfaction scores, and assists hospital management to design actionable strategies for improvement.

Keywords: Patient satisfaction · Quality of care · Hospital structure

1 Introduction

Quality of care has long been a key performance indicator in the healthcare industry. Although there is a lack of consensus on the definition of quality of care [26], most healthcare professionals believe that an important component of this metric is patient satisfaction [8, 9, 11], which refers to the opinions and attitudes of patients toward the health services they receive from their healthcare providers. In his seminal paper on healthcare quality assessment, Donabedian stated that the ultimate criterion for quality is about achieving and producing health and satisfaction [9].

The focus on patient satisfaction concurs with several recent trends in the healthcare industry. One of these trends is the growing acceptance of the concept and practice of patient-centered care. While continuing to maintain and improve clinical outcomes, healthcare providers also try to enhance patient experience and perceptions of the service quality. Meanwhile, healthcare regulators and associations have adopted a market-driven approach, which takes a consumer perspective, when evaluating the

© Springer International Publishing AG 2017
H. Chen et al. (Eds.): ICSH 2017, LNCS 10347, pp. 15–25, 2017.
https://doi.org/10.1007/978-3-319-67964-8_2

overall performance of healthcare institutions. Moreover, the rising patient expectations, growing medical expenses, and emerging medical technologies have spurred stronger competitions among healthcare organizations, which face constant evaluation and comparison. As result, hospital and clinic managements are striving to seek effective strategies and approaches to improve patient satisfaction and to achieve high quality of care. In the U.S., the Hospital Consumer Assessment of Health Plans Survey (HCAPHS) has been widely used as a tool for patient satisfaction assessment.

There have been a number of studies in the literature that examine patient satisfaction and its determinants. It has been found that in addition to patient individual characteristics, the process of service (e.g., how physicians and nurses interact with patients) and the outcome of service (e.g., hospital readmission rate) all have impact on how patients perceive the quality of care they receive. However, most of these studies have investigated the global satisfaction score without examining the multiple, individual dimensions of satisfaction. In the case of HCAPHS, for example, the majority of findings only concern the single survey question focusing on the overall patient satisfaction. Furthermore, although significant insights have been gathered into the roles of service process and outcome, little is known about how structural characteristics of a healthcare organization affect its patient satisfaction. Consequently, it is difficult for hospital management to utilize these research findings in practice and to design effective strategies for performance improvement.

We propose to bridge these research gaps in the study of patient satisfaction by addressing two research questions in this paper:

- RQ1: How are individual dimensions of patient satisfaction related to the overall satisfaction? What other information do these dimensions reveal in addition to the overall satisfaction?
- RQ2: How do the structural characteristics of a healthcare organization affect different dimensions of patient satisfaction?

The remainder of this paper is organized as follows. The next section reviews the literature on patient satisfaction. Section 3 presents our data and methods. The analysis and results are reported in Sect. 4. The Sect. 5 discusses the implications and limitations of this research and concludes the paper.

2 Literature Review

2.1 Patient Satisfaction

Patient satisfaction has been regarded as an important criterion in the assessment of quality of healthcare. Patient satisfaction scales provide feedback and information that can help performance improvement, strategic decision-making, and effective hospital management [2]. It has been found that patient satisfaction is associated with several healthcare quality indicators such as emergency department use and inpatient use, healthcare expenses, and mortality [11]. Various factors may have impact on patient satisfaction. Based on a meta-analysis of 221 studies, Hall and Dornan identified 11 factors related to patient satisfaction: overall satisfaction, humanness, technical competence, outcome, physical facilities, continuity of care, access, amount of information, cost, organization, and attention to psychological problems [14]. Cleary and McNeil categorized the determinants of patient satisfaction into four groups, which include patient characteristics and three characteristics of care: structure, process, and outcome [8]. Patient socio-demographics (e.g., age, gender, income, education, and health status) and patient expectations regarding the doctors, nurses, and treatments, etc. are individual characteristics of patients. The structure of care includes the organization and financing of care and the accessibility and continuity of care. The process of care refers to the technical aspect (e.g., the perceived competence, skills, and qualifications of the care provider) and interpersonal aspect (e.g. the communication and interaction between the patient and provider). Outcomes of care have been measured by readmission rate, mortality, and improvement of health condition.

A number of studies have examined the impacts of personal characteristics, care process, and care outcome on patient satisfaction. It has been found that age, gender, education, and health status were significantly correlated with patient satisfaction [7, 11, 15]. The fulfillment of expectation has also been shown to influence patient satisfaction [4]. Marley et al. proposed a causal model that focuses specifically on the role of hospital management's leadership, process of care, and outcome of care [20]. They found that the senior executives' participatory leadership had a stronger impact on the process quality, which was primarily concerning the patient-provider communication and interaction, than on clinical outcomes (e.g., readmission); and both the process and outcome quality influenced patient satisfaction. Boulding et al. reported that higher overall patient satisfaction and satisfaction with discharge planning were associated with lower 30-day readmission [5]. In terms of the interpersonal part of care process, Schoenfelder et al. found that, following the treatment outcome, the kindness of nurses was the second most salient predictor of patient satisfaction [24]. Being treated with courtesy by nurses and doctors has also been found to be the highest patient priority in other studies [21].

Although significant progress has been made in the research of patient satisfaction, only a limited number of studies have investigated the roles that the care structure plays in patient satisfaction and their findings are often mixed. Ghaferi et al. studied five hospital-level structural characteristics, including teaching status, hospital size, average daily census, nurse-to-patient ratios, and hospital technology, and found their significant impacts on the quality of care related to pancreatectomy [12]. However, another study reported that higher patient satisfaction was reversely associated with hospital size [3]. Hekkert et al. reported that hospital-level determinants (e.g., hospital size, hospital type) were less important for predicting patient satisfaction than individual characteristics of patients [15]. Similarly, some research shows that except for accessibility, other organizational features such as office staffing and visit-based continuity are not associated with any of the clinical quality indicators [25]. However, based on a survey of nurses and patients in a large number of European and U.S. hospitals, Aiken et al. recommended that improving nurse staffing (i.e., a higher nurse-to-patient ratio) could be a relatively low cost strategy to enhance healthcare quality and patient satisfaction [1]. In addition, Cheng et al. found that the associations between hospital accreditation status (e.g., medical center or regional hospital) with patient satisfaction were significant for diabetes related procedures, but not for other procedures (e.g., stroke, appendectomy) [7].

This research seeks to delve deeper into the impact of structural characteristics of healthcare organizations on patient satisfaction, which is measured using standard survey instruments such as the HCAHPS survey.

2.2   The HCAHPS Patient Satisfaction Survey

A relatively recent development in the measurement of patient satisfaction in the United States is the HCAHPS (Hospital Consumer Assessment of Healthcare Providers and Systems) survey (also known as the CAHPS survey). The HCAHPS survey was launched in 2006 on a voluntary basis, and became a national standard in 2008, when federal hospital payments were linked to survey outcomes and periodic public reporting of survey results was implemented [13]. According to publicly available fact sheets on the survey website (http://www.hcahpsonline.org), 2,421 hospitals reported survey results based on 1.1 million completed patient surveys. These numbers increased to 3,928 reporting hospitals and 3.1 million completed surveys in July 2013 and to 4,167 hospitals and more than 3.1 million completed surveys in April 2015. It is estimated that almost 90% of all eligible hospitals are reporting patient satisfaction data using HCAHPS [13].

The main purpose of HCAHPS is to provide uniform measurement and public reporting of patient's satisfaction with their hospital inpatient care, with the goal of improving the quality of care by providing feedback to hospitals regarding patient perceptions of different aspects of their care [13]. To this end, the current version of the survey reports seven composite measures (nurse communication, doctor communication, responsiveness of hospital staff, pain management, communication about medicines, patient understanding of the care needed after discharge, and discharge information), two individual measures (cleanliness of hospital environment, quietness of hospital environment), and two global measures of patient satisfaction (overall rating of hospital and willingness to recommend hospital). The results are reported as aggregates of individual scales in the following categories: strongly agree/agree/disagree or strongly disagree (understanding of care), yes/no (discharge information provided), yes definitely/yes probably/no probably (willingness to recommend), 9 or 10/7 or 8/6 or lower (overall rating), and always/usually/sometimes or never (all other measures).

The survey is administered to a random sample of eligible adult patients with at least one overnight inpatient stay and alive at discharge. The following categories are excluded from the sample: pediatric patients (under 18 years of age), psychiatric patients, prisoners, patients with a foreign home address, patients discharged to hospice or nursing care, and "no publicity" patients (i.e. patients who, at admission, opt out from information disclosure and from being surveyed). The survey can be administered directly by the hospital or using a survey vendor, and is available in four modes (mail, telephone, mail with telephone follow-up, or active interactive voice recognition). Finally, the survey results are adjusted for survey mode and hospital-specific patient characteristics, which are factors outside of a hospital's control that can affect the results, as well as for non-response bias [13, 19, 27].

Most existing studies based on HCAHPS data use only the global patient satisfaction measures (overall rating and willingness to recommend) [6, 23], a combination of these global measures and selected satisfaction items [16, 18], or a summary patient experience score combining all HCAHPS survey measures [10, 19]. These studies highlight the characteristics of top performing hospitals on the summary score [19], show how these summary scores increase over time [10], link staffing decisions for nurses and doctors to selected satisfaction measures [6, 16, 18], and investigate structural reasons (such as presence of psychiatric beds) for lower global satisfaction scores [23].

While global or summary patient satisfaction measures are useful in understanding trends across time or quickly identifying top performing hospitals, they do not offer actionable recommendations for improving quality of care. Instead, the nine HCAHPS measures of satisfaction with specific aspects of the hospital experience may be more useful. Preliminary studies conducted on the raw HCAHPS data show that despite some reliability and validity deficiencies, some of these specific satisfaction measures have significant positive impacts on the overall hospital rating, which in turn positively affects the willingness to recommend the hospital. However, some measures (such as quietness and discharge information) do not show significance, while others (cleanliness, communication about medicines, and responsiveness of hospital staff) only have significant impacts on overall satisfaction for some hospitals, but not others [27]. We believe there is a clear need for further studies using the multiple aspects of patient satisfaction, rather than only the global overall satisfaction measures.

3 Data

To examine the multiple aspects of patient satisfaction and the impact of hospital structural characteristics, we combined the latest available American Hospital Association (AHA) annual survey data (2013) with the corresponding HCAHPS survey data (2013–2014) for all reporting hospitals in the state of New York. The resulting sample contains 164 hospitals. All these hospitals are Medicare-certified by the U.S. Department of Health and Human Services.

Major hospital characteristics included in the analysis are number of full time nurses and doctors (per bed), total hospital expense, hospital's service area, and whether the hospital provides residency training or is the sole community provider. Patient satisfaction data include all measures available in the HCAHPS survey, including the two overall satisfaction scores (e.g., the star rating) and the nine specific satisfaction dimensions (e.g., room cleanness, doctor communication) (see Sect. 2.2). For each variable, we use the percent of patients whose answers are in the top reported level (always, strongly agree, 9 or 10, definitely yes, or yes, respectively, depending on scale). For example, if 60% of patients reported that "the room and bathroom were always clean", the hospital receives a measure of 60% for room cleanliness. Descriptive statistics for these hospital basic structure and patient satisfaction measures are shown in Table 1.

Table 1. Descriptive statistics for hospital structure and patient satisfaction

Hospital structural characteristics		Count	%	
Service area	Division	66	45	
	Metro	47	32	
	Micro	24	16	
	Rural	11	7	
Residency training (MAPP3)	1 yes	59	40	
	0 no	89	60	
Sole community provider (MAPP20)	1 yes	15	10	
	0 No	133	90	
	Mean	*Std*	*Max*	*Min*
Total hospital expense (EXPTOT, in million)	349.2	504.4	4062.4	8.28
Total hospital beds (HOSPBD, in hundreds)	3.2	3.0	23.6	0.04
Full time doctors (per bed)	1.8	4.7	30.7	0.00
Full time nurses (per bed)	1.3	0.7	3.2	0.16
Patient satisfaction	*Mean*	*Std*	*Max*	*Min*
Room/bathroom cleanliness (*roomclean*)	69.8%	0.081	100	51%
Quietness of hospital environment (*roomquiet*)	52.0%	0.075	78	37%
Nurse communication (*nurcom*)	75.3%	0.062	97	60%
Doctor communication (*doccom*)	77.4%	0.043	93	68%
Responsiveness of staff (received help as soon as wanted) (*response*)	61.2%	0.099	96	37%
Pain control (*paincon*)	66.9%	0.066	93	53%
Communication about medication before administration (*staffmed*)	60.7%	0.064	94	46%
Discharge information (*infohome*)	16.1%	0.048	29	6%
Understanding of care (*understood*)	46.8%	0.060	62	6%
Overall hospital rating (*hosrate*)	63.1%	0.099	91	42%
Willingness to recommend (*recom*)	65.5%	0.106	97	41%
Combined service quality dimensions	*Mean*	*Std*	*Max*	*Min*
Communication (combined nurse and doctor communication)	76.3%	0.049	90	64%
Environment (*roomevir*) (combined cleanliness and quietness)	60.9%	0.070	82	44%
Responsiveness (combined pain control and responsiveness of staff)	64.0%	0.079	95	47%

4   Analysis and Results

The analysis showed that all the nine specific satisfaction measures significantly correlate with the overall star rating. However, patients' satisfactions vary with different items. We found significant difference among levels of satisfaction for different aspects of the hospital experience, with the highest satisfaction achieved on nurse and doctor communication (75.3% and 77.4%) and the lowest satisfaction achieved on discharge information provision (16.1%) and explanation of medications before administration (46.8%) (see Table 1). Even the top rating hospitals did not achieve high satisfaction on all dimensions. A regression analysis shows that discharge information provision and medication explanation are negatively associated with the two overall satisfaction scores (all $ps < 0.001$).

Figure 1 presents a radar map that illustrates the differences among six selected hospitals' performance on these nine individual satisfaction items. These hospitals are represented by six colored polygons. Each polygon was constructed by connecting the nine satisfaction scores of a hospital using colored lines: blue, light green and light purple are three hospitals with recommendations great than 73% (i.e. over 73% of the patients said they would definitely recommend the hospital), and with the overall star rating equal to or greater than 4 out of 5. The red, green, and purple polygons are the other three hospitals with recommendations less than 50%, and with the overall rating less than or equal to 1 out of 5. This visual representation is fairly easy to interpret. In general, the bigger a polygon's size is, the higher the corresponding hospital's scores are. It can be seen that high rating hospitals performed very well on doctor and nurse communication, cleanliness, quietness, pain control, and communication about medication. However, the three low rating hospitals performed better than the high rating hospitals on patient's understanding of their care and discharge information.

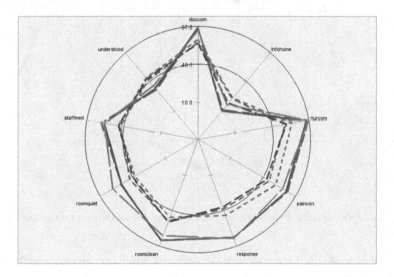

Fig. 1. Patient satisfaction dimensions for the highest rating and lowest rating hospitals. (Color figure online)

To generalize the patient satisfaction dimensions into more compact metrics, we grouped related items together according to the five dimensions of service quality: Reliability, Tangibles, Responsiveness, Assurance, and Empathy [22]. These service dimensions have been widely adopted and used in a variety of disciplines. This approach also complies with the categorization of the HCAHPS measures in the prior research [17, 27]. Three combined dimensions were generated by grouping doctor communication and nurse communication, with equal weights, into *Communication*; cleanliness and quietness into *Environment*; and pain control and responsiveness of hospital staff into *Responsiveness*. Table 1 includes descriptive statistics for these combined measures, and Fig. 2 compares the same six hospitals from Fig. 1 using the combined metrics.

Next, we examined the effect of hospital structural factors on these three combined dimensions (Communication, Environment, and Responsiveness) using the general linear models (GLM). The results show that, across the three care quality dimensions, hospitals in rural areas are better than hospitals in divisions, with all other variables controlled (see Table 2). Teaching hospitals are lower on satisfaction level than non-teaching hospitals especially in communications (b = −.027, p < .05) and responsiveness dimensions (b = −.053, p < .001). Being the sole community provider is associated with lower satisfaction level on responsiveness (b = −.045, p < .05) and room environment (b = −.027, p < .013). Finally, hospital size has a negative effect on all the three service quality dimensions (all ps < .01).

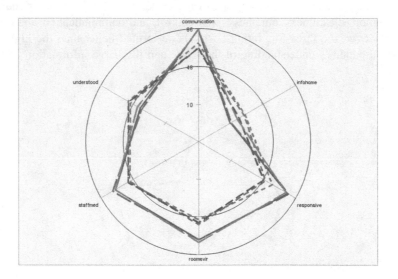

Fig. 2. Service quality dimensions for the highest rating and lowest rating hospitals.

Table 2. GLM model for Communication, Environment and Responsiveness (**bold** indicates significant values)

Parameters	Communication		Environment		Responsiveness	
	Estimates	P-value	Estimates	P-value	Estimates	P-value
Intercept	0.823	<.0001	0.689	<.0001	0.712	<.0001
Service area (Division)	−0.044	**0.015**	−0.055	**0.024**	−0.057	**0.017**
Service area (Metro)	−0.031	0.086	−0.067	**0.006**	−0.025	0.289

(*continued*)

Table 2. (*continued*)

Parameters	Communication		Environment		Responsiveness	
	Estimates	P-value	Estimates	P-value	Estimates	P-value
Service area (Micro)	−0.021	0.268	0.007	0.771	0.012	0.615
Residence training (MAPP3)	−0.027	**0.013**	−0.028	0.057	−0.053	**0.000**
Sole community provider (MAPP20)	−0.029	0.086	−0.059	**0.010**	−0.045	**0.039**
Total hospital beds (HOSPBD)	−0.010	**0.001**	−0.012	**0.003**	−0.015	**0.001**
Total hospital expense (EXPTOT, in million)	0.000	0.000	0.000	0.010	0.000	0.000

5 Discussion and Conclusions

Patient satisfaction is an important element in quality of care. With health care increasingly shifting to a patient-centered practice, understanding what patient satisfaction means and what drives it is becoming ever more important. This research takes the view that patient satisfaction has multiple dimensions that are relevant for managerial decision-making in practice. Thus, in order to provide actionable recommendations, research should focus not only on the overall patient satisfaction measures, but also on various facets of satisfaction with the care experience. By combining patient satisfaction (HCAHP) and hospital characteristics (AHA) data, our research shows that even the highest rating hospitals do not excel on all dimensions of satisfaction. While nurse and doctor communications with patients achieve high satisfaction, satisfaction levels with discharge information and explanation of medications could be significantly improved. Surprisingly, low rating hospitals are doing better than the high rating hospitals on these critical dimensions for the quality of care. Providing discharge information is essential for safe transition of care to a primary provider and successful recovery after the hospital stay. Similarly, properly communicating about medication before administration helps patients understand their care and reduces chances of medication administration errors (which can have many negative, and sometimes fatal, effects) and readmissions. One possible explanation why these measures are lower for top rating hospitals is that these dimensions of satisfaction may not always significantly impact the overall satisfaction [27]. As a result, if only the global satisfaction measures are used to incentivize hospitals (though payments for services) and compare hospitals, hospital administrators may choose to under-invest in specific care areas such as discharge information and medication communication efforts if their overall ratings are high. However, this may hide, in fact, lower levels of care, and generate opportunities for errors. Clearly, considering all satisfaction dimensions helps provide a more accurate picture of the care received by patients and is useful in pinpointing areas where hospitals are deficient and could improve.

In addition, the analysis of the impact of hospital structural factors on different satisfaction dimensions showed that these structural factors may have differential effects. For example, the type of hospitals (e.g., teaching vs. non-teaching) has a relatively small effect on the hospital room environment than on communication and responsiveness.

In this paper, we provide an initial attempt to examine the different dimensions of patient satisfaction, investigate how hospitals differ on these multiple dimensions, and analyze the differential effects of hospital structural factors on the satisfaction dimensions. Given the richness of the data available, future research could examine the effect of additional factors (such as facility characteristics or type of disease) on different dimensions of patient satisfaction, and investigate differences in these effects across multiple U.S. states. We believe these analyses could contribute to better understanding of patient satisfaction elements and better management of the care components that affect the different satisfaction dimensions.

References

1. Aiken, L.H., et al.: Patient safety, satisfaction, and quality of hospital care: cross sectional surveys of nurses and patients in 12 countries in Europe and the United States. BMJ **344**, e1717 (2012)
2. Al-Abri, R., Al-Balushi, A.: Patient satisfaction survey as a tool towards quality improvement. Oman Med. J. **29**, 3–7 (2014)
3. Baldin, E., et al.: Effect of organisational features on patient satisfaction with care in Italian multiple sclerosis centres. Eur. J. Neurol. **23**, 307–308 (2016)
4. Bjertnaes, O.A., Sjetne, I.S., Iversen, H.H.: Overall patient satisfaction with hospitals: effects of patient-reported experiences and fulfilment of expectations. BMJ Qual. Safety **21**, 39–46 (2012)
5. Boulding, W., Glickman, S.W., Manary, M.P., Schulman, K.A., Staelin, R.: Relationship between patient satisfaction with inpatient care and hospital readmission within 30 days. Am. J. Managed Care **17**, 41–48 (2011)
6. Chen, L.M., Birkmeyer, J.D., Saint, S., Jha, A.K.: Hospitalist staffing and patient satisfaction in the national medicare population. J. Hosp. Med. **8**, 126–131 (2013)
7. Cheng, S.-H., Yang, M.-C., Chiang, T.-L.: Patient satisfaction with and recommendation of a hospital: Effects of interpersonal and technical aspects of hospital care. Int. J. Qual. Health Care **15**, 345–355 (2003)
8. Cleary, P.D., McNeil, B.J.: Patient satisfaction as an indicator of quality care. Inquiry **25**, 25–36 (1998)
9. Donabedian, A.: The quality of care: How can it be assessed? J. Am. Med. Assoc. **260**, 1743–1748 (1988)
10. Elliott, M.N., et al.: Accelerating improvement and narrowing gaps: trends in patients' experiences with hospital care reflected in HCAHPS public reporting. Health Serv. Res. **50**, 1850–1867 (2015)
11. Fenton, J.J., Jerant, A.F., Bertakis, K.D., Franks, P.: The cost of satisfaction: A national study of patient satisfaction, health care utilization, expenditures, and mortality. Arch. Intern. Med. **172**, 405–411 (2012)

12. Ghaferi, A.A., Osborne, N.H., Birkmeyer, J.D., Dimick, J.B.: Hospital characteristics associated with failure to rescue from complications after pancreatectomy. J. Am. Coll. Surg. **211**, 325–330 (2010)

13. Giordano, L.A., Elliott, M.N., Goldstein, E., Lehrman, W.G., Spencer, P.A.: Development, implementation, and public reporting of the HCAHPS survey. Med. Care Res. Rev. **67**, 27–37 (2010)

14. Hall, J.A., Dornan, M.C.: Meta-analysis of satisfaction with medical care: description of research domain and analysis of overall satisfaction levels. Soc. Sci. Med. **27**, 637–644 (1998)

15. Hekkert, K.D., Cihangir, S., Kleefstra, S.M., van den Berg, B., Kool, R.B.: Patient satisfaction revisited: a multilevel approach. Soc. Sci. Med. **69**, 68–75 (2009)

16. Hockenberry, J.M., Becker, E.R.: How do hospital nurse staffing strategies affect patient satisfaction? ILR Rev. **69**, 890–910 (2016)

17. Huerta, T.R., Harle, C.A., Ford, E.W., Diana, M.L., Menachemi, N.: Measuring patient satisfaction's relationship to hospital cost efficiency: can administrators make a difference? Health Care Manage. Rev. **41**, 56–63 (2016)

18. Lasater, M.K., Sloane, D.M., Aiken, L.H.: Hospital employment of supplemental registered nurses and patients' satisfaction with care. J. Nurs. Adm. **45**, 145 (2015)

19. Lehrman, W.G., et al.: Characteristics of hospitals demonstrating superior performance in patient experience and clinical process measures of care. Med. Care Res. Rev. **67**, 38–55 (2010)

20. Marley, K.A., Collier, D.A., Goldstein, S.M.: The role of clinical and process quality in achieving patient satisfaction in hospitals. Decis. Sci. **35**, 349–369 (2004)

21. Otani, K., Herrmann, P.A., Kurz, R.S.: Improving patient satisfaction in hospital care settings. Health Serv. Manage. Res. **24**, 163–169 (2011)

22. Parasuraman, A., Berry, L.L., Zeithaml, V.A.: Understanding measuring and improving service quality: findings from a multiphase research program. In: Brown, S.W., Gummesson, E., Edvardsson, B., Gustavsson, B. (eds.) Service Quality: Multidisciplinary and Multinational Perspectives, pp. 253–268. Lexington Books, Lexington (1991)

23. Reese, M.L., Campbell, D.A., Kerr Jr., B.J., Alvarez, M.R., Smith, S.P.: The economic impact of Hospital Consumer Assessment of Healthcare Providers and Systems (HCAHPS) scores for hospitals providing inpatient psychiatric services. J. Health Care Financ. **42**, 1–14 (2015)

24. Schoenfelder, T., Klewer, J., Kugler, J.: Determinants of patient satisfaction: a study among 39 hospitals in an in-patient setting in Germany. Int. J. Qual. Health Care **23**, 503–509 (2011)

25. Sequist, T.D., et al.: Quality monitoring of physicians: linking patients' experiences of care to clinical quality and outcomes. J. Gen. Intern. Med. **23**, 1784–1790 (2008)

26. Thompson, A.G.H., Sunoi, R.: Expectations as determinants of patient satisfaction: Concepts, theory and evidence. Int. J. Qual. Health Care **7**, 127–141 (1995)

27. Westbrook, K.W., Babakus, E., Grant, C.C.: Measuring patient-perceived hospital service quality: Validity and managerial usefulness of HCAHPS scales. Health Mark. Q. **31**, 97–114 (2014)

Using Observational Engagement Assessment Method VC-IOE for Evaluating an Interactive Table Designed for Seniors with Dementia

Yuan Feng[1,2(✉)], Ruud van Reijmersdal[1], Suihuai Yu[2(✉)], Jun Hu[1],
Matthias Rauterberg[1], and Emilia Barakova[1]

[1] Department of Industrial Design, Eindhoven University of Technology,
Eindhoven, The Netherlands
{Y.Feng,j.hu,G.W.M.Rauterberg,E.I.Barakova}@tue.nl,
r.j.h.v.reijmersdal@student.tue.nl
[2] Department of Industrial Design, Northwestern Polytechnical University,
Xi'an, People's Republic of China
ysuihuai@vip.sina.com

Abstract. Seniors with dementia living in residential nursing homes are often lack of meaningful engagement and keeping them engaged in meaningful activities can help reduce boredom and improve their well-being. This paper presents an Interactive Table Design (ITD) for providing seniors with dementia meaningful engagements. An observational engagement assessment method, Video Coding – Incorporating Observed Emotion (VC-IOE), was adopted to further study the effectiveness of the intervention design. Qualitative data such as video recordings of four participants engaged with the ITD and comparison intervention Pim Pam Pet (PPP) in Vitalis Kelinschalig Wonen, were then analyzed following the video analysis protocols of VC-IOE. The results from video coding analysis provided an overview of participants' emotional responses and engagement situations through six dimensions of engagement including emotional, verbal, visual, behavioral, collective engagement and agitation. The results showed sufficient positive impacts of ITD on participants which indicate that the ITD has the potential to be an effective intervention for providing seniors with dementia with meaningful engagement while keeping them socially connected in a nursing home.

Keywords: Dementia · Engagement · VC-IOE · Video analysis · Design

1 Introduction

Dementia is an umbrella term for multiple variant disorders which affects the brain, impairing the cognitive function, the executive function including planning and problem-solving, as well as the independent function for a job or personal care. It can be divided into further categories according to the stage of the disease and have varied etiologies. The life expectancy after being diagnosed with dementia is eight years on average and has no known cure. Besides cancer and cardiovascular diseases, dementia is one of the main causes of senior deaths within the Netherlands [1].

© Springer International Publishing AG 2017
H. Chen et al. (Eds.): ICSH 2017, LNCS 10347, pp. 26–37, 2017.
https://doi.org/10.1007/978-3-319-67964-8_3

In early stages, persons with dementia encounter problems such as inhibited memory, language deficiencies, and difficulties in novel tasks. With the progression of dementia, the number of complications becomes greater and the affected behaviors are further exaggerated. A decline in neurological functions due to the progression of dementia may lead to disorientation in time and place which often results in confusion and conflicts with others [2]. The loss of functional abilities ultimately leads to complications with daily tasks such as eating or getting dressed, or any other personal-care activities. Therefore, seniors with dementia often need specialized care in the form of nursing homes or professional caregivers.

1.1 Engaging Seniors with Dementia in Social Activities

Since dementia is an age-related disease, seniors with dementia are faced with not only the challenges of the disease itself but also a decrease in their physical health as well as other age-related declines. A decrease in physical health such as the deterioration of mobility, hearing, and visual functions may disorient seniors further, leaving them feeling vulnerable and more emotional. This leads to their search for reassurance and attention from others [2]. The transition into residential nursing homes brings forth a new set of challenges for seniors with dementia as they can lose a sense of familiarity which is punctuated by participating in unplanned activities. This results in an increase in boredom and loneliness [3]. The prolonged lack of engagement increases the risk of behavioral and psychological symptoms of dementia such as apathy, depression, aggression and agitation [4].

In addition, due to their compounding conditions, seniors with dementia spend less time than their peers engaging in social activities and communication is crucial in daily lives since it provides a means for people to express their needs and feelings. Without communication, unmet needs can result in aggression or other complicated behaviors, further resulting in social isolation [5]. Engagement in social activities can help seniors with dementia improve one aspect of their quality of life by mitigating boredom and decrease depression, agitation, and aggression [6]. Also, engagement in social activities is beneficial for social connectedness and increases autonomy, which improves an individual's well-being [7]. Research in engagement is crucial for determining individual-centered activities for the betterment of their quality of life.

2 Assessing Engagement of Seniors with Dementia

The analysis of different forms of engagement that expected to help to define suitable interventions for increasing interests and positive emotions of persons with dementia has been done by researchers [8]. However, analyzing and assessing engagement can be challenging since seniors with dementia often have inhibited memory, deteriorated cognitive functions and degenerated language skills, which makes the evaluation through self-reflecting very difficult. Additionally, some dementia-affected seniors also have reduced emotionality which means they cannot express their facial emotions properly [2, 9]. This makes the analysis of the facial expression even more difficult.

The most notable work within the dementia engagement study is Cohen-Mansfield and her colleagues. They utilized a comprehensive model of five dimensions of engagement known as the Observational Method of Engagement (OME) [8]. It measures engagement through the rate of refusal of the stimulus, duration of the time that resident involved with the stimulus, level of attention to the stimulus, attitude toward the stimulus, and actions toward the stimulus. Unlike earlier research about dementia engagement that emphases on the effect of reducing agitation or agitated behaviors, OME specifically addresses the experience of engagement with measurable aspects, which provide a more comprehensive overview based on direct observation of engagement experience than simply studying the positive effect on agitation [10].

Most recently, Jones [11] proposed a video analysis method called Video Coding Incorporating Observed Emotion (VC-IOE) for assessing engagement of persons with dementia. VC-IOE is a video coding scheme based on theory integration of the Dual-channel hypothesis and the Comprehensive Process Model of Engagement framework [8], which integrates emotional and social aspects of the engagement experience as well. It is designed based on the OME and Lawton's commonly adopted the Observed Emotion Rating Scale (OERS) for assessing engagement and emotions [12]. By combining existing methods and adding verbal, emotional and collective engagement, VC-IOE provides a more comprehensive understanding of the engagement of dementia in order to study the effectiveness of interventions.

3   Design of an Interactive Table for Dementia

An interactive table was designed intended to be used as an intervention for providing meaningful activity and improving engagement among seniors with dementia living in care facilities [13]. The table figure was chosen since residents in nursing homes are already familiar and can interact with things placing on it naturally, therefore enables a simple level interaction based on former experience and cognitive function. Additionally, the table is already a physical connecting object since people sitting around often form a sense of connectedness.

The Interactive Table Design (ITD) (Fig. 1) consists of two basic elements which are the interactive feather ball sets placing two on each long side of the table and four symmetric leaf shape patterns embedded in the center of the table. The positioning of the interactive ball sets is formed by their daily sitting habits. The table design can support at most four users interacting at the same time, with each user have one set of interactive balls and a hollowed route link to the center leaf shape pattern filled with colored liquid. Ball sets were chosen as related research indicated that ball figure shows appealing feature to all levels of cognitive impairment of dementia [14, 15]. Four different colors are used for distinguishing user characters, and the same color is applied on both interactive ball set and the liquid inside leaf pattern interface in order to build a logic link in between. Feather feature provides an inviting gesture for different ways of interactions, such as stroking, petting, holding squeezing or slapping.

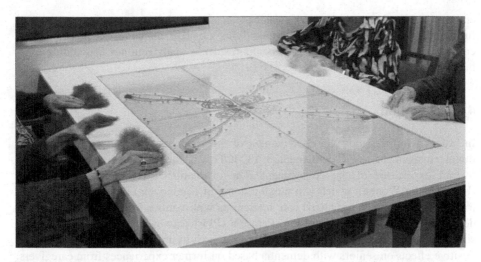

Fig. 1. The Interactive Table Design with four seniors with dementia from Vitalis Kelinschalig Wonen interacting with it (Color figure online)

Each ball set consists of three individual balls that are made of colored goose down with woven conductive wires, while still visually appears as an entity. Three separate balls are controlled by mechanics underneath the table individually so that together they can be programmed to mimic animal-like movements and respond to user gestures. For instance, when three balls are moving up and down gradually, they may appear like pulsing or alive and breathing in the perception of users. The conductive wires hidden in the feather are programmed for sensing different ways of contact, combining with force sensing in order to distinguish possible gestures. Different gestural interactions are defined so that ball set can respond correspondingly in order to provide an animal-like character. For example, when no engagement happens with the ball sets, they will show provoking reaction that is popping out the table surface now and then and acts like a curious and shy animal; when positive engaged such as stroking, holding, handling, or petting the feather balls, they will mimic a breath pattern by slowly moving; when negative engaged such as slapping or hitting, they will react hiding or diving back into the table to show a hurtful animal-like behavior.

Leaf shape patterns embedded in the center of the table were made of transparent acrylic-based resin plates. They are normally transparent and barely visible. When signals of continues positive interactions are detected from users' wrist by a pulse sensor installed near the ball sets on the table, a pump will start working to pump colored liquid towards the center along with the rhythm of users' heartbeat. The whole system consists of four sets of electronics. Each set of electronics contains one Arduino Uno board which controls all the sensors and actuators; three servomotors manipulate one interactive ball set through a motor controller; three groups of conductive wires that receive user's touch input through a breakout board; a pulse sensor for collecting pulse signals; a pump and a power converter. The ITD aims at providing meaningful engagement for keeping dementia residents in nursing homes occupied, in order to further preventing social isolation, magnifying positive affective effects and social connectedness without interfering dementia residents' daily routines and adding extra burdens on caregivers.

4   Evaluation

In order to further study the effectiveness of this designed intervention, an observational engagement assessment method VC-IOE was then adopted for acquiring an overall experience of the engagement. The evaluation was conducted in Vitalis (Kleinschalig Wonen), which is a nursing home in Eindhoven (The Netherlands) that focuses on providing specialized care for seniors with various forms and conditions of dementia. Additionally, a game Pim Pam Pet (PPP) was used for comparison study, since the game has already been used as a daily activity in Vitalis and proved to have positive effects on seniors with dementia based on former experiences from caregivers.

4.1   Participants

A sample contains four participants with a formal diagnosis of dementia were recruited from Vitalis. Residents with a functioning level of auditory, visual abilities and physically able for sitting and interacting with different stimulus were eligible to participate. All four participants are female due to the majority population living in Vitalis are female, and with the average age of 85 and different levels of cognitive functioning according to a diagnostic four-stage rating scale used in Vitalis. The same group of participants participated in both PPP and ITD evaluations. Participant demographics are shown in Table 1.

Table 1. Participant demographics

Participant	P1	P2	P3	P4
Gender	Female	Female	Female	Female
Age	75	84	88	93
Stage	2	2-3	2-3	3
Form of dementia	Vascular dementia	Vascular dementia	Vascular dementia	Vascular dementia
Marriage status	Widowed	Married	Widowed	Widowed
Cognitive function according to staff	Mild cognitive decline	Confused at times	Confused at times	Constantly confused

4.2   Procedure

Evaluations were agreed ahead with Vitalis and performed in different days during non-planned activity time from 14:30 until 16:00 inside a unit within Vitalis. Four participants were first invited to sit around a table in a living room formed by 7 residents of seniors with dementia and played with PPP for 20 min. The intervention session length was limited based on previous experience. The game PPP consists of a set of cards with questions and a turntable with letters from the alphabet. A registered nurse with extensive experience in dementia care as a facilitator to guide the game and read the questions on the cards, while participants take turns to roll the turntable then answer the questions on the cards start with the letter from the turntable. For instance, if the question is "what can you have on bread?" and if a participant rolls a letter "P", then "Peanut butter" should be one of the correct answers.

Participants were invited again another time for engaging with the ITD. As the intention of the design is to keep residents in nursing homes engaged with minimal involvement of caregivers, this evaluation was performed without a facilitator. Participants were first introduced to the table, then instructed to explore by themselves until loss of interest or left the table. Both evaluations were group sessions with the same four participants for better generating social connectedness and assessing collective engagement. Evaluations were documented using video cameras and cell phones for recording audios then transcribed into a manuscript and translated into English for further qualitative data analysis.

4.3   Assessing Engagement Using VC-IOE

A video coding protocol VC-IOE was used for video analysis according to the guidelines proposed by Jones [11]. The VC-IOE video coding protocol emphases on six dimensions of engagements, including emotional, verbal, visual, behavioral, collective engagement and signs of agitation. Each dimension will be assessed separately, and then considered jointly for providing a more comprehensive overview of the engagement experience.

The emotional engagement was assessed by observing facial responses and coded into three categories as pleasure, negative and neutral. The verbal engagement was assessed through conversations. It offers a context for understanding their engagement situations and behaviors toward stimulus. Visual engagement as an indicator of participants' non-verbal engagement was examined and coded according to the presence of the visual engagement, for instance, keeping eye contact with the stimulus, or no eye contact with the stimulus. Behavior engagement assessing was based on the relevant engagement study of Cohen-Mansfield et al. [16] and Kolanowski et al. [17]. Gestural interaction including petting, stroking, handling the stimulus properly were considered positive behavioral engagement, and hitting the table or pulling out the ball sets was considered negative behavioral engagement. The collective engagement was assessed when participants showed social connection such as introducing or instructing stimulus to others, encouraging others to interact with, or using stimulus as a communication tool for forming conversations. Agitation is coded based on Cohen-Mansfield's research on agitation and agitation behaviors (Cohen-Mansfield Agitation Inventory, CMAI) [18], both verbal and non-verbal aspects. The missing data was coded as no engagement. Table 2 presents and explains the video analysis protocols in details. Dedoose online platform (www.dedoose.com) was used for analyzing the qualitative data.

Table 2. Video coding protocols including six dimensions of engagement and observational signs used in evaluations

Engagement	Observation
Emotional engagement	
Positive emotions (Pleasure)	Smiling, laughing towards the stimulus
Negative emotions (Anger, Anxiety or fear, Sadness)	Physical aggression, yelling, cursing, drawing eyebrows together, clenching teeth, pursing lips, narrowing eyes; voice shaking, shrieking, repetitive calling out, line between eyebrows, lines across forehead, tight facial muscles; crying, frowning, eyes drooped, moaning, sighing, eyes/head turned down
Neutral	Relaxed or no sign of discrete facial expression
Verbal engagement	
Positive verbal engagement with stimulus or facilitator	Appreciating, praising the stimulus, making jokes, expressing happiness, fun experience, and participating and maintaining conversation, verbally responding to the stimulus
Negative verbal engagement	Verbalizes the desire to leave, refuses to participate in the activity anymore, makes repetitive generalized somatic complaints, cursing and swearing
No verbal engagement	Not participating and maintaining the conversation. Not responding or talking to the stimulus or facilitators
Visual engagement	
Visually engaged	Appears alerted and maintaining eye contact with the stimulus, including eyes following or looking at the stimulus
No visual engagement	Blank stare into space. Does not make eye contact with the stimulus
Behavioral engagement	
Positive behavioral engagement	Touching or attempting to touch the stimulus. Stroking, petting, holding and handling the stimulus appropriately
Negative behavioral engagement	Hitting, shaking and slapping the stimulus inappropriately, including Shoving it away and pulling it out
No behavioral engagement	No touching, physical contact and interacting with the stimulus
Collective engagement	
Evidence of collective engagement	Encouraging others to interact with the stimulus. Introducing stimulus to others. Using stimulus as a communication channel to interact and talk with others
No collective engagement	No sign of collective engagement
Agitation	
Evidence of agitation (verbal, vocal, motor activity)	Restlessness, repeated/agitated movement, picking and fiddling with clothes; repetitive rubbing own limbs or torso; appears anxious. Repeats words or phrases, abusive or aggressive toward self or other
No evidence of agitation	No sign of agitation as described above

5 Results

Coding result presented in Table 3 shows the duration of each participant engaged in six dimensions of engagement of two evaluations in seconds. The original coding results were converted and using 600 s as a unit of session duration of both evaluations for easier comparison purpose. Participants' emotional, verbal, behavioral responses to both PPP and ITD are summarized separately in Table 4.

Table 3. Session duration of each participant engaged in two evaluations in seconds

Evaluation	PPP				ITD			
Participant	P1	P2	P3	P4	P1	P2	P3	P4
Session duration	755	755	755	477	2832	1910	1399	1890

Table 4. Each participant's converted engagement duration using 600 s as a unit of both PPP and ITD evaluations in seconds

Evaluation	PPP				ITD			
Participant	P1	P2	P3	P4	P1	P2	P3	P4
Positive emotions	25.36	7.13	3.17	1.26	76.06	16.65	107.22	7.62
Negative emotions	1.59	0	0	0	5.08	13.19	2.14	11.11
Neutral	573.05	592.87	596.83	598.74	518.86	570.16	490.64	581.27
Visual engagement	529.46	397.09	493.79	435.22	261.86	394.87	208.00	330.16
Positive verbal engagement with stimulus or facilitator	88.77	40.42	9.51	5.03	323.31	37.70	258.18	54.29
Negative verbal engagement with stimulus or facilitator	0	4.76	0	0	22.46	0	14.15	8.89
Positive Behavioral engagement	3.17	9.51	0	0	167.80	385.13	88.78	203.17
Negative Behavioral engagement	0	0	0	0	0	0.63	2.14	0
Collective engagement	13.47	2.38	0	0	61.02	16.65	96.93	19.37
Agitation	3.17	5.55	0	40.25	0	6.28	4.29	38.41

5.1   Overall Observations in Six Dimensions of Engagement

It is obvious that the session duration of all participants when engaging with the ITD far surpasses the corresponding session duration of game PPP. They showed great interests towards the ITD. The attractiveness and aliveness of the design features, the inviting gesture for interacting, along with the calmness and connectedness brings by the ITD together shows a successful concept for residents with dementia in Vitalis. Longer positive emotional engagement towards the stimulus was also examined with the engagement of the ITD. Participants were found expressing emotions more often and with longer durations. Compared to the emotional engagement of PPP, ITD succeeded on provoking their emotional expressions. Both positive and negative emotional engagement experienced a rise, which suggested more brain activities regarding emotional expression were activated, and this may due to the rich multi-sensory stimulations and animal-like features of the ITD.

In addition, during evaluations, participants who expressed more verbally tend to have less behavioral and visual engagement. Their visual engagement is proportional to the behavioral engagement, as when they are behavioral engaged with the stimulus they usually also keep eye contact at the same time. Result also shows that seniors with advanced stage of dementia who have language deficiencies tend to be more engaged in behavioral engagement and find socially involved within collective engagement challenging.

Although evaluations of both evaluations are group sessions, engagement of all participants with the ITD shows much longer collective engagement duration. The results of qualitative video analysis present many clues on social inclusion. Participants helped each other on how to interact with the ball sets, how to make the liquid pumping works and guided each other's attention towards the stimulus. The interaction helped form conversations as well. Longer duration of verbal engagement was exhibited when engaged with the ITD. They were discussing the vibrant colored feather together and sharing past experiences. In addition, participants were found to be easily influenced by others during evaluations, for instance, petting behavior of one participant will trigger others' petting behaviors. No finding was found regarding the effect on ease of agitation.

5.2   Observations of Individual Cases

Results indicate that response varied between participants and overtime for each individual. Therefore, the below represents results of individual case studies, as case study method is advantageous for close inspection and exploration of the individual impacts when engaging with the stimulus.

Participant 1 (P1). Out of four participants, P1 attended the longest duration of both evaluations with PPP and the ITD and frequently showed positive expressions such as laughing and smiling. Also, longer positive emotional, verbal, behavioral engagement and collective engagement duration with the ITD was showed than with PPP. P1 verbally engaged well during both two evaluations. Her relatively high language skills, therefore, enabled more verbal expressions. The Result shows much more verbal engagement was provoked by ITD and both positive and negative verbal expressions were used. P1 also showed signs of collective engagement, such as verbally instructing others and encouraging other participants playing with the stimulus.

Participant 2 (P2). During both two tests, P2 spent the majority of time on behavioral engagement and visually focused with the stimulus instead of expressing herself verbally or emotionally. The highest positive behavioral engagement was exhibited that other participants, while few verbal languages and emotional changes were captured. She was very curious towards the stimulus distributed in front of her and connecting every element of the environment through touching, handling, stroking the stimulus, which created a profile that likely her way of expressing engagement is more through behavioral engaged than other sensory channels. About two-thirds of the time when interacting with the ITD was positively behavioral engaged and almost no negative engagement showed during the whole period. Improved collective engagement was found compared to engagement with PPP.

Participant 3 (P3). Different engagement situations were found when P3 playing with PPP and interacting with the ITD. When engaged with PPP, few emotional changes were showed and no behavioral engagement including positive and negative, no collective engagement or agitation was examined. The game almost didn't trigger any emotional and behavioral expressions. Although session duration with the ITD was the shortest compared to others, however a high level of positive emotions, positive verbal engagement, and collective engagement was exhibited. What notable is that among all participants P3 showed most signs of collective engagement.

Participant 4 (P4). The game session of PPP was planned for 20 min while participants' interests towards the game only last for about 12 min. P4 lost interests and left the table at about 8 min after the game started and began pacing in the room. During the whole session when engaged with PPP, P4 showed almost no positive or negative emotion but the neutral facial expression, which indicated that the game almost did not provoke any emotional engagement in general. While during the evaluation of the ITD, both positive and negative emotions were examined, and the participant can verbally respond to the design positively and negatively. Duration of verbal engagement, positive behavioral engagement, and collective engagement experienced a rise than with PPP. Besides, P4 also showed most of the agitated behaviors among all participants.

6   Concluding Remarks

We presented the design of an interactive table for providing dementia-affected seniors living in specialized nursing homes with meaningful social activities and leveled stimulations. The aim of the evaluation was intended to study the effectiveness of the ITD as an intervention. Cutting edge observational engagement assessment method, VC-IOE, was used for assessing engagement of seniors with dementia to provide critical analysis of the effectiveness of the intervention. Qualitative data such as video recordings of four participants engaged with two evaluations with the ITD and PPP in Vitalis were then analyzed following the video analysis protocols proposed by Jones.

The results from video coding analysis provided an overview of participants' emotional responses and engagement situations through six dimensions of engagement including emotional, verbal, visual, behavioral, collective engagement and agitation. The analysis of engagement with the ITD showed significant positive impacts such as improved emotional state of participants, activated behavioral engagement, and increased positive connections. These resulted in a reduction of boredom and loneliness, further improving well-being. All facts indicate that the ITD has the potential to be a more suitable and attractive intervention for improving the quality of life of seniors with dementia including their social interaction in nursing homes.

While Further evaluation of the ITD is needed and more research is required for its improvement. Also, a second coder is needed for enhancing the reliability and validity of the qualitative video data analysis. Long-term engagement with more participants should be considered for a more comprehensive investigation of the effectiveness of the ITD. A greater number of sessions are needed to obtain the average duration of the engagement. Furthermore, automatic interpretation of affective facial expression [19], qualitative measures of connectedness, and social inclusion should be included [20]. In addition, for studying effectiveness on agitation, participants' normal agitation state is needed in order to provide a baseline. As for the ITD, further design improvements based on evaluation feedbacks are necessary, and practical use scenarios should be taken into consideration as well.

Acknowledgments. The author would like to thank the Chinese Scholarship Council, T. Zuo from Jiangnan University, and Sylvia van Aggel, Helma Verstappel from Vitalis for their support on the study.

References

1. Alzheimer Netherland, Fact sheet about dementia, http://alzheimer.vps9.dolphiq.nl/media/30329/Factsheet%20dementie%20algemeen%20-%20publieksversie%2003-10-2016.pdf
2. James, I.A.: Understanding Behaviour in Dementia that Challenges: A Guide to Assessment and Treatment. Jessica Kingsley Publishers, London (2011)
3. von Kutzleben, M., Schmid, W., Halek, M., et al.: Community-dwelling persons with dementia: what do they need? what do they demand? what do they do? a systematic review on the subjective experiences of persons with dementia. Aging Ment. Health **16**(3), 378–390 (2012)
4. Moyle, W., Venturto, L., Griffiths, S., et al.: Factors influencing quality of life for people with dementia: a qualitative perspective. Aging Ment. Health **15**(8), 970–977 (2011)
5. Scherder, E.J., Bogen, T., Eggermont, L.H., et al.: The more physical inactivity, the more agitation in dementia. Int. Psychogeriatr. **22**(08), 1203–1208 (2010)
6. Cohen-Mansfield, J., Dakheel-Ali, M., Marx, M.S.: Engagement in persons with dementia: the concept and its measurement. Am. J. Geria. Psychiatry. **17**(4), 299–307 (2009)
7. Moyle, W., Jones, C., Sung, B., et al.: What effect does an animal robot called CuDDler have on the engagement and emotional response of older people with dementia? a pilot feasibility study. Int. J. Soc. Robot. **8**(1), 145–156 (2016)
8. Cohen-Mansfield, J., Marx, M.S., Freedman, L.S., et al.: The comprehensive process model of engagement. Am. J. Geria. Psychiatry. **19**(10), 859–870 (2011)

9. Perugia, G., Boladeras, M.D., Barakova, E.I., et al.: Social HRI for people with dementia: one size fits all? In: Proceedings of the Companion of the 2017 ACM/IEEE International Conference on Human-Robot Interaction, pp. 257-258. ACM, New York (2017)

10. Trahan, M.A., Kuo, J., Carlson, M.C., Gitlin, L.N.: A systematic review of strategies to foster activity engagement in persons with dementia. Health Educ. Behav. **41**(1), 70–83 (2014)

11. Jones, C., Sung, B., Moyle, W.: Assessing engagement in people with dementia: a new approach to assessment using video analysis. Arch. Psychiatr. Nurs. **29**(6), 377–382 (2015)

12. Lawton, M.P., van Haitsma, K., Klapper, J.: Observed affect in nursing home residents with alzheimer's disease. J. Gerontol. B Psychol. Sci. Soc. Sci. **51**(1), 3–14 (1996)

13. Feng, Y., Reijmersdal, R., Yu, S., et al.: Dynamorph: montessori inspired design for seniors with dementia living in long-term care facilities. In: 9th International Conference on Intelligent Technologies for Interactive Entertainment. Springer. (2017) (accepted)

14. Buettner, L.: Simple pleasures: a multilevel sensorimotor intervention for nursing home residents with dementia. Am. J. Alzheimer's Dis. **14**(1), 41–52 (1999)

15. Kolanowski, A., Buettner, L.: Prescribing activities that engage passive residents. Innovative Method. J. Gerontol. Nurs. **34**(1), 13–18 (2008)

16. Cohen-Mansfield, J., Marx, M.S., Dakheel-Ali, M., et al.: Can persons with dementia be engaged with stimuli? Am. J. Geria. Psychiatry. **18**(4), 351–362 (2010)

17. Kolanowski, A., Litaker, M., Buettner, L., et al.: A randomized clinical trial of theorybased activities for the behavioral symptoms of dementia in nursing home residents. J. Am. Geriatr. Soc. **59**(6), 1032–1041 (2011)

18. Cohen-Mansfield, J.: Conceptualization of agitation: results based on the cohen-mansfield agitation inventory and the agitation behavior mapping instrument. In. Psychogeriatr. **8**(3), 309–315 (1997)

19. Barakova, E.I., Gorbunov, R., Rauterberg, M.: Automatic interpretation of affective facial expressions in the context of interpersonal interaction. IEEE Trans. Hum. Mach. Syst. **45**(4), 409–418 (2015)

20. Hu, J., Frens, J., Funk, M., Wang, F., Zhang, Y.: Design for social interaction in public spaces. In: Rau, P.L.P. (ed.) CCD 2014. LNCS, vol. 8528, pp. 287–298. Springer, Cham (2014). doi:10.1007/978-3-319-07308-8_28

A Design to Reduce Patients' Cognitive Load for Cancer Risk Calculator

Binay Siddharth[1] ⓘ, Lyndal Trevena[2] ⓘ, and Na Liu[1](✉) ⓘ

[1] School of Information Technologies, Faculty of Engineering and IT,
The University of Sydney, Sydney, Australia
bina0004@uni.sydney.edu.au, liu.na@sydney.edu.au
[2] School of Public Health, The University of Sydney, Sydney, Australia
lyndal.trevena@sydney.edu.au

Abstract. Cancer was reported to be the chief killer in Australia by overtaking heart disease. Early detection of cancer aids in effective treatment. This poster paper proposes the design and implementation of an integrated cancer risk calculation tool to address the problem of diversified and unstandardized calculators for different types of cancer. Guided by cognitive load theory, the paper also proposes design features to reduce patients' cognitive load.

Keywords: Cancer risk calculation · System design · Cognitive load

1 Introduction

Cancer was reported to be the chief killer in Australia by overtaking heart disease (Vickery 2016). There has been steady growth in the number of patients in Australia across years where 130,446 are estimated to be diagnosed by cancer in the year 2016 (AIHW 2016). It is estimated that the total costs for cancer U.S in 2014 were $87.7 billion (American Cancer Society 2017).

Early detection of cancer aids in effective treatment. The most common types of cancers in Australia include breast cancer, ovarian cancer, bowel cancer, cervical cancer, lung cancer, prostate cancer and skin cancer. Many online websites, calculators and algorithms are available to project the risk percentage of an individual affected by cancer, and they are widely used by physicians for pre-consultation screening. However, these online cancer risk calculators are usually independent silos system, having different prerequisite questions and produce information based on momentary input. To utilize different tools, physicians or nurses have to input the same information several times, which causes data redundancy and may lead to data entry errors. Researcher also comment that current guidelines of cancer risk assessment are not sufficient and need a more comprehensive approach to determine risk.

To address the problem, the first objective of the project is to develop an integrated cancer risk prediction tool which gives the consulting doctor an insight to the probability of being prone to the seven types of most common cancer in Australia. A web-based tool will be designed for patients to enter their information before their first interaction with the physician. It will work as an umbrella solution with a single

H. Chen et al. (Eds.): ICSH 2017, LNCS 10347, pp. 38–41, 2017.
https://doi.org/10.1007/978-3-319-67964-8_4

clear view by integrating different silos. It will help in reducing the man hours of doctors by facilitating the patients to fill these questions and guides them in a user friendly way.

In order to calculate the risk of seven cancers at the same time, the integrated cancer risk calculator consists of 64 questions which may take more than 20 min to answer all. The long list of questions will impose cognitive loads to the patients when completing the questionnaire. Cognitive load is the mental effort devoted to solve a certain problem or learn something (Sweller 1994). In addition, patients with low health literacy may also find the questions hard to understand, which will impose additional cognitive burden to the patients. Thus, drawn on cognitive load theory, the second objective of the study is providing novel system designs to reduce the cognitive load of patients, shorten completion time, and improve the accuracy of data entry.

This research-in-progress paper will describe the theoretical background of the study and the initial design of the integrative cancer calculator.

2 Theoretical Background and Prototype Design

The first objective of the project is to build an integrative view of all the calculators and reduce the repetitive entry of some basic information, including age, gender, height and weight. A screen shots of the first page of the calculator is shown in Fig. 1 below. The list of cancer calculators will be filtered by gender type. The output of the calculator is a listed view of the possibility of all major types of cancers (Fig. 2).

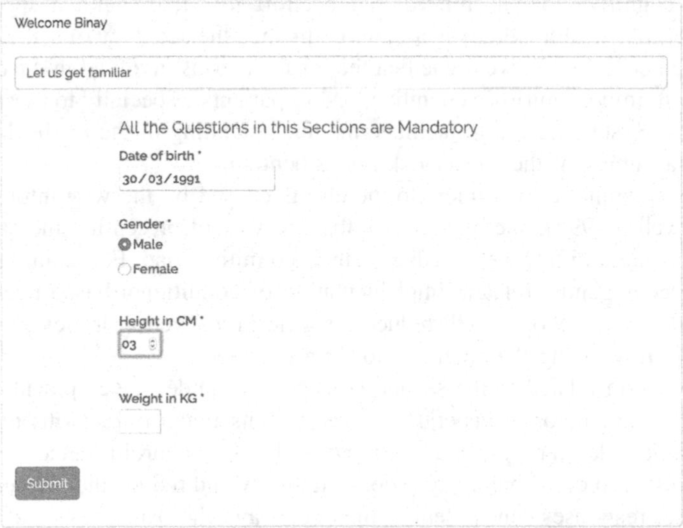

Fig. 1. Screen of the integrated cancer calculator tool

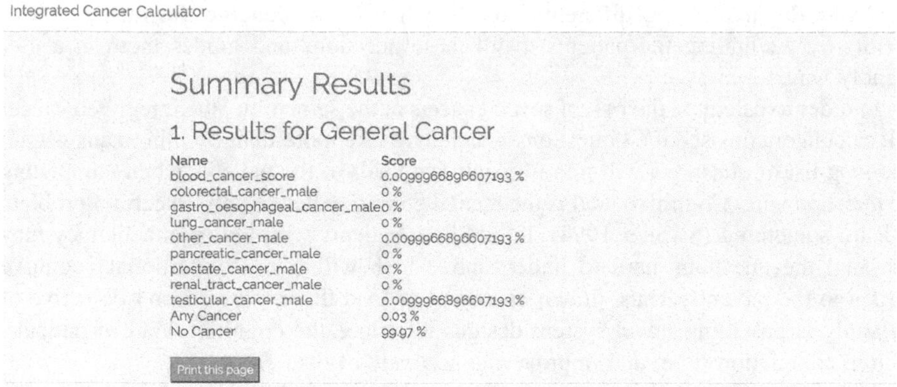

Summary Results

1. Results for General Cancer

Name	Score
blood_cancer_score	0.0099966896607193 %
colorectal_cancer_male	0 %
gastro_oesophageal_cancer_male	0 %
lung_cancer_male	0 %
other_cancer_male	0.0099966896607193 %
pancreatic_cancer_male	0 %
prostate_cancer_male	0 %
renal_tract_cancer_male	0 %
testicular_cancer_male	0.0099966896607193 %
Any Cancer	0.03 %
No Cancer	99.97 %

Print this page

Fig. 2. Screen of the integrated cancer calculator tool

The second objective of the study is to incorporate design features that reduce the cognitive loads for patients. The design is informed by the cognitive load theory, which was originally proposed to improve efficient learning and create long-term memory of knowledge. According to the theory, cognitive load refers to the amount of mental efforts required to solve a problem (Sweller 1994). There are three types of cognitive loads including intrinsic, extraneous, and germane. Germane cognitive load refers to the additional effort for creating permanent memory of knowledge, which is not relevant to this study.

Intrinsic cognitive load is related to the effort to comprehend a specific topic (Sweller 1994). As health literacy is found to influence the accuracy of self-rated health status (Bennett et al. 2009), we argue that the medical terms involved in the cancer risk assessment will impose intrinsic cognitive load to patients, especially to those with low health literacy. System design to facilitate the understanding of the medical terms will improve the accuracy of the cancer risk assessment.

Extraneous cognitive load refers to the efforts caused by the way information are presented (Sweller 1994). We hypothesize that the way of presenting the questions to patients will make a difference in reducing their cognitive load. For example, as some types of cancer is gender-related, implementation of conditional based questions that features gender based choices will reduce the time in answering irrelevant questions, and thus help in reducing the cognitive load on patients.

The features on related to the second objective are under development. However, this cancer risk calculator in general will maintain its integrity in terms of usage on different screens like laptops, iPad, iPhone and other android devices. This will facilitate the users to complete the questions on the fly and reduce their dependency on a device. Also, responses can be sent to the doctor and the patient as a pdf document which is required for consultation.

3   Next Step

We plan to implement the infrastructure and conduct pilot testing on different participants to understand the effect of cognitive load and tweak the presented design. Also, we plan to conduct a usability study (think aloud, a/b testing) on the acceptance of this website and implement the results.

We will collaborate with general practitioners to recruit patients to use the system for pre-consultation assessment. Half of the recruited patients will only use the general integrative calculator without cognitive load reducing features. Another half of the patients will use the calculator with our cognitive load reducing designs. The total completion time will be captured to compare the effectiveness of the design. Patients' feedback and evaluation on the cancer calculator will also be collected.

References

Vickery, K.: More Australians dying from cancer than heart diseases, new report from Australian Institute of Health and Welfare shows (2016). http://www.news.com.au/lifestyle/health/health-problems/more-australians-dying-from-cancer-than-heart-diseases-new-report-from-australian-institute-of-health-and-welfare-shows/news-story/cae4d17b17f2647e68fc570b1d8465aa. Accessed 12 Mar 2017

Australian Institute of Health and Welfare (2016). http://Aihw.gov.au. http://www.aihw.gov.au/cancers/all-cancers/. Accessed 13 Mar 2017

American Cancer Society (2017). Economic Impact of Cancer https://www.cancer.org/cancer/cancer-basics/economic-impact-of-cancer.html. Accessed 14 Mar 2017

Sweller, J.: Cognitive load theory, learning difficulty, and instructional design. Learn. Instr. 4(4), 295–312 (1994)

Bennett, I.M., Chen, J., Soroui, J.S., White, S.: The contribution of health literacy to disparities in self-rated health status and preventive health behaviors in older adults. Ann. Fam. Med. 7(3), 204–211 (2009)

The Impacts of Patients' Gift Giving Behavior on Physicians' Service Quality

Wei Zhao, Xitong Guo$^{(\boxtimes)}$, Tianshi Wu, and Jingxuan Geng

School of Management, eHealth Research Institute,
Harbin Institute of Technology, Harbin, China
weizhao9001@gmail.com, {xitongguo,wutianshi}@hit.edu.
cn, hitgengjingxuan@163.com

Abstract. The Online health community (OHC) provides convenience and benefits. Simultaneously, it also generates informal social moral problems regarding payment. However, few studies have explored the physicians' service delivery from the patients' perspective. Using unique interaction data between doctors and patients from an online health consultation community, we empirically examined how patients' gift giving behavior influences physicians' service delivery, and how this influence is being moderated by physicians' gift receiving ratio and social morality, using a difference-in-difference model. We find that the giving of gifts by patients has a positive impact on the physicians' service quality. Furthermore, this effect is significantly moderated by the physicians' gift receiving ratio and social morality. We discuss the implications of these findings for patients consulting in OHCs and for OHC designers.

Keywords: Online health community · Service quality · Gift giving

1 Introduction

Online health communities (OHCs) provide a convenient and economical approach for patients to obtain health information and health care resources [1–6]. Some OHCs provide patients with a function of gift-giving during the consultation process, and they claim that the function purely aims to open up a channel for patients to express gratitude. However, it could also generate social moral problems. Social media has exposed patients' complaints that the virtual gift giving is a form of disguised informal payment, and it may aggravate conflicts between doctors and patients. Is it a latent rule that patients give gifts to doctors during the consultation process? Although answering these questions is very important, few prior studies have explored the physicians' service delivery from the patients' perspective in OHCs.

Extant literature has studied online service quality. For example, researchers have developed a conceptual framework, e-SELFQUAL, to examine the quality of online self-services in e-retailing [7]. Furthermore, a recent study has examined the relationship between the physicians' service delivery process and patient satisfaction, but they have not studied the factors that impact the physicians' service delivery process [6]. Our study, rather, focuses on analyzing doctors' services in OHCs from the

© Springer International Publishing AG 2017
H. Chen et al. (Eds.): ICSH 2017, LNCS 10347, pp. 42–53, 2017.
https://doi.org/10.1007/978-3-319-67964-8_5

patients' perspective. This study aims to explore how patients' gift-giving behavior influences physicians' service delivery, and how this influence is moderated by the physicians' gift receiving ratio and social morality.

We use the interaction data from 242,585 patients to 825 doctors on two kinds of illnesses in a primary Chinese OHC. Our data also contains rich control variables, including demographic characteristics, online activity variables, and consultation variables. We rely on a natural experimental setup and employ a difference-in-difference econometric method to control both the physicians' and patients' endogeneity. The results demonstrate that patients' gift-giving has a positive impact on physicians' service quality. When a physician has a higher ratio of gift receiving, the impact of patients' gift giving on physicians' service quality will be less influential. We also found that when the ratio of gift receiving among physicians who belong to the same specialist category as a certain physician is higher, the impact of patients' gift-giving on this physician's service quality will be more influential.

Our paper aims to make a few contributions to extant literature. Our study contributes to OHC literature by exploring the impacts of patient behavior on physician service quality. In addition, our findings contribute to the literature on the gift theory, because we empirically investigate the moderation effects of social norms on the relationship between patients' gift-giving and physicians' service delivery. Moreover, our findings propose that OHC designers should specify that gift-giving is an instant and mutual benefit which purely aims to open up a channel for patients to express gratitude. Simultaneously, it is beneficial for patients to choose a physician who has a low ratio of gift receiving to maximize their gift-giving effectiveness.

In the next section, we review several extant studies to develop our hypotheses. In Sect. 3, we provide an overview of our research context and describe our empirical data set. Following this, we introduce our econometric model. In Sect. 4, we present our regression results and analyses. In Sect. 5, we discuss our study's implications. In Sect. 6, we end this study with a conclusion.

2 Theoretical Background and Hypotheses

In order to better understand this study and discuss the voids in the existing literature, we draw on several important streams of research: the online health community, service quality, the gift theory and reciprocity, as well as social influence and the social norm theory.

2.1 The Online Health Community

The online health community (OHC) provides a convenient and economic channel for patients to obtain health information and professional healthcare consultation services [1–5]. The patients can minimize healthcare costs and save time through using an online OHC [6]. Extant literature has explored the benefits and challenges facing stakeholders (Doctors, Patients, and Hospitals) when using OHCs [3, 4, 8, 9]. The website designs and their policies play an important role in the acceptance and use of OHCs [4]. According to a recent study, physicians have different views about whether and how to use social media to interact with patients on the Internet [9]. An extensive volume of research has examined the impacts of OHCs on physicians' performance and economic outcomes from the e-commerce perspective [10–12]. Customer satisfaction is a very important factor in commerce. The physician's service quality positively affects patients' satisfaction. If a physician has both a high response speed and response frequency during consultations, the patients are more likely to be satisfied [6].

Although a considerable volume of OHC literature has investigated the physicians' service or the physicians' performance in a commercial perspective, such research may not explore the service delivery from the patients' perspective. Our study will narrow this void by exploring the impacts of patient behavior on physicians' service quality.

2.2 Service Quality

Compared with tangible goods, service quality is more difficult to measure because of the absence of tangible evidence [13]. The measurement of service quality is a popular research topic. Extensive literature has focused on developing service quality measurement models. Many researchers have measured service quality by way of discrepancies between expectations and experience performance [13–15]. In many models, responsiveness is an important dimension for measuring physicians' service quality [13, 16, 17]. Responsiveness is one of the dimensions for measuring the quality of physicians' online service delivery in OHCs [6]. Therefore, our study uses responsiveness as the service quality measurement.

2.3 The Gift Theory and Reciprocity

Gift exchange is a very common phenomenon in social relationships. A considerable volume of literature has focused on the nature of gifts [18–24]. Some studies have regarded gift exchange as a kind of economic rationality behavior [25]. Gift givers frequently receive returned gifts because of the reciprocity norm [26]. The gift exchange process is considered as a continuous cycle of reciprocities [27]. Moreover, reciprocity is a moral norm and obligation [19]. Another study has proposed that gift exchange is bound by social rules and ethical principles. In a gift exchange process, while the giver does not expect feedback content, the giving and receiving have become potential obligations of a certain nature. As a result, the gift giving economy is regarded as a debt causing economy [18, 20]. For some patients, a gift is purely a goodwill gesture, but for others it is not so [28, 29]. Extant studies have suggested that gift-giving enables the improvement of workers' efficiency [23]. Gift giving enables the generation of externalities for third parties outside of bilateral relationships between the gift giver and the recipient in the medical context [30].

According to the gift theory, regardless of the motivations for patients' gift giving, the gifts provide physicians with economic and mental utility. Therefore, physicians constantly face the obligation and motivation to provide better service in order to reciprocate patients. According to the diminishing marginal utility theory, the more gifts physicians receive, the less the utility of these gifts. Furthermore, a physician's gift-receiving gift ratio indicates the probability of that physicians' receiving of gifts. If the physicians receive unexpected gifts, the influence of gift giving will be stronger. Therefore, we hypothesize that:

- Hypothesis 1. Patients' gift giving has a positive impact on physicians' response speed in OHCs.
- Hypothesis 2a. The impact of patients' gift giving on physicians' response speed decreases when the physicians' gift receiving ratio increases.

2.4   Social Influences and Social Norms

Social influences consist of normative and informational social influences. The normative influence refers to "an influence to conform to the positive expectations of others" [31]. An experimental study proposed that social influence can change individuals' attitudes and actions. This change is different from an individual's conformity. Compliance occurs when an "individual adopts the induced behavior in order to gain specific rewards and avoid specific punishments". Normative social influences lead to public compliance [32]. If patients' gift-giving is a common phenomenon in a group or community, the giving of gifts has become a social norm. Many empirical studies have suggested that social norms affect an individual's behavior [33, 34]. Therefore, we argue that when there is a higher tendency for patients to give gifts to physicians, and if a certain patient fails to comply with this norm, that patient may be punished. Otherwise, if a patient complies with this social norm, that patient will be rewarded with a better quality service. Therefore, we hypothesize that:

- Hypothesis 2b. The impact of patients' gift-giving on physicians' response speed increases when the existence of gift-giving social norm becomes clearer.

This study's theoretical framework is presented in Fig. 1.

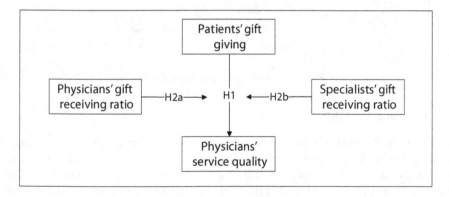

Fig. 1. Research model

3   Empirical Methodology

3.1   The Research Context

We obtained data from the Good Physician Online website (haodf.com) to empirically investigate the impacts of patients' gift-giving behavior on physicians' service quality. The Good Physician Online website was established in 2006, and is the biggest online healthcare community in China. There are more than 116,564 physicians providing consultation services. The patient can choose a physician and create a post to describe his/her health conditions and post questions by text or upload his/her medical records. The physicians can respond to the patients to provide a diagnosis or suggestions according to the patients' online text descriptions (see Fig. 2). The first three of the physician's answers are free of charge. If there are more than three responses, the physician will charge for online consultations, ranging from 1–20 RMB per response. The consultation price usually depends on a physician's rank and popularity. The patients can give digital gifts with a value ranging from 5–200 RMB to their physicians out of gratitude or for other purposes during consultation process (see Fig. 2). The Good Physician Online website is ideal for the purposes of our study because of the many interactions between physicians and patients.

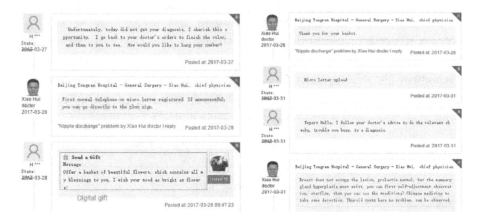

Fig. 2. Consultations and Digital gifts

3.2   Data and Variables

We randomly sampled 968 physicians who are specialists in coronary heart disease (CHD) and infertility diseases on www.haodf.com. The patients of these two specialties are common and suit our research context. We developed a Java program to collect data spanning from January 2015 to March 2016. Our dataset was constructed from two website function modules on a monthly basis. (1) Our primary patient-physician consultation interaction data was crawled from its "patient service function module". The consultation data included the descriptions of patients' conditions, physicians' reply texts, post time stamp charges and patients' gift giving records, all of which enable us to calculate physicians' response speeds and response attitudes to certain patients. (2) In order to control physicians' heterogeneity, we collected physicians' demographic data and online activity data from every physician's personal homepage. After clearing invalid data, we finally obtained the data of 621 physicians, 58,836 patients and 344,925 consultation texts.

- Dependent variables: Our dependent variable was the physicians' response speeds. The response speed was measured by the duration of the responses. A physician's response duration to a certain patient refers to the average interval between the patient's time of asking and the time a physician responds to a post. The smaller values represent the physician's faster response speeds. We used the following formulation to calculate the duration of the responses:

$$ResponseDuration_{ij} = \sum_{k=1}^{n_i} \left(AnswerTime_{ijk} - AskTime_{ijk}\right)/n_i \qquad (1)$$

In the above equation, $ResponseDuration_{ij}$ represents the duration of physician j response to patient i. n_i represents the total counts of the physician's response times to patient i. $AnswerTime_{ijk}$ and $AskTime_{ijk}$ respectively represent the answering point-in-time and consulting point-in-time between physician j and patient i.

- Independent variables: The primary independent variables of interest include patients' gift giving, the ratio of physicians' monthly gift receipts, and the ratio of monthly gift receipts of physicians of the same specialty. The patient's gift giving is a binary indicator for patients' gift-giving. $PatientGiftGiving_{ij} = 1$, if patient i gave a gift to physician j, zero otherwise. The formulas we used to the other two variables are shown as follows:

$$DocGiftRatio_{jt} = \frac{GiftPatientNum_{jt}}{PatientNum_{jt}} \qquad (2)$$

$$SpeGiftRatio_{st} = \frac{GiftPatientNum_{st}}{PatientNum_{st}} \qquad (3)$$

In the Eq. (2), $DocGiftRatio_{jt}$ represents the radio of physician j receiving gifts at month t. $GiftPatientNum_{jt}$ refers to the total number of patients giving gifts to physician j in month t. $PatientNum_{jt}$ refers to the total number of patients consulting physician j in month t, respectively.

In the Eq. (3), $SpeGiftRatio_{st}$ represents the radio of physicians of the specialty s receiving gifts in month t. The method to calculate $GiftPatientNum_{st}$ and $PatientNum_{st}$ is similar to the calculation of $DocGiftRatio_{it}$.

- To account for the unobserved physician heterogeneity and consultation conditions, we included physicians' demographic characteristics, online activity data, and consultations features (see Table 1).

Table 1. Description of control variables

	Variables	Definitions
Physicians' characteristics	Ranking	Physicians' ranking (director physician, associate director physician, chief physician, and physician)
Physicians' online activity data	Contribution	Contribution values
	Thank you letters	The number of thank you letters
	Essays	Quantity of essays
	Vote	Patients' votes
	Online lifespan	OHC use history
	Patient numbers	The number of patients
Consultation factors	Asking times	Patients' asking times
	Response times	The physicians' response times
	Asking words	The average number of text words for patients' questions
	Response words	The average number of text words for responses

Summary statistics of the dataset is provide in Table 2. We can found physicians' average of response duration is 23,258 s (about 6.46 h).

Table 2. Summary Statistics

Variable	Obs	Mean	Std. Dev.	Min	Max
ResponseDuration	117,454	23,258	28,469	0	143,096
DocGiftRatio	117,454	0.04	0.05	0	1
DepGiftRatio	117,454	0.04	0.02	0	0.06

Note: In order to conserve space, we only reported key variables for this study.

3.3 Econometric Model

Some patients give digital gifts to their physicians during healthcare consultations process on the OHC while others do not do so. This creates a natural experimental setting that enables us to compare the differences in physicians' service quality before and after patients' gift-giving. When a certain patient has given gifts to his/her physician, this patient belongs to a treatment group. If one patient did not give any gifts to the doctor, he/she belongs to a control group. Under these conditions, every consultation post represents each patient. We apply a difference-in-difference (DID) analysis to control physicians' and patients' endogeneity. The inclusion of DID and rich physicians' demographic variables and online activity variables enable control of the physicians' endogeneity and heterogeneity. We performed natural logarithm transformations on all variables except for the rankings and ratios to endorse the assumption of normality and eliminate the heteroscedasticity. We used ordinary least square regression to test our hypotheses.

DID Model: Main Effects of gift giving

$ResponseDuration_{ijt} = \alpha_{ij} + \alpha_1 \cdot Treat_{ij} + \alpha_2 AfterTreat_{ij} + \alpha_3 \cdot Treat_{ij} \cdot AfterTreat_{ij} + \alpha_4 \cdot PhysicianControl_{jt} + \varepsilon_{jt}$

In the above equation, i denotes a patient, j denotes a physician, and t denotes the time period. $Treat_{ij}$ equals 1 if the patient i is in the treatment group and 0 otherwise. $AfterTreat_{ij}$ is also a dummy variable. It takes the value 0 and 1 for periods prior to and post gift-giving. $PhysicianControl_{jt}$ represents the control variables for physician j at time t. α_{ij} is the patient fixed effects that control time-invariant differences across patients. The coefficient α_3 is the difference-in-difference estimate of the effects of gift giving on service quality. Because the unobservable of patients belonging to the same physician will be correlated, we conducted a cluster standard error on physician level.

DDD approach: Moderating Effects of Hypothesized Variables

$$ResponseDuration_{ijt} = \alpha_{ij} + \alpha_1 \cdot Treat_{ij} + \alpha_2 \cdot AfterTreat_{ij} + \alpha_3 \cdot Treat_{ij} \cdot AfterTreat_{ij}$$
$$+ \alpha_4 \cdot Treat_{ij} \cdot AfterTreat_{ij} \cdot DocGiftRatio_{jt} + \alpha_5 \cdot Treat_{ij} \cdot$$
$$AfterTreat_{ij} \cdot SepGiftRatio_{kt} + \alpha_6 \cdot PhysicianControl_{jt} + \varepsilon_{jt}$$

The meaning of variables in this equation is the same as denoted in the former equation. The difference of this equation from the previous one is that this formulation includes three-way interactions between patients' gift-giving, the time of gift-giving and one of the moderating variables, including the ratio of physicians' monthly gift receipts, and the ratio of monthly gift receipts of physicians of the same specialty. The key parameters of interest are those three coefficients ($\alpha_3, \alpha_4, \alpha_5$), which estimate the moderating effects of gift giving on a physician's service quality.

4   Results

Table 3 records the results of our model. Model 1 records the estimates from the baseline DID model with no additional controls. Model 2 includes all physicians' control variables. In Model 3, we added two interaction items to estimate the moderating effects of DocGiftRatio and SepGiftRatio on the relationship between patients' gift-giving and physicians' response speeds. The results indicate that the adjusted R-Square increases gradually along with the adding of control variables and interaction items. Moreover, models are stable from Models 2 to 3. No VIF (variance inflation factor) statistics for the variables were greater than 2, which indicates the absence of multicollinearity.

Table 3. OLS regression

Variable	Model 1	Model 2	Model 3
Intercept	2.259(0.014)***	3.499(1.223)***	3.900(1.156)***
Treat	0.033(0.012)***	0.224(0.075)***	0.128(0.133)
AfterTreat	0.035(0.004)***	0.321(0.032)***	0.286(0.047)***
Treat × AfterTreat	−0.051(0.006)***	−0.454(0.051)***	−0.216(0.111)*
DocGiftRatio	–	–	2.914(0.889)***
SepGiftRatio	–	–	−13.286(2.546)***
Treat × AfterTreat × DocGiftRatio	–	–	2.572(0.882)***
Treat × AfterTreat × SepGiftRatio	–	–	−7.950(2.627)***
Controls	N	Y	Y
Adj. R square	0.006	0.122	0.131

Note: In order to conserve space, we only reported variables of interest for this study. Signif. codes: 0 '***' 0.01 '**' 0.05 '*' 0.1

The coefficients of the DID item were negative and statistically significant (In Model 2, this estimate is −0.454), which means that patients' gift-giving has a negative impact on physician's response duration. In other words, a patient who gives gifts will obtain a faster response speed. It supports Hypothesis 1. For practical significant, physician' response speed to a patient who gave gifts will increase by 36.5% (about 2.38 h). In Hypothesis 2a, we aimed to test the moderating effects of physicians' gift receiving ratio on the relationship between patients' gift giving and physicians' response speeds. The results show that the coefficient of the DocGiftRatio interaction item is positive and statistically significant, indicating that when a physician has a higher ratio of gift receiving, the impacts of patients' gift giving on physicians' response speeds will be less influential. In Hypothesis 2b, we aimed to test the moderating effects of the ratio of gift receiving among physicians of the same specialty on the relationship between patients' gift giving and physicians' response speeds. The results show the coefficient of the SepGiftRatio interaction item is negatively and statistically significant, indicating that when the physicians of the same specialty exhibit a higher ratio of gift receiving, the impacts of patients' gift giving on physicians' response speeds will be more beneficial.

5   Discussion

This study provides several insights. First, the results demonstrate that patients' gift-giving has positive impacts on physicians' response speeds. If a patient give gifts to a doctor during a consultation, he/she is more likely to receive better service quality. In other words, patients' gift giving is effective in obtaining a faster physicians' response. The result is consistent with the gift theory. When a patient exerts effort and money in giving a digital gift to a doctor, the physician is obliged to reciprocate to that patient by providing a better service because of the reciprocity norm [19, 26]. Therefore, gift-giving in OHCs is mutually beneficial rather than being perceived as compulsive behavior. Simultaneously, we also found that when a physician has a higher ratio of gift receiving, the impacts of patients' gift giving on physicians' service quality will be less influential. In other words, the higher the probability of physicians' receiving gifts, the lower will be the effects of patients' gift giving. According to the diminishing marginal utility theory, the receiving of gifts is more effective for doctors who rarely receive gifts. Our results suggest that choosing a physician with a low ratio of gift-giving will maximize the gift-giving effects. Moreover, our findings indicate that patients' gift-giving has a greater influence on physicians' service quality, as well as resulting in a higher ratio of gift receiving among physicians of the same specialty. As we mentioned in Sect. 2.4, when patients' gift-giving become a common phenomenon in OHCs, gift-giving will be regarded as a social norm. It will affect the members' behavior [33, 34]. If the members comply with this social norm, they will be rewarded with better service quality [32].

We emphasize two theoretical implications of our study. First, our results show that patients' gift-giving has a significant effect on doctors' service delivery. Second, our findings contribute to the literature on the gift theory. This paper empirically investigated the moderate effects of social norms on the relationship between patients' gift-giving and physicians' service delivery. In addition, our study has provided two practical suggestions. First, in order to maximize the effectiveness of gift-giving, patients ought to choose a physician with a low ratio of gift receiving. Second, our findings propose that the OHC website ought to make gift-giving transparent and normative to distinguish it from the traditional hospitals' red envelopes (the informal payment). It is also beneficial for patients to obtain better services in OHCs and the relationship between patients and doctors.

6 Conclusion

In this paper, we investigated the relationship between patients' gift giving and physicians' service delivery by using interaction data between doctors and patients from an online health consultation community. We constructed a difference-in-difference model to empirically examine how patients' gift-giving influences physicians' service delivery and how this influence was moderated by the ratio of physicians' gift receipts and social morality. The results demonstrate that patients' gift-giving has a positive impact on physicians' service quality. In addition, we found that the ratio of physicians' gift-receiving has negative moderation effects on the relationship between patients' gift giving and physicians' service quality. Moreover, the effects of patients' gift giving on physicians' service quality were positively moderated by social norms.

References

1. Denecke, K., Nejdl, W.: How valuable is medical social media data? Content analysis of the medical web. Inf. Sci. **179**(12), 1870–1880 (2009)
2. Kitchens, B., Harle, C.A., Li, S.: Quality of health-related online search results. Decis. Support Syst. **57**, 454–462 (2014)

3. Househ, M., Borycki, E., Kushniruk, A.: Empowering patients through social media: the benefits and challenges. Health Inform. J. **20**(1), 50–58 (2014)
4. Frost, J., Vermeulen, I.E., Beekers, N.: Anonymity versus privacy: selective information sharing in online cancer communities. J. Med. Internet Res. **16**(5), e126 (2014)
5. Yan, L., Peng, J., Tan, Y.: Network dynamics: how can we find patients like us? Inform. Syst. Res. **26**(3), 496–512 (2015)
6. Yang, H., Guo, X., Wu, T.: Exploring the influence of the online physician service delivery process on patient satisfaction. Decis. Support Syst. **78**, 113–121 (2015)
7. Ding, D.X., Hu, P.J.-H., Sheng, O.R.L.: e-SELFQUAL: a scale for measuring online self-service quality. J. Bus. Res. **64**(5), 508–515 (2011)
8. Fischer, S.H., David, D., Crotty, B.H., Dierks, M., Safran, C.: Acceptance and use of health information technology by community-dwelling elders. Int. J. Med. Informatics **83**(9), 624–635 (2014)
9. Brown, J., Ryan, C., Harris, A.: How doctors view and use social media: a national survey. J. Med. Internet Res. **16**(12), e267 (2014)
10. Liu, X., Guo, X., Wu, H., Wu, T.: The impact of individual and organizational reputation on physicians' appointments online. Int. J. Electron. Commer. **20**(4), 551–577 (2016)
11. Yan, Z., Wang, T., Chen, Y., Zhang, H.: Knowledge sharing in online health communities: a social exchange theory perspective. Inf. Manag. **53**(5), 643–653 (2016)
12. Wu, H., Lu, N.: How your colleagues' reputation impact your patients' odds of posting experiences: evidence from an online health community. Electron. Commer. Res. Appl. **16**, 7–17 (2016)
13. Parasuraman, A., Zeithaml, V.A., Berry, L.L.: A conceptual model of service quality and its implications for future research. J. Mark. **49**(4), 41–50 (1985)
14. Brown, S.W., Swartz, T.A.: A gap analysis of professional service quality. J. Mark. **53**, 92–98 (1989)
15. Bolton, R.N., Drew, J.H.: A multistage model of customers' assessments of service quality and value. J. Consum. Res. **17**(4), 375–384 (1991)
16. Bowers, M.R., Swan, J.E., Koehler, W.F.: What attributes determine quality and satisfaction with health care delivery? Health Care Manage. Rev. **19**(4), 49–55 (1994)
17. Johnston, R.: The determinants of service quality: satisfiers and dissatisfiers. Int. J. Serv. Ind. Manag. **6**(5), 53–71 (1995)
18. Mauss, M., Halls, W.D.: The Gift: The Form and Reason for Exchange in Archaic Societies. WW Norton & Company, New York (2000)
19. Gouldner, A.W.: The norm of reciprocity: a preliminary statement. Am. Sociol. Rev. **25**, 161–178 (1960)
20. Cheal, D.: The gift economy. (1988)
21. Giesler, M.: Consumer gift systems. J. Consum. Res. **33**(2), 283–290 (2006)
22. Komter, A.: Gifts and social relations the mechanisms of reciprocity. Int. Sociol. **22**(1), 93–107 (2007)
23. Kube, S., Maréchal, M.A., Puppea, C.: The currency of reciprocity: gift exchange in the workplace. Am. Econ. Rev. **102**(4), 1644–1662 (2012)
24. Romele, A., Severo, M.: The economy of the digital gift: from socialism to sociality online. Theory Cult. Soc. **33**(5), 43–63 (2016)
25. Bronislaw, M., George, F.S.J.: Argonauts of the Western Pacific (1922)
26. Komter, A.E.: Reciprocity as a principle of exclusion: gift giving in the Netherlands. Sociology **30**(2), 299–316 (1996)
27. Sherry, J.F.: Gift giving in anthropological perspective. J. Consum. Res. **10**(2), 157–168 (1983)

28. Drew, J., Stoeckle, J.D., Billings, J.A.: Tips, status and sacrifice: gift giving in the doctor-patient relationship. Soc. Sci. Med. **17**(7), 399–404 (1983)
29. Lyckholm, L.J.: Should physicians accept gifts from patients? JAMA **280**(22), 1944–1946 (1998)
30. Currie, J., Lin, W., Meng, J.: Social networks and externalities from gift exchange: evidence from a field experiment. J. public Econ. **107**, 19–30 (2013)
31. Deutsch, M., Gerard, H.B.: A study of normative and informational social influences upon individual judgment. J. Abnorm. Soc. Psychol. **51**(3), 629 (1955)
32. Kelman, H.C.: Compliance, identification, and internalization three processes of attitude change. J. Conflict Resolut. **2**(1), 51–60 (1958)
33. Teo, T.S., Pok, S.H.: Adoption of WAP-enabled mobile phones among Internet users. Omega **31**(6), 483–498 (2003)
34. Hsu, C.-L., Lin, J.C.-C.: Acceptance of blog usage: the roles of technology acceptance, social influence and knowledge sharing motivation. Inf. Manag. **45**(1), 65–74 (2008)

Utilizing Social Media to Share Knowledge of Healthcare and Improve Subjective Wellbeing of Aging People

Yumeng Miao[✉], Rong Du, and Shizhong Ai

Xidian University, Xi'an 710126, China
ymmiao@stu.xidian.edu.cn

Abstract. In recent decades, many healthcare service providers embrace social media to spread knowledge to the public and communicate with them. However, elderly people are not paid much attention. As we know, more and more countries have to face the challenge of rapidly aging and it is vital to meet their demands of healthcare such as how to manage their chronic diseases by themselves. Information technology (IT) may provide solutions and studies on IT use in different contexts of aging have emerged. However, research relating IT use to healthcare knowledge sharing and wellbeing of aging people is limited. This study aims to examine relations among social media use, healthcare knowledge sharing, and seniors' wellbeing in the context of China. For this purpose, we use a mixed method to test our conceptual model, which consists of both quasi-experiment and questionnaire survey conducted with retired elderly people. Our research can give healthcare service providers suggestions about how to use social media to increase seniors' knowledge of self-management and to improve their wellbeing.

Keywords: Healthcare · Knowledge sharing · Social media · Subjective wellbeing · Senior care

1 Introduction

In recent years, with rapid population aging in many countries, greater attention has been paid to the issues of senior care. As a result, the development of information technology (IT) has provided some solutions, specifically, in China, "internet+" was proposed in the report on the work of the government. For example, when a retailer sells his products on Taobao platform, we think he is using internet to sell products. It is a kind of application of "internet+" combining internet with traditional retailing. "Internet+" has put emphasis on the essential role of the internet in developing various industries. Decidedly, through the internet, social media provide a platform for people to create and share opinions and experience. For healthcare service providers, social media are used as a platform to spread related information and interact with people. For example, many hospitals have official accounts of social media platforms such as WeChat and MicroBlog to post their information (Kordzadeh and Young 2015). For patients, social media are used as a source of healthcare information and a platform for seeking and offering support. For instance, people can consult a physician online on

Haodf.com (an online health community for people to consult physicians) instead of going to a hospital. Undoubtedly, young people are so familiar with different kinds of social media that they can use them easily. Nevertheless, for elderly people (between 50 to 65 years old), social media are often regarded as new technologies. To use or not to use depends on people's age, gender, education and family composition. Moreover, social environment and psychological characteristics are also important factors (Deursen and Helsper 2015). Negative attitudes towards IT lack of IT experience are obstacles for older adults (Wagner et al. 2010; Lee et al. 2011). However, reports show that more and more elderly people tend to use internet in China (Fig. 1). Thus, we target elderly people who are familiar with basic operations of computers or mobile phones through internet. As for people who will retire or have retired, they may become more and more worried about their health, especially when left alone. Hence, we seek to explore the impacts of social media on seniors' wellbeing.

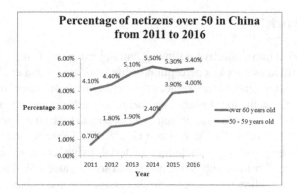

Fig. 1. Percentage of netizens over 50 years old in China from 2011 to 2016.

Although the relationship between social media and knowledge sharing has been excessively studied, healthcare knowledge sharing is distinct from other knowledge sharing. It is closely linked to individuals' health status, treatments and privacy. Some are unwilling to share related knowledge to others for they may feel painful when recalling bad memories. Healthcare knowledge is categorized into general healthcare knowledge (public medical and health knowledge) and specific healthcare knowledge (private knowledge) (Yan et al. 2016). The latter is more difficult to contribute and obtain, but it is particularly important, especially for those who have the same or similar diseases. The majority of seniors are more likely to have some similar chronic diseases, so it is considerable to stimulate their healthcare knowledge sharing.

We can assume that social media use for senior people can influence their quality of life and affect their wellbeing. Apparently, senior people can benefit from social media in their healthcare to acquire healthcare knowledge for preventing themselves from some diseases and managing themselves better. However, there is very little literature addressing the impacts of social media use and IT-enabled healthcare knowledge sharing on aging people's wellbeing. We seek to reduce this gap by investigating the relationship between social media use, IT-enabled healthcare knowledge sharing and seniors' wellbeing. Our research questions are as follows:

RQ1:   How social media use can have an impact on seniors' subjective wellbeing?

RQ2:   How healthcare knowledge sharing acts as a mediator between social media use and seniors' subjective wellbeing?

Specifically, WeChat are used quite frequently in China as a kind of social applications, thus in this research, we plan to use WeChat as the specific social media for seniors and conduct a mixed research approach composed of quasi-experiment and questionnaire surveys.

The rest of the paper is organized as follows: in the next section we present the related work. Then, we propose a research model and relevant hypotheses. After that, we introduce our methodology, i.e., the design of quasi-experiment and survey questionnaire. In the concluding part, we give discussions and extensions for further study.

2 Related Work

Wellbeing is divided into subjective wellbeing and objective wellbeing while subjective wellbeing is identified as people's perception of life satisfaction and evaluation of happiness. Scholars often understand subjective wellbeing from three different types, including evaluative wellbeing, hedonic wellbeing and eudemonic wellbeing (Steptoe et al. 2015). Some scholars measure subjective wellbeing to understand people's feelings or experiences directly (Chen 2013; Wei and Gao 2017). There are volumes of factors influencing subjective wellbeing including material living conditions, gender, age, income, education and culture, subjective needs and social values (Wei and Gao, 2017).

As the aging population increases, researchers have become interested in the topics of elderly people's subjective wellbeing and their health. For example, Angus Deaton, the 2015 Nobel Prize winner in economics, has made great contributions to this stream of research. He explored the relationships between age, gender, religion and health through data from the Gallup World Poll (Deaton 2011). Empirical evidence revealed the relevance of injustice about health inequalities and education, income and status (Deaton 2013). His study also explained the differences in life evaluation and the experience of happiness among the elderly. On the basis of his research, the relationship between seniors' subjective wellbeing and health has been studied (Steptoe et al. 2015). The findings indicate that subjective wellbeing and health are closely related to each other, especially for elderly people. Therefore, it is important to find the ways to improve seniors' subjective wellbeing. According to Angus Deaton's research, subjective wellbeing and health are very closely related especially among seniors and are important for seniors to maintain their wellbeing.

Taking characteristics of the elderly people into consideration, a great number of researchers have made contributions to the literature. People can get information more conveniently through internet and there are many social media like online health communities providing information for patients (Whitten et al. 2004). Prior research shows that patients can be managers of their own information to realize self-management of health and diseases with the help of IT tools (Seckin 2010). Hence, social media help individuals to get health information or knowledge quickly (Anderson 2004; Whitten et al. 2004). That is why knowledge sharing is so important. Knowledge sharing is defined as a process of communication among several parties including the contribution and acquisition of knowledge (Usoro et al. 2007). In this paper, within the context of healthcare, knowledge sharing refers to the information/knowledge exchange behavior of participants, such as posting, browsing, and transferring as well as sharing (Zhou et al. 2014). We can depict knowledge-sharing from two angles, i.e. knowledge acquisition and knowledge contribution. Several studies have explored knowledge-sharing from different perspectives. For example, some have focused on the factors influencing individuals' willingness to share knowledge (Bock et al. 2005; Kankanhalli et al. 2005; Wasko and Faraj 2005; Chiu et al. 2006; Hsu et al. 2007). When exploring individuals' behavior about knowledge sharing, social cognitive theory (SCT) has been applied widely. According to the findings in SCT (Bandura 1986), knowledge sharing behavior is affected by both personal factors and environment.

Besides, many studies have considered the role of media. For instance, people's choices are affected by social influence such as peer effects (Agarwal et al. 2009). Previous research has indicated that traditional media, new media and internet are related to people's subjective wellbeing because of, for example, social engagement and social integration (Wei and Gao 2017). Social media may improve senior people's quality of life. So it is important to do research into the relevance of social media use for older people's healthcare and wellbeing.

3 Research Model and Hypotheses

To explore the new ways that facilitate elderly people produce subjective wellbeing, we propose a research model as shown in Fig. 2. In the model, social media use, senior people's healthcare knowledge sharing (including knowledge acquisition and knowledge contribution) and subjective wellbeing are considered.

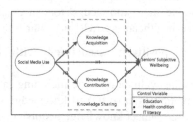

Fig. 2. Research model.

According to the mandatory age for retirement in China (the retirement age of male workers is 60 years old and that of female workers is 50 years old), in this paper, we limit elderly people to those older than 50 but younger than 65. For those people, they have enough time and energy to experience more things. The majority of them are at higher risk of chronic diseases, so they often pay close attention to healthcare. It means that they are likely to use social media if there is a lot of healthcare knowledge on social media. Therefore, we target people ranging from 50 to 65 years of age.

We believe that social media exert great influences on people's subjective well-being, which is always associated with their health, especially for seniors. First, seniors could improve their wellbeing by making friends with others and engaging in several activities through social media to improve quality of life and increase happiness. Second, seniors can get emotional support through social media. Communicating with people who have similar experience will help seniors reduce their frustration and panic for their chronic diseases. It has been manifested that patients' wellbeing is influenced by their use of the online community maintained by a doctor (Liu et al. 2016). Similarly, in the era of internet+, we suggest that social media are related to their subjective wellbeing within the context of senior care:

H1. Social media use positively improves seniors' subjective wellbeing
It has been demonstrated that social media serve as a platform for knowledge collaboration and crowd-sourced knowledge (Aghili et al. 2015). Namely, people can query healthcare information, offer some related knowledge through social media including virtual communities, forums and some applications. Social media have a potential to arouse people's engagement and interact with others. For seniors, they pay close attention to their health and often read some materials about healthcare, especially those with chronic illness. Social media provide a source for them to obtain more healthcare knowledge. Therefore, we posit:

H2. Social media use is positively associated with healthcare knowledge acquisition
When seniors obtain more healthcare knowledge, they may want to share it to their friends and family members, particularly those who suffer from some diseases same to them. Moreover, when seniors find it interesting to interact with others through social media, they may feel happy and are more willing to share some of their own experience. For example, cancer patients always feel desperate and have a negative attitude toward cancer treatment. It means that they need support from people who have similar experience to them. Social media provides such a platform. Others can tell fighting diseases stories and contribute their knowledge to cancer patients. Thereby, social media use will increase their healthcare knowledge contribution:

H3. Social media use is positively associated with healthcare knowledge contribution
Subjective wellbeing covers the evaluation of life including satisfaction and happiness. Prior studies on virtual communities have linked knowledge sharing to hedonic value of people (Liao 2016). We also connect knowledge acquisition with hedonic wellbeing, which is one dimension of subjective wellbeing. Obtaining healthcare knowledge may make seniors much happy and feel a sense of safety. That is to say, seniors who obtain healthcare knowledge may feel satisfied. Accordingly, we hypothesize that:

H4. Healthcare knowledge acquisition positively affects seniors' subjective wellbeing

When contributing healthcare knowledge to others through social media, seniors have chances to give emotional and information supports to other people, especially fellow sufferers and they may feel happy when contributing useful or needed disease experience and some exercise or diet suggestions to others. Besides, there are both scientific and unscientific knowledge on the social media, however, seniors often share some knowledge they think credible. After that, they are likely to be more confident and deem that they play an important role among their friends or family. It can be inferred that knowledge contribution can enhance seniors' subjective wellbeing positively. Therefore, we assume that:

H5. Healthcare knowledge contribution positively affects seniors' subjective wellbeing

In addition to the factors above, we consider three control variables including education, health condition and IT literacy. Senior respondents in our study are all familiar with basic WeChat online activities; that is, they all have a reasonable level of education and IT literacy. Furthermore, it is obvious that a person's health condition can influence one's social media use, knowledge sharing and subjective wellbeing. Therefore, we regarded education, health condition and IT literacy as control variables in our proposed model.

4 Methodology

We plan to test our hypotheses with a quasi-experiment and surveys after interviewing seniors who are familiar with WeChat. We need to interview seniors who will take part in our research to identify what kind of knowledge they really need. After that, a pilot study needs to be conducted among some seniors to help us do some adjustments.

4.1 Quasi-Experimental Design and Procedures

The first step in the quasi-experimental design is to select several participants. For this, we will collaborate with a local hospital and recruit 100 seniors who will be paid RMB 50. As health condition will affect the willingness to share information, we will select seniors who have hypertension or those are recognized to be at risk of hypertension.

We plan to create a WeChat official account to push some healthcare knowledge and create a WeChat group which is composed of 50 senior participants to communicate with each other. The other 50 participants are regarded as a control group. They will not use WeChat to share healthcare knowledge. There are some reasons why we choose WeChat. First, it is easy for people to use mobile phones whenever and wherever, which is not limited to computers and internet. WeChat is an application on mobile phones and it is so popular among Chinese people no matter how old they are. Besides, seniors always transfer or share some passages related to healthcare, especially for elderly people in WeChat. These provide advantages of WeChat for us to do this research.

It will be necessary to recruit several volunteers to help with the quasi-experiment and it will last 6 weeks to give seniors enough time to adapt to it. For the control group, we will require them obtain hypertension healthcare knowledge in other ways instead of WeChat. For the treatment group, the process is as follows:

Post hypertension healthcare knowledge for seniors every day. A specific researcher will post healthcare information about hypertension through WeChat every day during the experimental phase. It is important for seniors to know about the knowledge about hypertension. So we can post relevant knowledge to them, such as about diet and exercise.

Promote seniors' absorption of knowledge about hypertension healthcare. The most important thing is how to promote those seniors' absorption of hypertension healthcare knowledge. Some measures must be taken. For instance, we can post multiple forms of knowledge including pictures and videos. In addition, a pattern like 'quick quiz' may be useful. Our volunteers will ask questions about hypertension healthcare knowledge that have been posted on the day, and offer rewards to people who first answer the questions correctly.

Check seniors' knowledge about hypertension healthcare every week. We need to know the effects of our knowledge sharing. So we should check seniors' hypertension healthcare knowledge and record their grades every week. An online test might be carried out. Combined with such a test, the follow-up investigation might be more convincing.

Build a knowledge-sharing system of hypertension healthcare to provide services for seniors. Finally, a knowledge sharing system of hypertension healthcare will be built to offer healthcare service to seniors. Linking the system to seniors in the community can help them to relieve their stress of hypertension healthcare concerns, and provide a more convenient service for them. For example, we may collect data about seniors' healthcare and combine this with analyses of patients in community hospital, with their cooperation. Then we could give suggestions to seniors about their healthcare. So here comes the question: how to collect these data? In addition to seniors' own description and their records in community hospital, something like Mi Band might be useful. Mi Band is a kind of wearable health devices which can record information of motion, sleep, and heart rate. Combined with physicians' guidelines, our study will be more helpful with practical significance.

4.2 Survey Design and Development

We designed a survey to measure seniors' social media use, healthcare knowledge sharing (knowledge acquisition and knowledge contribution) and subjective wellbeing. Before the quasi-experiment, a first-stage survey will be carried out with about 100 seniors to explore the relationship among social media use, knowledge acquisition and knowledge contribution and seniors' wellbeing. Then, after the quasi-experiment is conducted, that is, after the healthcare knowledge sharing system is built, we will do a second-stage survey which we can compare outcomes of the two surveys.

In this study, social media use is measured by the intensity of social media use and the activities conducted on social media (Wei and Gao 2017). We make some adjustments and understand the intensity of social media use from the length of using WeChat (in years), average time spent on social media WeChat every day (in hours), number of friends on WeChat, and the reliance on social media, which is measured by six questions. We measure activities on social media by how often seniors conducted 12 different activities on social media.

We measure knowledge sharing through eight items based on instruments of knowledge acquisition and knowledge contribution (Zhou et al. 2014), which were developed in the context of virtual communities (VC), and SCT was applied to analyze factors of VC users' behavior. Because of the comparability between VC and WeChat, a communication application tool and the context of this study, the measurements of knowledge acquisition and knowledge contribution for VCs are suitable for this research.

We divide seniors' subjective wellbeing into evaluative wellbeing, hedonic wellbeing and eudemonic wellbeing. Evaluative wellbeing, i.e., life satisfaction, refers to people's evaluations of how satisfied they are with their lives. Evaluative wellbeing is measured using a 'Cantril ladder' (Cantril 1965; Tinkler and Hicks 2011). Hedonic wellbeing concentrates on people's feelings such as happiness, pain, anger, sadness and other moods. We assess hedonic wellbeing by the Positive and Negative Affect Schedule (PANAS) used in the research of Watson et al. (Watson et al. 1988), which is highly accepted (Crawford and Henry 2004). Eudemonic wellbeing is defined as people's judgements about value or purpose of life. It is measured by nineteen items using a self-enumerated scale of quality of life called CASP-19 (Hyde et al. 2003; Wiggins et al. 2008).

Existing instruments can be applied to our present study. Most of these questions will have to be adapted to our research context, and several of them may need to be modified. Because our respondents are Chinese, we must investigate them in the Chinese language. We will employ in our study several international students in our university who know both English and Chinese well. Following the translation-back translation procedure, these international students will help us translate these English questionnaires into Chinese versions. Moreover, these Chinese questionnaires will be sent to other professionals to translate back into English. A pre-test will be conducted which can help us modify our questionnaires when we receive the feedback. We will use existing instruments because most questions are adapted to our context and we just make slight modifications (Table 1).

Our hypotheses need to be test by data collected in the quasi-experiment and survey. We intend to recruit students in our university as our volunteers to guide senior participants finish questionnaires. These students must be trained by our researchers with background of our study and they have knowledge on survey administration. With regard to respondents, we plan to seek 100 seniors who are familiar with mobile phones.

Table 1. Construct measures.

Constructs		Items	Item Scales	Sources
Social media use	The intensity of social media use	1. The length of using WeChat (in years) 2. Average time spent on WeChat every day (in hours) 3. Number of friends on WeChat 4. Visiting WeChat is my daily routine 5. I am proud to tell others that I am using WeChat 6. Using WeChat has already been my everyday habit 7. I'll feel unconnected if I do not use WeChat 8. I am a member of WeChat communities 9. I'll feel pitiful if WeChat is shut down	1 = never to 5 = very often	Modified from Wei and Gao (2017)
	The activities on social media	1. Posting 2. Re-posting 3. Commenting 4. Sharing pictures and video related to healthcare 5. Searching for healthcare knowledge 6. Discussing healthcare news with others on WeChat 7. Interacting with friends about healthcare 8. Using WeChat to kill time 9. Getting to know new friends 10. Joining groups/communities online 11. Initializing or participating in online activities on WeChat 12. Following healthcare official accounts		

(*continued*)

Table 1. (*continued*)

Constructs		Items	Item Scales	Sources
Knowledge sharing	Knowledge acquisition	1. I always seek knowledge in WeChat 2. I always seek information in WeChat 3. I always carefully read others' posting 4. I always carefully learn knowledge in WeChat	1 = Strongly disagree to 5 = Strongly agree	Modified from Zhou et al. (2014)
	Knowledge contribution	1. I always contribute knowledge in WeChat 2. I always contribute information in WeChat 3. I frequently participate in the knowledge contribution activities in WeChat 4. I spend a lot of time on knowledge contributing activities in WeChat	1 = Strongly disagree to 5 = Strongly agree	Modified from Zhou et al. (2014)
Seniors' subjective wellbeing	Evaluative wellbeing	Cantril's Self-anchoring Ladder of Life Satisfaction	From 0 to 10	Adopted from Cantril (1965)
	Hedonic wellbeing	Positive and Negative Affect Schedule (PANAS)	1 = very slightly or not at all, 2 = a little, 3 = moderately, 4 = quite a bit, 5 = extremely	Adopted from Watson et al. (1988)
	Eudemonic wellbeing	1. My age prevents me from doing the things I would like to 2. I feel that what happens to me is out of my control 3. I feel free to plan for the future 4. I feel left out of things 5. I can do the things that I want to do 6. Family responsibilities prevent me from doing what I want to do 7. I feel that I can please myself what I can do	1 = never to 5 = very often	Adopted from Hyde et al. (2003)

(*continued*)

Table 1. (*continued*)

Constructs	Items	Item Scales	Sources
	8. My health stops me from doing the things I want to do 9. Shortage of money stops me from doing the things that I want to do 10. I look forward to each day 11. I feel that my life has meaning 12. I enjoy the things that I do 13. I enjoy being in the company of others 14. On, balance, I look back on my life with a sense of happiness 15. I feel full of energy these days 16. I choose to do things that I have never done before 17. I feel satisfied with the way my life has turned out 18. I feel that life is full of opportunities 19. I feel that the future looks good for me		

5 Discussion and Planned Extensions

This paper has proposed a conceptual model to explore the relationship among elderly people's social media use, knowledge sharing (including knowledge acquisition and knowledge contribution), and their subjective wellbeing within the context of healthcare. We are using both quasi-experiment and questionnaire survey to do the research. Data will be collected among the retired seniors in collaborated community, Xi'an, China. Future work will mainly focus on the conduct and analysis of the quasi-experiment as well as survey. Hopefully the findings of this research can provide suggestions not only for elderly people to improve their subjective wellbeing, but also for healthcare service providers to facilitate seniors' healthcare activities and increase their knowledge of self-management and self-control through social media.

References

Agarwal, R., Animesh, A., Prasad, K.: Social interactions and the 'digital divide': explaining variations in Internet use. Soc. Sci. Electron. Publishing **20**(2), 277–294 (2005)

Aghili, G., Lapointe, L., Vaast, E.: Apparatuses of knowledge delivery to patients: the role of social media in vaccine controversies. In: Thirty Sixth International Conference on Information Systems, Fort Worth (2015)

Ahn, M., Beamish, J.O., Goss, R.C.: Understanding older adults' attitudes and adoption of residential technologies. Family Consum. Sci. Res. J. **36**(3), 243–260 (2008)

Anderson, J.G.: Consumers of e-health: patterns of use and barriers. Soc. Sci. Comput. Rev. **22**(2), 242–248 (2004)

Bandura, A.: Social foundations of thought and action: a social cognitive theory. Prentice-Hall Inc., NJ (1986)

Bock, G.W., Zmud, R.W., Kim, Y.G., Lee, J.N.: Behavioral intention formation in knowledge sharing: examining the roles of extrinsic motivators, social-psychological factors, and organizational climate. MIS Q. **29**(1), 87–111 (2005)

Cantril, H.: The Pattern of Human Concerns. Rutgers University Press, New Brunswick (1965)

Chen, J.: Perceived discrimination and subjective well-being among rural-to-urban migrants in China. J. Sociol. Soc. Welfare **40**(1), 131–156 (2013)

Chiu, C.M., Hsu, M.H., Wang, E.T.G.: Understanding knowledge sharing in virtual communities: an integration of social capital and social cognitive theories. Decis. Support Syst. **42**(3), 1872–1888 (2006)

Crawford, J.R., Henry, J.D.: The positive and negative affect schedule (PANAS): construct validity, measurement properties and normative data in a large non-clinical sample. Br. J. Clin. Psychol. **43**(3), 245–265 (2004)

Deaton, A.: Aging, Religion, and Health. Explorations in the Economics of Aging, pp. 237–262. University of Chicago Press, Chicago (2011)

Deaton, A.: What does the empirical evidence tell us about the injustice of health inequalities. In: Eyal, N., Hurst, S., Norheim, O.F., Wikler, D. (eds.) Inequalities in Health: Concepts, Measures and Ethics, pp. 263–281. Oxford University Press, Oxford (2013)

Guo, X., Sun, Y., Yan, Z., Wang, N.: Privacy-personalization paradox in adoption of mobile health service: the mediating role of trust. In: Pacific Asia Conference on Information Systems (PACIS), Paper 27 (2012)

Hsu, M.H., Ju, T.L., Yen, C.H., Chang, C.M.: Knowledge sharing behavior in virtual communities: the relationship between trust, self-efficacy, and outcome expectations. Int. J. Hum Comput Stud. **65**(2), 153–169 (2007)

Hwang, Y.C.: Design healthcare service for senior citizens: a case of personalized stoke-precaution service with social network. J. Convergence Inform. Technol. **6**(4), 352–360 (2011)

Hyde, M., Wiggins, R.D., Higgs, P., Blane, D.B.: A measure of QoL in early old age: the theory, development and properties of a needs satisfaction model (CASP-19). Aging Mental Health **7**(3), 186–194 (2003)

Wei, L., Gao, F.: Social media, social integration and subjective well-being among new urban migrants in China. Telematics Inform. **34**(3), 786–796 (2017)

Kankanhalli, A., Tan, B., Wei, K.K.: Contributing knowledge to electronic knowledge repositories: an empirical investigation. MIS Q. **29**(1), 113–143 (2005)

Lee, B., Chen, Y., Hewitt, L.: Age differences in constraints encountered by seniors in their use of computers and the Internet. Comput. Hum. Behav. **27**(3), 1231–1237 (2011)

Liao, T.H.: Developing an antecedent model of knowledge sharing intention in virtual communities. Univ. Access Inform. Soc., 1–10 (2016)

Liu, X., Liu, Q., Guo, X.: Patients' use of social media improves doctor-patient relationship and patient wellbeing: evidence from a natural experiment in China. In: Thirty Seventh International Conference on Information Systems, Dublin, Ireland (2016)

Kordzadeh, N., Young, D.K.: Understanding how hospitals use social media: an exploratory study of Facebook posts. In: Americas Conference on Information Systems (2015)

Seckin, G.: Patients as information managers: the Internet for successful self-health care & illness management. Open Aging J. 4, 36–42 (2010)

Steptoe, A., Deaton, A., Stone, A.A.: Subjective wellbeing, health, and ageing. Lancet 385 (9968), 640–648 (2015)

Tinkler, L., Hicks, S.: Measuring Subjective Well-Being. Office for National Statistics, London (2011)

Usoro, A., Sharratt, M.W., Tsui, E., Shekhar, S.: Trust as an antecedent to knowledge sharing in virtual communities of practice. Knowl. Manag. Res. Pract. 5(3), 199–212 (2007)

van Deursen, Alexander J.A.M., Helsper, E.J.: A nuanced understanding of Internet use and non-use among the elderly. Eur. J. Commun. 30(2), 171–187 (2015)

Wagner, N., Hassanein, K., Head, M.: Computer use by older adults: a multi-disciplinary review. Comput. Hum. Behav. 26(5), 870–882 (2010)

Wasko, M.L., Faraj, S.: Why should I share? Examining social capital and knowledge contribution in electronic networks of practice. MIS Q. 29(1), 35–57 (2005)

Watson, D., Clark, L.A., Tellegen, A.: Development and validation of brief measures of positive and negative affect-the PANAS scales. J. Pers. Soc. Psychol. 54(6), 1063–1070 (1988)

Whitten, P., Notman, M., Maynard, C., Henry, R., Glandon, R.: Interactive health communication technologies in the public health sector: positive perceptions still outpace actual utilization. J. Technol. Hum. Serv. 22(3), 25–40 (2004)

Wiggins, R.D., Netuveli, G., Hyde, M., Higgs, P., Blane, D.: The evaluation of a self-enumerated scale of quality of life (CASP-19) in the context of research on ageing: a combination of exploratory and confirmatory approaches. Soc. Indic. Res. 89(1), 61–77 (2008)

Yan, Z., Wang, T., Chen, Y., et al.: Knowledge sharing in online health communities: A social exchange theory perspective. Inf. Manag. 53(5), 643–653 (2016)

Yang, H., Guo, X., Wu, T.: Exploring the influence of the online physician service delivery process on patient satisfaction. Decis. Support Syst. 78, 113–121 (2015)

Zhang, X., Guo, X., Guo, F., Lai, K.H.: Nonlinearities in personalization-privacy paradox in mHealth adoption: the mediating role of perceived usefulness and attitude. Technol. Health Care 22(4), 515–529 (2014)

Zhou, J., Zuo, M., Yu, Y., Chai, W.: How fundamental and supplemental interactions affect users' knowledge sharing in virtual communities? A social cognitive perspective. Internet Res. 24(5), 566–586 (2014)

How Out-of-Pocket Ratio Influences Readmission: An Analysis Based on Front Sheet of Inpatient Medical Record

Luo He[1(✉)], Xiaolei Xie[2], Hongyan Liu[1], and Bo Li[1]

[1] School of Economics and Management, Tsinghua University, Beijing, China
{hel.16,liuhy,libo}@sem.tsinghua.edu.cn
[2] Department of Industrial Engineering, Tsinghua University, Beijing, China
xxie@tsinghua.edu.cn

Abstract. Readmission is often an important indicator of care quality, which also accounts for a major proportion of medical expenses. In this paper, we study the relationship between out-of-pocket ratio in medical cost and readmission. Apart from out-of-pocket ratio, we also consider other factors such as demographic features of patients, medical expenses, and variables about diseases. As there are a large number of diseases and operations, for better interpretation, we adopt data mining method to identify discriminative features. Our study is based on the front sheet of inpatient medical record from 150 hospitals in Beijing from year 2012 to 2014. In the records with primary diagnoses being rectal malignant tumor, we find out that when out-of-pocket ratio is low or high, the readmission is relatively high. Meanwhile, discriminative features found based on group difference mining method are helpful to gain understanding of the results.

Keywords: Out-of-pocket ratio · Readmission · Logistic regression · Group difference mining

1 Introduction

Although there are some limitations [1], readmission is regarded as a marker for quality of hospital care [2,3]. Gerard F. Anderson et al. point in [4] that over $2.5 billion were spent per year on readmission between 1974 and 1977, and in 1984, such expenditures approached $8 billion. Lee Park et al. show that by the fiscal year 2015, penalty by readmissions will increase to 3% of reimbursement for inpatient services [16]. Besides, governments usually use readmissions as an important indicator to measure the quality of a hospital. Therefore, how to reduce readmission rate is an important issue for all hospitals. An effective way to achieve this goal is to find out the associated factors that influence readmissions. Some factors regrad to the attributes of the patients; some factors relate to the health care process; some factors associate with medicine the patients take. However, little research has been done about the relationship between the payment for medical cost and readmissions. Medical cost may influence the incentive of patients'

© Springer International Publishing AG 2017
H. Chen et al. (Eds.): ICSH 2017, LNCS 10347, pp. 67–78, 2017.
https://doi.org/10.1007/978-3-319-67964-8_7

and hospitals' behavior, thus influence the readmissions [18]. The work regarding to medical care performance and medical cost is little and mainly model-based, therefore we try to study the relationship between readmission and out-of-pocket ratio in a data based view in this paper. As diagnosed diseases and operations may also be factors influencing readmission and the number of diseases and operations is large, we adopt a data mining approach, group difference mining, to identify discriminative patterns among patients with different readmissions. Our dataset comes from the front sheet of inpatient medical record data of 150 hospitals in Beijing from year 2012 to 2014 with 679,243 discharge records, including diseases about digestive system, liver, gallbladder and pancreas. And our study concentrate on one specific disease, rectal malignant tumor, which is a very common cancer in China. The main result is that the relationship between out-of-pocket ratio and readmissions is like a bowl-shape, which indicates when out-of-pocket ratio is low or high, the corresponding readmissions is relatively high.

The remainder of the paper is organized as follows. Section 2 is the literature review. In Sect. 3, we describe our study sample in detail. Section 4 introduces the variables and models. Results are included in Sect. 5. We conclude this article in Sect. 6. The last Section is the Acknowledgements.

2   Literature Review

Our work is related to the research regarding to discovering the factors that influence readmissions. So we organize literature review as two parts: literatures that relate to medical cost and literatures that don't relate to medical cost. Many work relate to the non-cost factors of readmissions. As in Sect. 1, Some factors regard to the patients' attributes. For example, Mortensen et al. [5] and Chan et al. take demographic features into consideration; In Howell et al.'s model, co-morbidities are included to identify patients at risk of hospital readmission [7]; Ayyagari et al. study the association of obesity with 30-day readmission rates in [8]. Some factors are about the health care process. Rayner et al. compare the differences of hospital readmission rates with different outpatient review practices in [9], while Damiani et al. take hospital discharge planning and continuity into consideration in [10]. Whether compliance with hospital accreditation is also studied in [11]. Factors associated with medicine are also an important aspect for consideration. Rehospitalization after discontinuation of paliperidone in patients with schizophrenia has been studied by Bae et al. in [12]. Olson et al. [13] and Han et al. [14]. consider patients with the same diagnosis but taking different medicine, and find out that it will lead to different readmission rates. Factors related with people who provide medical service are also studied. Han et al. have found that higher number of registered nurses or neurosurgeons shows inverse relation with early readmission [15]. Some other novel factors like seasons [16] and geography [17] are also well explored.

While medical cost being a vital factor concerning readmissions, little research has been done about this relationship. Medical cost can influence the behavior of patients or health care service provider, thus influence the health care outcome. Some theoretical statements have appeared in Thomas H. Lee et al. [18]. Thomas H. Lee et al. show that enrollees in high-deductible health plans are likely to receive common conservative services and tend to have health problems as a result of avoiding seeing a physician because of cost. In [22], Elodie Adida et al. focus on the incentives of health care providers across several payment mechanisms. They point out that hospitals are encouraged to provide more services which are not always necessary with fee-for-service payment, while with fee-for-performance payment, hospitals tend to provide the minimum service that are suitable for the patients. Elodie Adida et al.'s work is based on a model view, which is different from our work that is based on a data view.

3 Study Sample

The dataset we use comes from the front sheet of inpatient medical record data of 150 Beijing hospitals from the year 2012 to 2014 with 679,243 discharge records. Each record of the dataset includes detailed information of expenses in hospital, payment type, demographic features, number of days in hospital, diagnosed disease, operations, in hospital date and out hospital date. For readmission, we choose 30-days-readmission, which represents the readmissions within 30 days from the index discharge, as many researches do [15,16,19]. Therefore, in our study, we discard records in December of 2014 for reasonable 30-days-readmission. After obtaining 30-days-readmission, we select the records with primary diagnosis being rectal malignant tumor as our study sample.

4 Variables and Methods

4.1 Variables

To avoid confounding effects in the logistic regression model, we refer to many researches to include as many control variables as we can. Here, we list all independent variables that we take into consideration.

Out-of-pocket Ratio. Out-of-pocket ratio is the proportion of medical cost patients really pay by themselves. We put patients whose out-of-pocket ratios are zero in 0-out-of-pocket-ratio group. Medical cost of this group is usually paid by government or insurance companies. Similarly, those who pay for the medical cost totally by themselves are in the 1-out-of-pocket-ratio group. In this paper, we count the number of readmissions for each patient in our dataset. We divide all patients into non-readmission group and readmission group. Patients with zero readmission in 30 days after discharge are in non-readmission group. Patients with at least one readmission in 30 days after discharge are in readmission group. The relationship between readmissions and out-of-pocket ratio may not be linear. In our preliminary data analysis, we find out that the support of readmission (the number of records with non-zero readmission) is high in both groups of 0-out-of-pocket-ratio and 1-out-of-pocket-ratio groups. It is reasonable to suppose that there may be quadratic term in the relationship between the number of readmissions and out-of-pocket ratio. So we add the square of out-of-pocket ratio in our model. We guess that when out-of-pocket ratio is low or high, the probability of readmissions is relatively high. This variable and its square are the key variables in this analysis. There are some research considering the impact of out-of-pocket ratio on medical care quality, but without data analysis [18].

Demographic Features. The demographic features we can obtain are age and gender. Many researches regarding to readmission include demographic features in their model, such as age, gender, occupation and location [5,6].

Medical Process. Medical process has four variables: types of discharge, hospital grade, and the number of operations, number of days in hospital.

There are 6 types of discharge: discharged upon doctor's advice, discharged not upon doctor's advice, inter-hospital transfer upon doctor's advice, transferred to community hospital upon doctor's advice, death and others. Similar factors also appear in the literature, such as outpatient review practice after discharge, hospital discharge planning and continuity [9].

Hospital grade represents hospital's level of quality. In China, hospitals are classified into three grades. Each grade is divided into three classes. Hospital grade implies the functions, facilities and technique conditions of a hospital. As readmission is an important indicator for medical care quality, we regard hospital grade as a factor that influences readmissions.

The number of operations conducted on a patient represents the treatment for a patient. More operations may represent more complicated conditions of a patient. Besides, the number of days in hospital is also an important metric for hospital's performance.

Medical Expense. Six types of medical expense are included in our model. They are medical care expense, nursing care expense, medical technique expense, management expense, medicinal expense, and consumptive material expense.

Disease Factors. The number of diseases diagnosed may imply the health status of a patient. With more confirmed diseases, the probability of a patient with worse health status is higher. So a reasonable guess is that with more confirmed disease diagnosis, the readmission risk of a patient is higher. Some researches have confirmed the relationship between number of diseases diagnosed and readmissions [20].

As the front sheet of inpatient medical record data provides detailed diagnosis information of patients, we can include all diseases diagnosed in our model. Usually, a patient is diagnosed with more than one disease, even up to more than 50 diseases. In our dataset, there are more than 4,000 diseases in total. Not all diseases are necessary to be included in the model, otherwise our model would be too complicated to be interpretable and would also suffer from overfitting problem. We adopt a data mining method to select the key diseases to our model, which will be introduced in detail later.

4.2   Method

In this study, we first use a data mining approach, group difference mining method, to select discriminative disease diagnosis patterns. Since diseases of a patient may be influential factors of readmissions, while we cannot code all 4,000 diseases in the model. Therefore, we need to identify the most influential diseases. Out of the same motivation, we wish to discover the most influential operations conducted on a patient. Group difference mining method is proposed to detect differences between groups. We adopt an algorithm named DIFF [21] to identify the difference patterns of disease diagnosis. An itemset I (here represents a set of diseases or operations) is regarded as a difference pattern across two groups if it satisfies the following conditions [21]:

$$|Support(I|Group1) - Support(I|Group2)| \geq min\_dif \tag{1}$$

$$\frac{min(Support(I|Group1), Support(I|Group2))}{max(Support(I|Group1), Support(I|Group2))} \leq min\_ratio \tag{2}$$

$$P(I|Group1) \neq P(I|Group2) \tag{3}$$

We use the group difference mining method to discover both disease difference patterns and operation difference patterns between non-readmission group and readmission group.

After identifying these disease difference patterns and operation difference patterns, we include them in the logistic regression model. Because only few patients have more than one readmissions within 30 days from the index discharge, we model readmission as a binary variable. Readmission equaling to 0 implies no admission happens within 30 days from the index discharge. Readmission equaling to 1 represents at least one admission happens within 30 days from the index discharge. The independent variables we are interested in are out-of-pocket ratio, its square, demographic features, medical process variables, medical expense, disease and operation factors. To guarantee that our model is robust, we add each group of variables in order. In detail, we first conduct logistic regression analysis between readmission and out-of-pocket ratio and its square. Then we add demographic features into the model, and adding other groups of variables into the model in turn. At last, we obtain a full model, containing all variables. If the outputs of the five models are consistent, we have great confidence in our result.

5   Results

5.1   Data Review

Our analysis is based on the front sheet of inpatient medical record data of 150 hospitals in Beijing. The recorded time is from the year 2012 to 2014. We extract a subset from the dataset, which includes the records with the primary diagnosed diseases as Rectal malignant tumor. This dataset contains 14,955 records, with 9,153 males and 5,802 females. The number of non-readmission patients is 14,049, and the number of readmissions patients is 906. The age distribution and out-of-pocket ratio distribution are presented in Fig. 1(a) and (b) respectively.

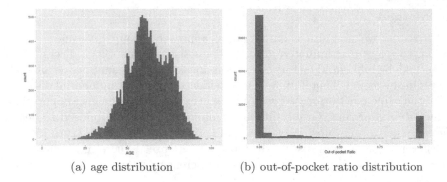

(a) age distribution   (b) out-of-pocket ratio distribution

Fig. 1. distribution of age and out-of-pocket ratio

5.2   The Difference Pattern of Key Disease

To contain discriminative disease diagnosis in our model, we adopt DIFF to identify the key disease difference patterns distributed differently between the group with zero readmission and the group with one or more than one readmissions in 30 days from the index discharge. The result of rectal malignant tumor is shown in Table 1. Support 1 is the support in non-readmission group, and Support 2 represents the support in readmission group. Support difference and support ratio are the absolute difference and ratio between Support 1 and Support 2 respectively. However, no operation difference pattern is found using DIFF, which implies no major differences of operation between non-readmission group and readmission group.

Table 1. Disease difference patterns found for rectal malignant tumor patients

Difference patterns	Support 1	Support 2	Support difference	Support ratio
Maintenance chemotherapy for malignant tumor	0.0478	0.0080	0.0398	0.1674
Radiotherapy for malignant tumor	0.0564	0.0120	0.0444	0.2129
Hypertension III	0.0521	0.0120	0.0401	0.2302
Preoperative chemotherapy of malignant tumor	0.0466	0.0140	0.0326	0.3006
Mixed hemorrhoids	0.0441	0.0140	0.0301	0.3173
Postoperative chemotherapy of malignant tumor	0.0613	0.0220	0.0393	0.3590
Pulmonary infection	0.0542	0.0240	0.0302	0.4428
Hypoproteinemia	0.1057	0.0620	0.0437	0.5864
Type 2 diabetes mellitus	0.1191	0.0700	0.0491	0.5878

We code each disease difference pattern as a binary variable. Namely, if a record in the dataset contains disease difference pattern A, we code it as 1, otherwise we code it as 0.

5.3 Logistic Regression Results

We conduct logistic regression five times for different groups of variables. In each regression, the coefficients of out-of-pocket ratio square are all significant and range from 1.34 to 1.56, showing that the relationship between readmission and out-of-pocket ratio is a bowl shape. Moreover, five of the nine disease difference patterns are remarkably significant, which implies the effectiveness of group difference mining method in indentifying the discriminative disease patterns. The detailed results are shown in Tables 2, 3, 4, 5 and 6. And Table 7 is the meaning of the variables used in the regression models.

Table 2. Logistic regression result 1

Variables	Estimate	Std. Error	z value	$Pr(> |z|)$
OOPR	−0.94419	0.67725	−1.394	0.1633
OOPR square	1.34765	0.67642	1.992	0.0463*

Table 3. Logistic regression result 2

Variables	Estimate	Std. Error	z value	$Pr(> |z|)$
OOPR	−1.154017	0.683065	−1.689	0.0911
OOPR square	1.559965	0.682047	2.287	0.0222*
Age	0.013677	0.00274	4.982	6.29e-07***
Male	0.106325	0.071310	1.491	0.1360

Table 4. Logistic regression result 3

Variables	Estimate	Std. Error	z value	$Pr(> |z|)$
OOPR	−1.113018	0.699669	−1.591	0.111660
OOPR square	1.448206	0.697878	2.075	0.037972*
Male	0.129235	0.072775	1.776	0.075764
LOS	−0.030138	0.003743	−8.052	8.15e−16***
DUDA	−1.980903	0.390971	−5.067	4.05e-07***

(*continued*)

Table 4. (*continued*)

Variables	Estimate	Std. Error	z value	$Pr(> |z|)$
TCHUDA	−13.288903	304.981485	−0.044	0.965245
IHTUDA	−2.018511	0.584736	−3.452	0.000556***
Death	−3.155066	0.422995	−7.459	8.73e−14***
DNUDA	−2.452975	0.454137	−5.401	6.61e−08***
Class 3-C hospital	0.613073	0.438145	1.399	0.161739
Class 3-B hospital	−11.710939	348.999009	−0.034	0.973231
Class 3-A hospital	−0.823580	0.433457	−1.900	0.057429
Class 2-C hospital	0.851481	0.585049	1.455	0.145558
Class 2-B hospital	1.605420	0.947362	1.695	0.090147
Class 2-A hospital	0.174818	0.439389	0.398	0.690729
#Operations	−0.064332	0.015363	−4.187	2.82e−05***

Table 5. Logistic regression result 4

Variables	Estimate	Std. Error	z value	$Pr(> |z|)$
OOPR	−1.090e+00	6.959e−01	−1.567	0.117207
OOPR square	1.378e+00	6.935e−01	1.987	0.046966 *
Age	9.873e−03	2.844e−03	3.472	0.000517***
Male	1.046e−01	7.357e−02	1.422	0.155029
LOS	−1.318e-02	4.553e−03	−2.894	0.003803**
DUDA	−1.796e+00	3.898e−01	−4.607	4.09e-06***
TCHUDA	−1.361e+01	3.074e+02	−0.044	0.964696
IHTUDA	−2.011e+00	5.833e−01	−3.448	0.000565***
Death	−3.165e+00	4.225e−01	−7.493	6.73e-14***
DNUDA	−2.465e+00	4.525e−01	−5.448	5.11e-08***
Class 3-C hospital	8.421e−01	4.382e−01	1.922	0.054613
Class 3-B hospital	−1.157e+01	3.492e+02	−0.033	0.973572
Class 3-A hospital	−3.546e−01	4.345e−01	−0.816	0.414510
Class 2-C hospital	8.838e−01	5.847e−01	1.512	0.130636
Class 2-B hospital	1.451e+00	9.391e−01	1.546	0.122186
Class 2-A hospital	3.161e−01	4.388e−01	0.720	0.471239
#Operations	2.027e−02	1.642e−02	1.234	0.217080
EXPENSE_YL	3.853e−06	3.486e−06	1.105	0.269035
EXPENSE_HL	−8.045e−05	1.111e−04	−0.724	0.468811
EXPENSE_YJ	−3.583e−05	1.713e−05	−2.092	0.036429 *
EXPENSE_GL	2.261e−05	8.715e−06	2.595	0.009472**
EXPENSE_YP	2.736e−06	3.515e−06	0.778	0.436334
EXPENSE_YP_HC	−5.568e−05	6.701e−06	−8.309	<2e−16***

Table 6. Logistic regression result 5

Variables	Estimate	Std. Error	z value	$Pr(> |z|)$
OOPR	−1.173e+00	7.011e−01	−1.674	0.094207
OOPR square	1.501e+00	6.983e−01	2.149	0.031655*
Age	5.374e−03	2.968e−03	1.811	0.070172
Male	1.204e−01	7.411e−02	1.625	0.104214
LOS	−1.009e−02	4.670e−03	−2.161	0.030682*
DUDA	−1.883e+00	3.907e−01	−4.819	1.44e−06***
TCHUDA	−1.348e+01	3.053e+02	−0.044	0.964798
Death	−3.735e+00	4.313e−01	−8.659	<2e−16***
DNUDA	−2.550e+00	4.542e−01	−5.613	1.99e−08***
Class 3-C hospital	6.874e−01	4.400e−01	1.562	0.118192
Class 3-B hospital	−1.155e+01	3.354e+02	−0.034	0.972522
Class 3-A hospital	−3.816e−01	4.355e−01	−0.876	0.380899
Class 2-C hospital	7.661e−01	5.863e−01	1.307	0.191309
Class 2-B hospital	1.375e+00	9.569e−01	1.437	0.150773
Class 2-A hospital	2.187e−01	4.401e−01	0.497	0.619239
#Operations	2.336e−03	1.688e−02	0.138	0.889929
EXPENSE_YL	−3.373e−06	4.349e−06	−0.776	0.437888
EXPENSE_HL	−1.270e−04	1.119e−04	−1.134	0.256595
EXPENSE_YJ	−3.814e−05	1.725e−05	−2.211	0.027048*
EXPENSE_GL	1.770e−05	8.898e−06	1.989	0.046681*
EXPENSE_YP	−1.943e−06	3.714e−06	−0.523	0.600842
EXPENSE_YP_HC	3.905e−05	7.094e−06	−5.504	3.70e−08***
#Diseases	6.261e−02	1.452e−02	4.313	1.61e−05***
Disease1	5.580e−01	2.126e−01	2.625	0.008667**
Disease2	4.643e−01	2.506e−01	1.853	0.063863
Disease3	3.227e−01	1.406e−01	2.296	0.021672*
Disease4	6.640e−01	2.061e−01	3.222	0.001274**
Disease5	1.625e−01	1.948e−01	0.834	0.404263
Disease6	9.184e−02	1.960e−01	0.469	0.639387
Disease7	3.194e−01	1.657e−01	1.928	0.053890
Disease8	4.103e−01	1.362e−01	3.011	0.002603**
Disease9	−6.687e−02	1.133e−01	−0.590	0.555158

Table 7. Variable's meaning

Variables	Variable's meaning
OOPR	$out-of-pocket\ ratio$
OOPR square	$out-of-pocket\ ratio\ square$
AGE	$Patient's\ age\ when\ discharge$
LOS	$Length\ of\ stay$
MALE	
DUDA	$Discharged\ upon\ doctor's\ advice\ or\ not$
TCHUDA	$Transferred\ to\ community\ hospital\ upon\ doctor's\ advice$
IHTUDA	$Inter-hospital\ transfer\ upon\ doctor's\ advice$
DEATH	$Dead\ when\ discharge$
DNUDA	$Discharged\ not\ upon\ doctor's\ advice$
Class 3-C hospital	$Class\ 3-C\ hospital\ or\ not$
Class 3-B hospital	$Class\ 3-B\ hospital\ or\ not$
Class 3-A hospital	$Class\ 3-A\ hospital\ or\ not$
Class 2-C hospital	$Class\ 2-C\ hospital\ or\ not$
Class 2-B hospital	$Class\ 2-B\ hospital\ or\ not$
Class 2-A hospital	$Class\ 2-A\ hospital\ or\ not$
EXPENSE_YL	$medical\ care\ expense$
EXPENSE_HL	$nursing\ care\ expense$
EXPENSE_YJ	$medical\ technique\ expense$
EXPENSE_GL	$management\ expense$
EXPENSE_YP	$medicinal\ expense$
EXPENSE_YP_HC	$consumptive\ material\ expense$
#Diseases	$The\ number\ of\ diseases\ diagnosed$
#Operations	$The\ number\ of\ operations\ conducted$
Disease1	$Maintenance\ chemotherapy\ for\ malignant\ tumor$
Disease2	$Radiotherapy\ for\ malignant\ tumor$
Disease3	$Hypertension\ III$
Disease4	$Preoperative\ chemotherapy\ of\ malignant\ tumor$
Disease5	$Mixed\ hemorrhoids$
Disease6	$Postoperative\ chemotherapy\ of\ malignant\ tumor$
Disease7	$Pulmonary\ infection$
Disease8	$Hypoproteinemia$
Disease9	$Type\ 2\ diabetes\ mellitus$

6 Discussion and Conclusions

The results indicate that when out-of-pocket ratio is either low or high, the probability of readmission is relatively high.

When out-of-pocket ratio is high, patients pay for most of medical bills by themselves. In this case, they may seek for low price medical treatment and medicine, which may affect the medical care quality.

When out-of-pocket ratio is low, patients' choices to receive better medical service is limited. For example, some effective imported medicines are not paid by insurance or government, which leads to poor medical care for these patients.

From our conclusion, we can obtain some insights into how we should design medical insurance to maximize the medical care quality. In the future, we would like to explore the relationship between out-of-pocket ratio and readmissions in the hospital level, which may offer a different view in hospital management.

Acknowledgements. This work is supported in part by the National Natural Science Foundation of China (NSFC) with grant numbers 71432004 and 71490724.

References

1. Hasan, M.: Readmission of patients to hospital: Still ill defined and poorly understood. Int. J. Qual. Health Care **13**(3), 177–9 (2001)
2. Milne, R., Clarke, A.: Can readmission rates be used as an outcome indicator? BMJ **301**(6761), 1139–40 (1990)
3. Ashton, C.M., Del Junco, D.J., Souchek, J., et al.: The association between the quality of inpatient care and early readmission: a meta-analysis of the evidence. Med. Care **35**(10), 1044 (1997)
4. Anderson, G.F., Steinberg, E.P.: Hospital readmissions in the medicare population. N. Engl. J. Med. **311**(21), 1349–1353 (1984)
5. Mortensen, P.B., Eaton, W.W.: Predictors for readmission risk in Schizophrenia. Psychol. Med. **24**(1), 223–232 (1994)
6. Chan, F.W.K., Wong, F.Y.Y., Yam, C.H.K., et al.: Risk factors of hospitalization and readmission of patients with COPD in Hong Kong population: analysis of hospital admission records. BMC Health Serv. Res. **11**(1), 186 (2011)
7. Howell, S., Coory, M., Martin, J., et al.: Using routine inpatient data to identify patients at risk of hospital readmission. BMC Health Serv. Res. **9**(1), 96 (2009)
8. Ayyagari, R., Revol, C., Tang, W., et al.: PSS41 Association of Obesity with 30-day readmission rates among patients Hospitalized with Acute Bacterial Skin and Skin-Structure Infections (ABSSSI). Value Health **18**(3), A186 (2015)
9. Rayner, H.C., Temple, R.M., Marshall, T., et al.: A comparison of hospital readmission rates between two general physicians with different outpatient review practices. BMC Health Serv. Res. **2**(1), 12 (2002)
10. Damiani, G., Federico, B., Venditti, A., et al.: Hospital discharge planning and continuity of care for aged people in an Italian local health unit: does the care-home model reduce hospital readmission and mortality rates?[J]. BMC Health Serv. Res. **9**(1), 22 (2009)
11. Falstiejensen, A.M., Nrgaard, M., Hollnagel, E., et al.: Is compliance with hospital accreditation associated with length of stay, acute readmission? A Danish nationwide population-based study. Int. J. Qual. Health Care **27**(6), mzv070 (2015)

12. Wu, J.H., Mao, L., Pesa, J., et al.: Rehospitalization after discontinuation of paliperidone er in patients with Schizophrenia. Value Health **11**(3), A110 (2008)
13. Bae, J.P., Faries, D.E., Ernst, F.R., et al.: PCV8 Assessment of 30-day rehospitalization for Acute Myocardial Infarction in patients with acute coronary syndrome who received percutaneous coronary intervention: a comparative effectiveness study of Clopidogrel and Prasugrel. J. Am. Coll. Cardiol. **60**(17), B16 (2012)
14. Olson, W.H., Ma, Y.W., Lefebvre, P., et al.: Effect of Prasugrel vs Clopidogrel on hospital readmission among Acute Coronary Syndrome patients treated with Prasugrel. Value Health **17**(3), A102 (2014)
15. Han, K.T., Lee, H.J., Park, E.C., et al.: Length of stay and readmission in lumbar intervertebral disc disorder inpatients by hospital characteristics and volumes. Health Policy **120**(9), 1008 (2016)
16. Park, L., Andrade, D., Mastey, A., et al.: Institution specific risk factors for 30 day readmission at a community hospital: a retrospective observational study. BMC Health Serv. Res. **14**(1), 40 (2014)
17. Yang, C., Torabi, M., Forget, E.L., et al.: Geographical variation analysis of all-cause hospital readmission cases in Winnipeg, Canada. BMC Health Serv. Res. **15**(1), 1–7 (2015)
18. Lee, T.H., Zapert, K.: Do high-deductible health plans threaten quality of care? N. Engl. J. Med. **353**(12), 1202–1204 (2005)
19. Helm, J.E., Alaeddini, A., Stauffer, J.M., et al.: Reducing hospital readmissions by integrating empirical prediction with resource optimization. Prod. Oper. Manage. **25**(2), 233–257 (2016)
20. Emmanuel, J., Ma, L., Saleh, S., et al.: PHS147 what determinants help predict readmission in a teaching hospital. Value Health **17**(3), A150 (2014)
21. Liu, H., Yang, Y., Chen, Z., et al.: A tree-based contrast set-mining approach to detecting group differences. Informs J. Comput. **26**(2), 208–221 (2014)
22. Adida, E., Mamani, H., Nassiri, S.: Bundled payment vs. fee-for-service: impact of payment scheme on performance. Manage. Sci. **63**(5), 1606–1624 (2016)

Wearable and Mobile Health

Fall Detection Using Smartwatch Sensor Data with Accessor Architecture

Anne Ngu[3], Yeahuay Wu[1], Habil Zare[3], Andrew Polican[2(✉)],
Brock Yarbrough[3], and Lina Yao[4]

[1] Department of Computer Science, Temple University, Philadelphia, USA
tuf02038@temple.edu
[2] Department of Computer Science, Arizona State University, Tempe, USA
adpolican@gmail.com
[3] Department of Computer Science, Texas State University, San Marcos, USA
{angu,zare,bcy3}@txtate.edu
[4] School of Computer Science and Engineering,
University of New South Wales, Kensington, Australia
lina.yao@unsw.edu.au

Abstract. This paper proposes using a commodity-based smartwatch paired with a smartphone for developing a fall detection IoT application which is non-invasive and privacy preserving. The majority of current fall detection applications require specially designed hardware and software which make them expensive and inaccessible to the general public. We demonstrated that by collecting accelerometer data from a smartwatch and processing those data in a paired smartphone, it is possible to reliability detect (93.8% accuracy) whether a person has encountered a fall in real-time. By wearing a smartwatch as a piece of jewelry, the well-being of a person can be monitored in real-time at anytime and anywhere as contrasted to being confined in a particular facility installed with special sensors and cameras. Using simulated fall data acquired from volunteers, we trained a fall detection model off-line that can be composed with a data collection accessor to continuously analyze accelerometer data gathered from a smartwatch to detect minor or serious fall at anytime and anywhere. The accessor-based architecture allows easy composition of the fall-detection IoT application tailored to heterogeneity of devices and variation of user's need.

1 Introduction

Internet of Things (IoT) is a domain that represents the next most exciting technological revolution since the Internet [2]. IoT will bring endless opportunities and impact every corner of our planet. In the healthcare domain, IoT promises to bring personalized health tracking and monitoring ever closer to the consumers. This phenomena is evidenced in a recent Wall Street Journal (June, 29, 2015) article entitled "Staying Connected is Crucial to Staying Healthy". IoT applications represents a new trend of softwares that involve interaction with

© Springer International Publishing AG 2017
H. Chen et al. (Eds.): ICSH 2017, LNCS 10347, pp. 81–93, 2017.
https://doi.org/10.1007/978-3-319-67964-8_8

everyday internet connected physical objects. Previous work in IoT fall detection applications required specialized hardware and software. This translated to buying an expensive vendor-specific device and creating a new native application for each type of device, which is not scalable. Moreover, the privacy aspect of data collection is not being addressed in the sense that data is being automatically collected and transmitted to the vendor's designated server without user's permission or input. Our fall detection IoT application is created using accessor-based architecture [1] which is based on Javascript and is designed to be device agnostics.

The laborious process in creating IoT application is the design of a set of experiments to collect and label data reliability and pre-processing of the data to gain an intuition of the most significant features. For our fall detection application, we recruited six volunteers and set up a robust methodology to systematically collect and label fall data. We used the support vector machine (SVM) algorithm to train a fall detection model using mainly resultant acceleration data over a sliding window. Our model has 93.8% precision and 97.2% recall. We showed how a model trained off-line could be easily integrated with a data collection accessor running on an Android compatible phone that supports Bluetooth Low Energy (BLE) communication protocol and used to detect falls in real-time.

By wearing a smartwatch as a piece of jewelry, the well being of an elderly person can be monitored in real-time at anytime and anywhere. The application can be set up to compose with other accessors such that customized functionalities can be incorporated, e.g., further confirmation from the user, sending a text message to a trusted family member or friend, or calling 911 in the event of a fall being detected. Currently, there are no known fall-detection IoT applications that leverage data from commodity-based wearable devices to monitor the well-being of patients non-invasively, in real-time, and with privacy preserving. The later refers to the fact that personal daily activities data of the elderly person can be stored locally or archived to a secure storage of choice by the user. The main contributions of the paper are:

– An Android IoT platform that supports composition of IoT applications using the accessor design pattern that is reusable across heterogeneous devices.
– A fall detection model that leverages a commodity-based smartwatch and smartphone which provides full mobility and full control of collected data for the users.
– A methodology for collecting simulated fall data from volunteers and annotating them for model training.

The remainder of this paper is organized as follows. In Sect. 2, we present the current work on daily activities detection, emphasize on research work that specifically address the fall detection and also briefly discuss the need for adopting accessor framework for building this style of IoT application. In Sect. 3, we provide a detailed description of the accessor framework and the implementation of an Android accessor host. In Sect. 4, we outline the methodology we used to collect training data for fall detection. In Sect. 5, we discuss the generation and the evaluation of the model and finally in Sect. 6, we present our conclusion and future work.

2   Related Works

The World Health Organization (WHO) reported that 28%–35% of people aged 65 and above fall each year. This rate increases to 32%–42% for those over 70 years of age. Thus, a great deal of research has been conducted on fall detection and prevention. The early researches in this area were concentrated on specially built hardware that a person could wear or installed in a specific facility. The fall detection devices in general try to detect a change in body orientation from upright to lying that occurs immediately after a large negative acceleration to signal a fall. However, modern smartphones and related devices now contain more sensors than ever before. Data from those devices can be collected more easily and more accurately with the increase in the computing power of those devices. Moreover, smartwatches and smartphones are becoming more pervasive in this 21st century. There is thus a dramatic increase in the research on smartphone based fall detection and prevention in the last few years. This is highlighted in the survey paper [6]. The smartphone-based fall detection solutions in general collect accelerometer, gyroscope and camera sensor data for fall detection. Among the collected sensor data, the accelerometer is the most widely used. The collected sensor data were analyzed using two broad type of algorithms. The first is the threshold-basted algorithm which is less complex and requires less computation power. The second is the machine learning based fall detection solutions. We will review both type of work below.

A threshold-based algorithm using a trunk mounted bi-axial gyroscope sensor is described in [3]. Ten young healthy male subjects performed simulated falls and the bi-axial gyroscope signals were recorded during each simulated-fall. Each subject performed three identical sets of 8 different falls. Eight elderly persons were also recruited to perform Activity of Daily Life (ADL) that could be mistaken for falls such as sitting down, standing up, walking, getting in and out of the car, lying down and standing up from bed. The paper showed that by setting three thresholds that relate to the resultant angular velocity, angular acceleration, and change in truck angle signals, a 100% specificity was obtained. However, there was no discussion on the practicality of attaching a trunk mounted sensor on a patient for a prolonged period of time. The restriction on the mobility of the patients and the privacy issue of data storage were not discussed as well.

The use of machine learning algorithms is recently presented by John Guirry in [5] for classifying ADLs with 93.45% accuracy using SVM and 94.6% accuracy using C4.5 decision trees. These ADLs include: running, walking, going up and down stairs, sitting and standing up. Their setup include a Samsung Nexus Galaxy smartphone and the Motorola Moto Actv smartwatch. Data was collected from the accelerometer, magnetometer, gyroscope, barometer, GPS, and light sensors. They synthesized a total of 21 features from all the sensors. They did not specifically address the fall detection. Our choice to use SVM as the machine learning algorithm for our fall detection was first inspired by Guirry's work on using smartwatch paired with smartphone for ADL detection.

SVM have been used for fall detection by other scholars [9]. They used a trunk-mounted tri-axial sensor (a specialized hardware) to collect data. They were able to achieve 99.14% accuracy with four features using only high-pass and low-pass accelerometer data. They used a 0.1 s sliding window to record minimum and maximum directional acceleration in that time period for a feature. We drew inspiration from this approach as it allowed us to have temporal data within each sampling point rather than having to choose a generalized feature for the whole duration.

Jantaraprim et al. also used SVM on fall detection for the elderly people [7]. They defined the "critical phase" for a fall sequence as a sudden drop in resultant acceleration followed by an immediate increase, and ending with an increase in the maximum acceleration value for the interval. That is, S_{min} was the value of the initial decrease in acceleration, S_{max} was the value of the corresponding increase, while $max(A_{res})$ was the value of the maximum resultant acceleration for the phase. They obtained fall detection results with a sensitivity of 91.1% and a specificity of 99.2% using the maximum peak feature. Their SVM models were trained with both the Radial Basis Function (RBF) kernel and the Linear Kernel, which achieved the same results in their study. We adopted the same set of features as them for our fall detection model.

None of the existing work addressed the ease of composition and development of IoT application which falls under the general category of ambient data collection and analytics type. This category of applications is growing rapidly especially in the healthcare domain where personalized health tracking and monitoring has become vital to improved and affordable healthcare. We built this category of IoT applications from ground up in our earlier work for prediction of Blood Alcohol Content (BAC) using smartwatch sensor data [10]. We learnt that the creation of this category of IoT applications can be done in three phases. The first phase involves data collection, the second phase deals with pre-processing of data and training of a model, and the third phase involves creating a native application with the trained model for prediction. Out of the three phases, the second phase is application specific and there is not much opportunity for a complete automation abielt we can use existing tools such as R to streamline the pre-processing of the data and analysis of significant features. Existing machine learning algorithms available via Weka or Matlabs can be leveraged for model training. The first phase, the data collection and the third phase are almost identical across the ambient data collection and analytic IoT applications and can benefit from reuse and sharing of existing codes via wrapping them as accessors [8] which can be deployed and executed on a light-weight accessor host.

3   System Architecture

Figure 1 shows the main infrastructure used for real-time analysis of fall detection using smartwatch sensor data. It consists of a smartwatch paired with a smartphone, a cloud persistence storage, and data analysis packages such as R and

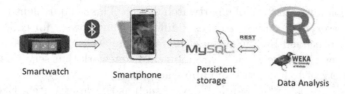

Fig. 1. Infrastructure for data collection and analysis

Weka. Figure 2 shows the overall solution expressed as accessors. The data collection accessor is running on the smartphone that has a working accessor host. The data collection accessor provides an abstraction over the low-level details of data collection process such as managing the various threads for reading the sensor values at specified sampling rate from the MS Band smartwatch.

The fall detection accessor predicts "FALL" or "NOT FALL" based on a model trained offline using the collected data in phase one as discussed in Sect. 4. An alert accessor informs the carer in the event of a fall. In fall detection, it is critical that data can be stored locally to preserve privacy and is in close proximity to the fall detection accessor for real time prediction. However, initial data analytics/training phase usually needs to be performed on a high performance server to build an accurate model by experimenting with different machine learning algorithms. There is thus a need to transfer the collected sensor data to a cloud server securely for initial analysis and this is done by the database accessor. Our long term goal is to set up a protocol where participating users' smartphones (with consent) transmit sensor information via a REST-based web service periodically. The archived sensor data can be visualized and analyzed. The archived sensor data can be aggregated and displayed on a map to examine health and lifestyles across a region. The true positive samples can be used for re-training of the model and adapt the fall detection accessor dynamically.

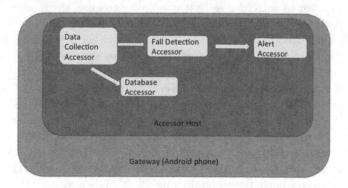

Fig. 2. Overall solution for fall detection IoT application

We could have implemented a custom native Android app for the fall detection that encompassed the functionalities provided by all the above accessors combined. This will result in a monolithic native application for data collection and prediction for each type of smartwatch device. This is equivalent to the scenario where every IoT device requires a different web browser for connection to the Internet as echoed by Zachariah et al. [11]. The accessor-based architecture provides an open, lightweight IoT development framework that serves as a bridge across a variety of IoT devices and applications.

An accessor encapsulates an IoT device such as the smartwatch. Each accessor has an interface and an implementation. The accessor interface specifies the input and output ports, the parameters and the communication protocol used for device's interaction. We implemented an Android accessor host leveraging J2V8, a Java binding for the V8 JavaScript engine. Our Android accessor host enables execution of accessors in various Android hardware and external services (Microsoft Band smartwatch) in simple script.

An accessor can run in any environment where there is a working accessor host. This is similar to the Java programming motto of "compiled once and run everywhere" paradigm. Accessors can be easily strung together in order to create an IoT application. For example, In the case of a more advanced fall detection system, the output of fall detection accessor could be routed to a text messaging accessor or a phone call accessor. The flexibility of the accessor paradigm enables various hardware and services to be interchanged with only minor adjustments.

4   Data Collection Methodology

We designed a robust methodology for collecting test data for the initial model training. Six subjects of good health were recruited. Their ages ranged from 19 to 29. We choose young healthy subjects because they are more versatile and no injuries can occur. Each subject was told to perform a pre-determined set of ADLs (Activities of daily life). Examples of ADLs that were performed include: running, walking, picking things off the ground, and throwing objects. We picked these set of activities so that it is easier to label them later. The data was collected via smartwatch through a data-collection accessor. The sensor data that we were interested in was the accelerometer. Because it was difficult to label activities for our training set based solely on the raw data we collected, we also had a stopwatch in hand to record the time stamp of each fall as it occurred.

Each ADL sequence occurred over a period ranging from 60 to 90 s. In some sequences, falls would be incorporated within the sequences of ADLs. Each subject was told to fall for a total of 8 times: 2 left side falls, 2 right side falls, 2 back falls, and 2 front falls. There were no restrictions placed on the subjects in regards to the number of times that they could fall within one sequence although it never exceeded two times. Subjects were also instructed to vary the intensity of the falls between each type of fall: one "soft" fall and one "hard" fall in order to capture a larger variety of falls. The hard fall was defined as a fall with faster run-up speed than the soft one. When participants in our experiment fell, their falls were padded by a twin-sized mattress in order to prevent any injuries. One issue with this method is that none of the falls collected include the "real impact" from falling directly on the ground. However, this is not critical to our labeling methodology because it is focused on identifying the "critical phase" that occurs *before* the initial impact of falling on the ground. From the raw data, we computed the values of the four features as the input to the SVM algorithm: (1) length of the acceleration vector at the time of sampling (A_{res}), (2) minimum resultant acceleration in a 750 ms sliding window (S_{min}), (3) maximum resultant acceleration in a 750 ms sliding window (S_{max}), and (4) the euclidean norm of the difference between maximum and minimum acceleration in a 750 ms sliding window (ΔS). More detailed descriptions for the features along with our methods for selecting them are further explained in the next section.

We then labeled each sample point as either *not falling* or *falling*. The determination of these categories was influenced by the concept of a critical phase of a fall in [7]. We defined the beginning of a fall sequence as the beginning of the critical phase and the ending of the critical phase as the occurrence of $\max(A_{res})$. This parameter, $\max(A_{res})$, is defined as the maximum resultant velocity within the critical phase. Figure 3, which is taken from [7], illustrates where the critical phase of a fall lies.

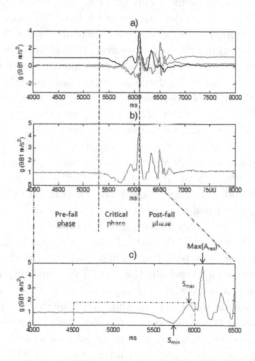

Fig. 3. "Critical phase" of a fall within an entire fall sequence, (a) Break down of the fall sequence in terms of the x, y, and z acceleration, the dotted lines denote where the critical phase occurs (b) Fall sequence in terms of resultant acceleration, once again the critical phase is within the dotted lines (c) Enlargement of the fall sequence from the beginning of the pre-fall phase up until the beginning of the post fall phase, defines where S_{min} and S_{max} are within the critical phase.

5   Training and Evaluation

Our goal is to be able to detect accurately whether someone has fallen in real time based on the motion sensed by the smartwatch that a person is wearing. We decided to use Weka, an open source Java package that covers many machine learning algorithms for training and prediction of falls. The Android accessor host supports Java binding. Both LibSVM 1.0.8 and libsvm-3.21 libraries had to be added to the accessor host in order to use the Support Vector Machine (SVM) algorithm in Weka. The total training set consisted of 1,934 samples.

We choose to use SVM because previous studies had used SVM with a tri-axial trunk-mounter sensor (a specialized hardware) with good results. We wanted to test if these results could translate to a commercial wearable device such as a smartwatch. When formulating feature selection for smartwatch, we realized that specialized trunk mounted sensors have a couple of critical advantages over wrist mounted smartwatch sensors. The main one being the ability to record data for features that relate to a subject's posture. Since the sensor is trunk-mounted, its point of data collection is from the torso of the subject, allowing the posture of the subject to be recorded. This was described in [9], where a parameter defined as Φ_z called the "posture angle" was utilized. This feature was derived by taking the angle between the vertical acceleration and the gravitational component, $|G|$. Creating a feature like this from the smartwatch's accelerometer data is extremely difficult because there is little relation between wrist position and the overall posture. However, we noticed that by combining features from previous research in [7,9], it is possible to capture the balance between features that could reflect the state of the subject at the exact time of sampling, just before, and just after the sampling. This intuition captures the notion of critical phase of a fall very well. We used the principle component analysis to check the viability of this combination of features and ended up with four core features. Details of feature selection is described in the next section.

Our SVM model is trained to predict falls on a sample by sample basis, categorizing each sample taken every 250 ms as a fall or not a fall. This method does not necessarily suit the nature of the activity we are trying to detect as detecting a fall constitutes finding a pattern from a succession of points. Since this is the case, we must determine a threshold (or range) of consecutive fall predictions that would constitute a sequence of 2–5 samples as a fall. We experimented with the model in real life using actions that could be defined in two categories: (1) short term spikes in acceleration and (2) long term increase in acceleration. Actions that could be categorized as (1) are various hand and arm gestures such as waving, throwing an object, and punching. An action that would belong in category (2) would be running, which is demarcated by a sudden increase in acceleration that is maintained over a duration of time over three seconds.

We determined from experiments involving these two categories of actions that the ideal threshold for the number of consecutive predictions in one fall sequence that could be constituted as falls would be between 2 and 5. The reasoning for this is if the number of consecutive predictions is over 5, then the action would be a long term increase in acceleration such as running. In the case where it is below 2, the action would most likely be a short spike in acceleration such as arm waving. For example, if the fall sequence consisted of 8 samples and our algorithm detected only 2 of these samples, we would count all 8 samples as "correct predictions" since 2 is within our threshold. Likewise, if our algorithm only detects 6 of the 8 as falls, all the 8 samples would be counted as "wrong predictions", specifically false negatives. This occurs because 6 is over our threshold of 5. Now, if our fall sequence consisted of 8 samples and our algorithm only classified 1 of them as fall, all 8 samples would also be counted as "wrong predictions" since 1 is below our threshold of 2. To our knowledge, no other paper on fall detection has used such a method of threshold detection based on a consecutive position prediction sample within a range.

5.1 Feature Selection

We used the Euclidean norm to measure the length (magnitude) of acceleration and velocity vectors. That is, for any vector r in R^3, we used:

$$\|r\|_2 = \sqrt{r_x^2 + r_y^2 + r_z^2}. \tag{1}$$

The original features that we defined were A_{res}, ΔS, S_{min}, S_{max}, V_{res}, and ΔV, which are defined the following.

A_{res}, resultant acceleration, is defined as the magnitude of the acceleration vector at the time of collection. Using Eq. 1, we defined:

$$A_{res} = \|A\|_2. \tag{2}$$

ΔS, adapted from Liu and Cheng's paper in [9], is the magnitude of the difference between minimum and maximum acceleration in a sliding window. That is, using Eq. 1, we defined:

$$\Delta S = \|S_{max} - S_{min}\|_2. \tag{3}$$

where S_{min} and S_{max} adapted from Jantaraprim et al.'s paper [7] are defined as the minimum and maximum resultant acceleration in a sliding window of 750 milliseconds. In the original implementation by Jantaraprim et al. and Liu and Cheng's, the sliding window was designated to be 0.1 s.

V_{res}, the resultant velocity, is defined as the magnitude of velocity for each sample taken every 250 milliseconds, i.e.,

$$V_{res} = \|V\|_2. \tag{4}$$

Similar to ΔS, ΔV is defined as the magnitude of the difference between minimum velocity (V_{min}) and maximum velocity (V_{max}) for the same sliding window of 750 milliseconds, i.e.,

$$\Delta V = \|V_{max} - V_{min}\|_2. \tag{5}$$

We started off with six features. However, after running Principal Component Analysis (PCA), we reduced the number of features to four. We noticed that the addition of the velocity derived features: ΔV and V_{res} decreased the weights of all the features in the first two principal components to values below 0.01. With the removal of the velocity features, we found that the first two principal components contained 98% of the variance in the features. The first principal component vector, PC1, puts a lot of weight on resultant acceleration and S_{max} while the second principle component, PC2, puts a lot of weight on ΔS and resultant acceleration. In the first two components, S_{min} takes on low weights (i.e., 0.00872 and 0.1897 for PC1 and PC2 respectively).

5.2   Algorithm Testing

We tested our SVM classifier with a testing set that contained 569 samples. Since we trained it with an RBF Kernel, the weights of each of the 4 features could not be retrieved. The number of samples was chosen because it consisted of approximately 1/3 of our total data set of 1934 samples. Each sample was collected at a rate of 4 Hz (every 250 ms). The other 2/3 of the total data set was set aside as training data. With this data set we achieved an accuracy of 98%, specificity of 99%, a precision of 93.6%, and a recall of 80%. The confusion matrix detailing our results is in Table 1. TP stands for True Positive, this means we predict that it is not a fall and indeed it is not a fall. FN stands for False Negative, this means we predicted that it is not a fall, but it is a fall. FP stands for False Positive, this means we predicted a fall, but it is not a fall. TN stands for True Negative, this means we predicted that there is a fall and indeed there is a fall. We also ran a lazy learning algorithm, k-Nearest Neighbors (KNN), in order to better gauge the performance of our SVM. The KNN was ran with a rectangular kernel with k = 4. The distance parameter and the kernel were adjusted to the get result with the highest sensitivity and specificity. The algorithm achieved an accuracy of 96.13%, a specificity of 99%, a precision of 88%, and a recall of 69%. The confusion matrix detailing our results is in Table 1. Most of the mislabeled samples were the same between KNN and SVM, with KNN having more false negatives.

Table 1. Confusion matrices for SVM with RBF kernel and KNN with rectangular kernel and $k = 4$. A sample is considered to be true positive (TP) if it is correctly predicted to be "not fall".

Method	SVM		KNN		
Prediction	Not fall	Fall	Not fall	Fall	Total
Actual not fall	511 (TP)	3 (FN)	509 (TP)	5 (FN)	514
Actual fall	11 (FP)	44 (TN)	17 (FP)	38 (TN)	55
Total	522	47	526	43	559

The following table compares the performance of KNN and SVM. SVM performs better in all the classification metrics that we accounted for. The SVM model takes around six seconds to make a prediction. This is due to the fact that the conversion of accelerometer data to the four features we used in the model incurs some overhead (Table 2).

Table 2. Fall detection classification results by algorithm

Algorithm	Accuracy	Recall	Precision	Specificity
SVM	98%	80%	93.6%	99%
KNN	96.13%	69%	88%	99.2%

6 Conclusions

A custom development of a native application for each type of IoT application running on different IoT devices is not scalable. Accessor based architecture has the advantage that it is light-weight and is analogous to the Java programming environment of "compile once and run everywhere" paradigm. We demonstrated the feasibility of developing an Android accessor host (a.k.a. a virtual accessor machine) based on J2V8 engine that serves as the bridge across a variety of IoT devices and applications. This accessor host is used to prototype a real-time fall detection application that utilizes an MS Band smartwatch paired with a Google smartphone. The accessor-based fall detection application can be easily configured to run on other IoT devices such as Moto 360 smartwatch and Samsung smartphone without additional programming. This framework can be used as the foundation for developing reusable accessors for IoT applicationss. The accessor-based fall detection application can run continuously for 12 hours with 20% of battery power left intact.

We have experimented with bother eager (SVM) and lazy (KNN) machine learning techniques for fall detection, and we showed that SVM model is more reliable. While our model has an average sensitivity of 81.8%, it classifies with a high specificity and precision at values of 99% and 93.8%, respectively. In other words, our true positive rate is average while our true negative rate is high. These results show that our model has some trouble distinguishing between sudden arm gestures and actual falls. A suggestion for the future is to leverage the accelerometer sensor in the phone whenever it is possible as a trigger for the prediction. That is, fall detection should only begin when the accelerometer on the phone detects an acceleration above some threshold, assuming that the user will carry the cellphone in a certain fixed orientation (the user's pocket or a purse for women). We have developed an intuitive procedure of classifying fall data on a sequence basis rather than just a point by point basis. This procedure allowed us to extend the results of our predecessors, which used specialized sensors for activity recognition, into the realm of commercially available sensors with comparable results. An immediate future work in improving our classification is to apply dynamic Bayesian network [4], which is known to perform well for sequence data.

We acknowledge that the model is trained using data from young and healthy volunteers, which might not reflect the actual fall data from elderly people. Currently, there is no publicly available fall data of elderly people. It is impossible to collect simulated fall data from the elderly group of people because of higher likelihood of injuries. To address that, we plan to use the system to collect ADL data from elderly and verify how many of ADL activities are falsely classified as falls to fine tune our initial model. Currently, we have obtained permission to do a trial on senior citizens in a nursing home at San Marcos regarding wearing smartwatches and carrying smartphones. We will recruit eight seniors for the trial. In particular, we want to know (1) How long seniors will wear smartwatches? (2) How much ADL activity data we can collect in a week? (3) How ADL activities affect our fall detection model? (4) What are seniors' main concerns regarding wearing smartwatches over a long period of time? The collected activity data from our senior volunteers can be used to measure the false positive rate and gauge the practically of using resultant acceleration (A_{res}), ΔS, S_{max} and S_{min} for fall prediction.

Acknowledgement. We thank the National Science Foundation (NSF) for funding the research under the Research Experiences for Undergraduates Program (CNS-1358939) and the Infrastructure grant (NSF-CRI 1305302) at Texas State University.

References

1. What are Accessors? https://www.terraswarm.org/accessors/
2. Internet of Things (2016). https://en.wikipedia.org/wiki/Internet_of_thing
3. Bourke, A.K., Lyons, G.M.: A threshold-based fall-detection algorithm using a bi-axial gyroscope sensor. Med. Eng. Phys. **30**(1), 84–90 (2008)
4. Dagum, P., Galper, A., Horvitz, E.: Dynamic network models for forecasting. In: Proceedings of the Eighth International Conference on Uncertainty in Artificial Intelligence, pp. 41–48. Morgan Kaufmann Publishers Inc. (1992)
5. Guiry, J.J., van de Ven, P., Nelson, J.: Multi-sensor fusion for enhanced contextual awareness of everyday activities with ubiquitous devices. Sensors **14**(3), 5687–5701 (2014)
6. Habib, M.A., Mohktar, M.S., Kamaruzzaman, S.B., Lim, K.S., Pin, T.M., Ibrahim, F.: Smartphone-based solutions for fall detection and prevention: challenges and open issues. Sensors **14**(4), 7181–7208 (2014)
7. Jantaraprim, P., Phukpattaranont, P., Limsakul, C., Wongkittisuksa, B.: Fall detection for the elderly using a support vector machine. Int. J. Soft Comput. Eng. (IJSCE) **2**, March 2012
8. Latronico, E., Lee, E.A., Lohstroh, M., Shaver, C., Wasicek, A., Weber, M.: A vision of swarmlets. IEEE Internet Comput. **19**(2), 20–28 (2015)
9. Liu, S.H., Cheng, W.C.: Fall detection with the support vector machine during scripted and continuous unscripted activities. Sensors **12**(9), 12301 (2012). http://www.mdpi.com/1424-8220/12/9/12301

10. Gutierrez, M.A., Fast, M.L., Ngu, A.H., Gao, B.J.: Real-Time prediction of blood alcohol content using smartwatch sensor data. In: Zheng, X., Zeng, D.D., Chen, H., Leischow, S.J. (eds.) ICSH 2015. LNCS, vol. 9545, pp. 175–186. Springer, Cham (2016). doi:10.1007/978-3-319-29175-8_16
11. Zachariah, T., Klugman, M., Campbell, B., Adkins, J., Jackson, N., Dutta, P.: The internet of things has a gateway problem. In: HotMobile. ACM, Santa Fe, New Mexico, USA, February 2015

Implementation of Electronic Health Monitoring Systems at the Community Level in Hong Kong

Wai Man Chan, Yang Zhao$^{(\boxtimes)}$, and Kwok Leung Tsui

Department of Systems Engineering and Engineering Management,
City University of Hong Kong, Kowloon Tong, Hong Kong
{wmcha3,yangzhao9,kltsui}@cityu.edu.hk

Abstract. Rapid advances in information and sensor technology have led to the development of tools and methods for individual health monitoring. These techniques support elderly health management by tracking the vital signs and detecting physiological changes for the target population, such as the elderly and patients with chronic diseases. Two pilot studies were conducted to demonstrate the implementation of electronic wearable wellness devices and an all-in-one station-based health monitoring device at the community level in Hong Kong. Real-time and daily changes of key vital signs in elderly people recruited from a nursing home and a geriatric daycare center were collected. Preliminary analysis of the collected data provided insights into the characteristics of vital signs of the elderly from two centers, which could bring benefits to the management of healthcare services. Additionally, a personalized wellness forecasting system was built to identify the factors influencing the personal wellness of the elderly, by aggregating historical daily vital signs.

Keywords: Smart elderly care · Sensors · Health monitoring systems

1 Introduction

Hong Kong faces the challenge of a rapidly aging population, like most other developed regions. The proportion of elderly people aged 65 and over is projected to rise significantly from 15% in 2014 to 36% in 2064 [1]. Elderly care has therefore become an important concern in government policy planning [2], including improving elderly services and medical services. In addition, the dramatic growth of the elderly population in Hong Kong is creating an extra burden on its healthcare system. In Hong Kong, although both public and private healthcare sectors have been providing numerous and high quality medical services, the burden is shifting to public healthcare sector due to highly uneven costs of the services provided. In addition, the portion of the elderly using medical services provided by public healthcare sector has been found to be much higher compared with younger population [3, 4]. Heavy reliance on public healthcare sector is affecting the quality of the services. For example, long waiting time for follow-up checking has been observed in many public healthcare sectors at Hong Kong, which may delay the detection on the deterioration of health condition. It

© Springer International Publishing AG 2017
H. Chen et al. (Eds.): ICSH 2017, LNCS 10347, pp. 94–103, 2017.
https://doi.org/10.1007/978-3-319-67964-8_9

is even worse if insufficient resource fails to meet the increasing demands. These challenges highlight a need for an extremely reliable integrated system of personalized health management that enables real-time health monitoring, early disease detection and medical intervention, and resource allocation optimization. Currently, many elderly with chronic diseases only receive insufficient and minimum care from the government or through various non-government organizations. The quality of elderly care is believed to be getting worse, as there is no significant increase of resources combined with a lack of any dramatic improvement in terms of efficiency and effectiveness in the elderly care service, as the proportion of the elderly population increases. Hong Kong is therefore facing unprecedented challenges in seeking solutions for efficient management of individual healthcare for the elderly in its healthcare system.

The rapid development of information technology, together with automated sensor-based data collection and abundant storage capability with minute physical size, has led to a rapid growth in the development of various types of sensor-based personal health monitoring devices, for either continuous or discrete measurements of different physiological variables. Many studies and publications have focused on discussions of the technologies involved in health monitoring devices and the challenges faced, but the research trend has started to shift to the application level, such as the potential application of health monitoring technology to the elderly and patients suffering from chronic diseases in home and community contexts [5–13]. An Australian research team has developed an all-in-one station-based health monitoring device for home telehealth monitoring of the elderly, and the results of the trials have been encouraging [14, 15]. Alongside doctor's visits, the implementation of health monitoring systems at a community level could be an easier and quicker way for the elderly to understand more about their own health conditions. It could also be beneficial to improving the quality of healthcare services provided, and ease the heavy burden on local healthcare systems.

The idea of integrated health monitoring via sensor-based devices for elderly care is, as far as we know, new to Hong Kong. In this study, two pilot studies were conducted to demonstrate the implementation of electronic wearable wellness devices and an all-in-one station-based health monitoring device at a community level in Hong Kong. The preliminary analysis illustrated the potential benefits of these devices through the implementation of health monitoring systems with personal healthcare monitoring and management of healthcare services.

2 Pilot Study 1

2.1 Research Methodology

The aim was to evaluate the effectiveness of using electronic wearable wellness devices for real-time continuous measurements on vital signs of the elderly, in terms of health monitoring and management in nursing homes. Sixteen elderly people with a mean age of 81.13 years from a local nursing home were invited to participate in this pilot study. They were asked to wear a commercial electronic wearable wellness device, the Sony Smartband 2 [16], continuously for 28 days. Twenty-four-hour real-time heart rates (HR) levels were monitored automatically with optical sensors included in the device.

Daily step counts could be measured and the types of activities were further classified as either walking or running with a 3-axis accelerometer. Sleep data, including sleeping duration and sleeping states, further classified into light or deep sleeping states, were also collected on a daily basis. The real-time data were then aggregated into daily measurements for each participant, and the mean values of these measurements over the 28-day observation period were calculated. To illustrate the common characteristics of the collected vital sign data of the elderly from the nursing home, 34 elderly people (mean age = 78.65 years old) were recruited from a local geriatric daycare center, and their vital signs were measured with the same device for comparison.

2.2 Preliminary Analysis

A summary of the aggregated heart rates, step data and sleep data is given in Table 1.

Table 1. Comparison of the aggregated vital signs of the elderly from different centers

		Nursing home (n = 16)	Elderly geriatric center (n = 34)	P value (Chi-square test)
Demographic				
Mean age (S.D.)		81.13 (13.38)	76.56 (7.62)	0.500
Gender	Male	8 (50.00%)	5 (14.71%)	*0.008
	Female	8 (50.00%)	29 (85.29%)	
Heart rates (HR)				
Mean HR (S.D.)		68.63 (7.69)	68.56 (6.50)	0.973
Max HR (S.D.)		149.06 (26.06)	122.91 (14.79)	*<0.001
Min HR (S.D.)		46.13 (3.56)	44.12 (3.56)	0.069
Step data				
Daily No. of steps (S.D.)		3,050 (1,891)	9,532 (3,619)	*<0.001
Daily No. of walking steps (S.D.)		1,464 (1,009)	5,729 (2,708)	*<0.001
Ratio (%) (S.D.)		47.43 (16.20)	57.75 (11.11)	*0.031
Daily No. of running steps (S.D.)		139 (290)	405 (419)	*0.013
Ratio (%) (S.D.)		3.64 (5.17)	4.40 (5.04)	0.621
Sleep data				
Daily duration (hrs) (S.D.)		9.06 (4.11)	6.77 (1.55)	*0.025
Deep sleep states (hrs) (S.D.)		3.26 (1.37)	2.88 (0.92)	0.089
Ratio (%) (S.D.)		37.47 (11.01)	42.21 (9.63)	0.253
Light sleep states (hrs) (S.D.)		5.80 (3.10)	3.90 (1.04)	*0.020
Ratio (%) (S.D.)		62.53 (11.01)	57.79 (9.63)	0.127

The aggregated HR data, mean HR and minimum HR of the participants from the two centers showed no significant difference while the maximum HR of the participants of the nursing home were significantly higher than those from the elderly geriatric center (Max. HR: nursing home = 149.06 bpm vs. elderly geriatric center = 122.91 bpm, $p = < 0.001$) (Fig. 1). For the step data, the average daily number of steps of the elderly from the nursing home was significantly lower than those from the geriatric center ($p < 0.001$) (Fig. 2). In addition, the proportion of the average walking steps over the average number of step counts was tested with a significant lower value (p = 0.031), while the difference in proportions of the running steps was tested with an insignificant value (p = 0.621). Those from the nursing home were found to have a longer average sleeping duration than those from the elderly geriatric center (p = 0.025) (Fig. 3), but the pattern of light and deep sleeping showed no statistically significant difference between the two groups.

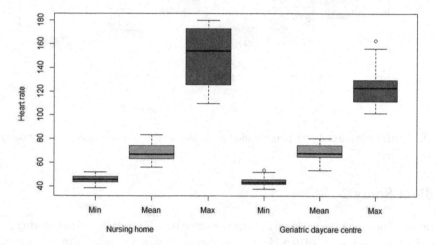

Fig. 1. Variation in the daily mean, minimum and maximum heart rates of the elderly from the two centers in pilot study 1

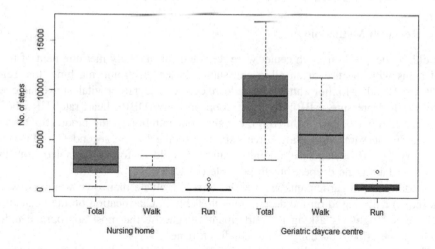

Fig. 2. Variation in the daily step counts of the elderly from the two centers in pilot study 1

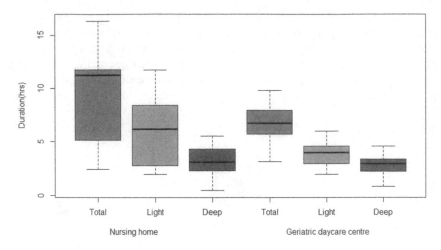

Fig. 3. Variation in the daily sleeping duration of the elderly from the two centers in pilot study 1

3   Pilot Study 2

The aims of this pilot study were (1) to demonstrate the effectiveness of monitoring data related to the vital signs of the elderly to determine their wellness with the use of a commercial all-in-one station-based health monitoring machine and (2) to build a decision support system with essential personalized rules for forecasting the wellness of each elderly person. This pilot study was also conducted in one nursing home and one geriatric daycare center where elderly people with various chronic diseases were cared for.

3.1   Research Methodology

Ten elderly people from each center were recruited for the daily measurement of their vital signs with the use of an all-in-one station-based electronic machine, the Tele-MedCare Health Monitor (http://telemedcare.com/). The target vital signs included systolic blood pressure (SBP), diastolic blood pressure (DBP), heart rate (HR), body temperature (BT), body weight (BW), oxygen concentration in the blood (SpO$_2$) and spirometric measures (including force expired volume in one second (FEV1), peak expiratory flow (PEF) and the amount of air that could be forcibly exhaled from the lungs after taking the deepest breath possible (FVC).

In addition, the participants were asked to self-evaluate their own wellness (wellness index) daily based on the descriptions in Table 2. Clarification on the evaluation results was sought via asking the participants to choose the most appropriate index which can describe their daily health condition if necessary.

The regression tree method proposed by Sparks and Okugami [15] was applied to forecast the wellness of the elderly based on the lagged vital sign measures (one day before) and the previous day's wellness measure as determinants. In the regression tree,

Table 2. Self-evluation of wellness

Wellness index	Description of wellness of the elderly
1	Feeling terrible
2	Feeling very unwell but not terrible
3	Feeling worse than average
4	Feeling a little worse than usual
5	Feeling very slightly off but close to usual
6	Feeling very slightly better than usual
7	Feeling a little better than usual
8	Feeling better than usual
9	Feeling much better than usual but not terrific
10	Feeling terrific

the daily collected wellness index and vital sign measures are regarded as response variables and covariates, respectively. The chosen time lag was only one day, shorter than that in the work by Sparks and Okugami. A more conservative approach was chosen, as the expected trends on the vital signs were not clearly shown. With the aid of an R software package, "rpart" [17], the first 30-consecutive-day data were considered as the training dataset to create the personalized classification rules, which were then further tested with the remaining daily data to evaluate their precision when forecasting personal wellness.

3.2 Preliminary Analysis on Individual Wellness Monitoring

As the target population was elderly people with chronic illnesses, any adverse conditions remaining untreated could have resulted in a higher chance of hospitalization and a longer recovery time. Theoretically, this negative health outcome can be prevented by early detection and treatment. Forecasting the wellness of the elderly based on identified personalized rules may be a useful indicator in early anomaly detection and potential treatment. In Table 3, we demonstrate the wellness analysis using the identified personalized rules of two selected elderly people. The rules identified are unique to each person.

The bolded vital sign measurements are the key splitters found in the regression tree and are the main predicted rules for the forecasting on wellness, while the others are the summarized characteristics of the nodes. Figures 4 and 5 are the graphical presentations of the fitted regression tree models of the two participants. The validation results of the identified rules are summarized in Table 4. Taking the validation results of participant 8 in Table 4 as an example, the wellness indexes are further categorized into three main classes for evaluating the prediction accuracy of wellness. The precision and detection accuracy of the corresponding wellness class were calculated. A larger value in precision and detection accuracy indicated better prediction capability.

Table 3. Identified rules and results of selected elderly people (Participants 8 and 9)

Participant		Identified rules	
8	Rule 1 (Mean wellness index = 4.429)	Rule 2 (Mean wellness index = 5)	Rule 3 (Mean wellness index = 5.286)
	BW (the day **before) < 69.78** BT (the day before) < 35.65 Wellness index (the day before) < 4.5	**BW (the day** **before) >= 69.78** **HR (the day** **before) < 56.5** SBP (the day before) < 110 FEV1 (the day before) < 0.715 SpO2 (the day before) < 97.5	**BW (the day** **before) >= 69.78** **HR (the day** **before) >= 56.5** FVC (the day before) < 1.475
9	Rule 1 (Mean wellness index = 5.143)	Rule 2 (Mean wellness index = 6)	Rule 3 (Mean wellness index = 6.8)
	FVC (the day **before) >= 2.215** Wellness index (the day before) < 5.5 Body temperature (the day before) < 35.65	**FVC (the day** **before) < 2.215** **Wellness index (the** **day before) < 6.5** FVC (the day before) < 1.875 PEF (the day before) < 1.155 FEV1 (the day before) < 1.065 BW (the day before) < 65.125	**FVC (the day** **before) < 2.215** **Wellness index (the** **day before) > 6.5**

Table 4. Validation results of the identified rules of selected elderly people (Participants 8 and 9)

Participant	Wellness index	Applied rule	Predicted No. of date with corresponding wellness	Actual No. of date with corresponding wellness	Pr (Precision)	Pr (Detection accuracy)
8	<5	1	2	1	0/2 = 0	0/1 = 0
	5	2	6	13	5/6 = 0.83	5/13 = 0.38
	>5	3	6	0	0/6 = 0	0
9	<6	1	0	5	0/0 = 0	0/5 = 0
	6	2	9	9	9/9 = 1	9/9 = 1
	>6	3	2	3	2/2 = 1	2/3 = 0.66

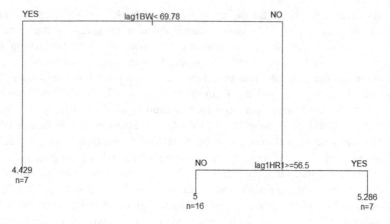

Fig. 4. Fitted regression tree model showing the rules for forecasting the wellness of participant 8

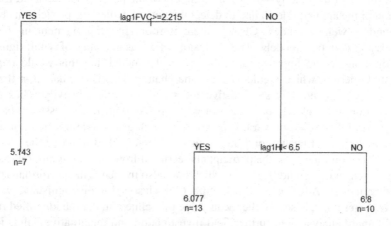

Fig. 5. Fitted regression tree model showing the rules for forecasting the wellness of participant 9

4   Discussion and Future Research

The findings of the first pilot study provided a general picture of the differences in the lifestyles of the elderly recruited from different centers. Elderly people who lived in the nursing home usually slept longer and had a lack of physical activities, while those recruited from the geriatric daycare center showed a more active lifestyle, lower sleeping duration and more physical activities. Clearly, the living environment of the elderly influenced their health, but to what extent was not revealed in this pilot study. Another significant finding was that the maximum heart rates of the elderly recruited from the nursing home were higher on average than those from the geriatric daycare center. This could be an important sign reflecting the wellness of the elderly, and it deserves further analysis to identify potential influential factors. The aggregated results provide informative guidance for the management of healthcare services provided by the centers. For example, the sleeping patterns and activity levels of the participants recorded by the wearable device were useful in terms of micro-monitoring health, which could not have been previously achieved, if manpower was limited.

The ranges of the collected real-time heart rates, sleep data and step data showed high variations among the elderly from both centers. The variations found were believed to be due to different personal factors such as medical history and lifestyle. Further analysis could be conducted to evaluate the extent of the influence of these factors. The analyzed results could also be beneficial to the quality of the healthcare service provided, in terms of meeting the individual demands of the elderly.

The second pilot study demonstrated that the wellness of the elderly with different health conditions could potentially be forecast with the aid of machine learning algorithms, based on daily measurements of vital signs and self-evaluations of wellness. The identified rules could be informative, mainly in terms of indicating the key vital measurements affecting wellness and the corresponding threshold values on causing shifts in wellness, but some of the rules failed to give precise predictions of the future wellness of the elderly—either the wellness of the participants deviated from the prediction or the applied rules failed to detect the date on which the participants had the corresponding wellness index. Clearly, there is room for improvement in the forecasting regression tree models. The inclusion of measurements of vital signs with longer time lags could improve the accuracy of the model, but this would require a longer study period, which would increase the chances of missing data. On the other hand, the wellness index is a subjective measurement, which heavily relies on the self-perception of the elderly on their own wellness. An objective assessment based on the integrated information on various parameters, such as lifestyle information, mental wellness and physical health conditions, has great potential to improve the prediction accuracy. The compliance of the participants recruited from the community in terms of daily health checking would be lower, which may also influence the performance of the forecasting model. Additionally, the number of classes for distinguishing wellness levels was determined based on the mean value of wellness under the identified rules in our preliminary analysis, but further field investigation and quantitative validation are required to obtain a more precise categorization of wellness.

In the two pilot studies, real-time health monitoring data and daily vital signs measurements were collected and analyzed separately. How to integrate these data to improve elderly wellness assessment and prediction is a challenge. In the future, we will investigate the correlations between elderly wellness and multiple factors, including summarized real-time health monitoring data, daily vital sign measurements and personalized health information. Assessment models incorporating these correlations at a very granular level will be developed, and could be applied to predict individual health risks given specific factor inputs.

Acknowledgements. This work was supported in part by the RGC Theme-Based Research Scheme (TBRS) No. T32-102/14-N and the National Natural Science Foundation of China (NSFC) No. 71420107023.

References

1. Census and Statistics Department. Hong Kong Population Projections 2015–2016 (2015). http://www.statistics.gov.hk/pub/B1120015062015XXXXB0100.pdf. Accessed 3 July 2016
2. The 2016 policy address, Chapter 4 - Medical Services, Public Health and Elderly Care (2015). http://www.policyaddress.gov.hk/2016/eng/pdf/Agenda_Ch4.pdf. Accessed 3 July 2016
3. Food and Health Bureau. My Health My Choice – Healthcare Reform Second Stage Public Consultation – Consultation Document, Appendix C – Hong Kong's Current Private Healthcare Sector (2010). http://www.myhealthmychoice.gov.hk/pdf/appendixC_eng.pdf. Accessed 1 May 2017
4. Food and Health Bureau. Consultation Document on Voluntary Health Insurance Scheme, Chapter 8 – Implications from Hong Kong's Healthcare System (2014). http://www.vhis.gov.hk/doc/en/full_consultation_document/consultation_full_eng.pdf. Accessed 1 May 2017
5. Patel, S., Park, H., Bonato, P., Chan, L., Rodgers, M.: A review of wearable sensors and systems with application in rehabilitation. J. Neuro Eng. Rehabil. 9(1), 21 (2012)
6. Anliker, U., Ward, J.A., Lukowicz, P., et al.: AMON: a wearable multiparameter medical monitoring and alert system. IEEE Trans. Inf. Technol. Biomed. 8, 415–427 (2004)
7. Pandian, P.S., Mohanavelu, K., Safeer, K.P., Kotresh, T.M., Shakunthala, D.T., Gopal, P., Padaki, V.C.: Smart Vest: Wearable multi-parameter remote physiological monitoring system. Med. Eng. Phys. 30, 466–477 (2008)
8. Sloboda, J., Manohar, D.: A simple sleep stage identification technique for incorporation in inexpensive electronic sleep screening devices. In: Proceedings of the 2011 IEEE National Aerospace and Electronics Conference (NAECON), pp. 21–24 (2011)
9. Rebolledo-Nandi, Z., Chavez-Olivera, A., Cuevas-Valencia, R.E., Alarcon-Paredes, A., Alonso, G.A.: Design of a versatile low cost mobile health care monitoring system using an android application. In: 2015 Pan American Health Care Exchanges (PAHCE), pp. 1–4 (2015)
10. Pallavi, M., Dharma, P.A.: A hybrid key management scheme for healthcare sensor networks. In: 2016 IEEE International Conference on Communications (ICC), pp. 1–6 (2016)
11. Moser, L.E., Melliar-Smith, P.M.: Personal health monitoring using a smartphone. In: 2015 IEEE International Conference on Mobile Services (MS), pp. 344–351 (2015)
12. Hughes, E., Masilela, M., Eddings, P., Rafiq, A., Boanca, C., Merrell, R.: VMote: a wearable wireless health monitoring system. In: 2007 9th International Conference on e-Health Networking Application and Services, pp. 330–331 (2007)
13. Patrick, C., Vallipuram, M.: Using smart phones and body sensors to deliver pervasive mobile personal healthcare. In: 2010 Sixth International Conference on Intelligent Sensors Sensor Networks and Information Processing (ISSNIP), pp. 291–296 (2010)
14. Sparks, R., Celler, B., Okugami, C., Jayasena, R., Varnfield, M.: Telehealth monitoring of patients in the community. J. Intell. Syst. 25, 37–63 (2015)
15. Sparks, R., Okugami, C.: Tele-health monitoring of patient wellness. J. Intell. Syst. 25(4), 515–528 (2015)
16. https://www.sonymobile.com/global-en/products/smart-products/smartband-2/
17. Therneau, T., Atkinson, B., Ripley, R.: rpart: Recursive partitioning and regression trees. Ver 4.1-10 (2015). http://cran.r-project.org/web/packages/rpart/index.html

Influence of Technology Affordance on the Adoption of Mobile Technologies for Diabetes Self-management

Ramakrishna Dantu[1(✉)], Radha Mahapatra[2], and Jingguo Wang[2]

[1] College of Business Administration, California State University, Sacramento,
6000 J Street, Sacramento, CA 95819, USA
dantu@csus.edu
[2] Information Systems and Operations Management Department,
College of Business, University of Texas at Arlington,
701 S Nedderman Dr., Arlington, TX 76019, USA

1 Introduction

Diabetes is a costly chronic disease, and a leading cause of death and disability worldwide. According to a report from the Center for Disease Control, diabetes cost an estimated \$245 billion to the US economy in 2012 [12]. Like other chronic conditions, such as hypertension, heart disease, and cancer, there is no cure for diabetes. However, the debilitating effects of the disease can be slowed down and the patient's quality of life improved by proper care management. In this context, self-management practices that enable a patient to play an active role in managing his/her health condition have been found to be very effective in improving the patient's quality of life while lowering the overall healthcare cost [5, 35, 46]. Therefore, encouraging diabetes patients to adopt self-management practices has become a part of the best practices in diabetes care management [7, 24, 51]. Diabetes self-management practices include activities, such as, eating healthy food, exercising regularly, monitoring and maintaining blood sugar level, etc. In recent times, mobile technology-based interventions, including apps and devices, have been developed to help diabetics follow self-management practices. Several studies have found such interventions to be helpful in promoting diabetes self-management [23, 30]. However, the adoption of such mobile technology-based interventions are very limited [2, 19]. The goal of this study is to understand what facilitates adoption of mobile technologies for diabetes self-management.

Technology adoption has been extensively studied in the information systems literature, with the technology acceptance model (TAM) and its related research forming a mature research stream [37, 59, 60]. This large body of research has resulted in a parsimonious model to explain individual's intention to adopt information technologies and has clearly established the efficacy of perceived usefulness (PU) and perceived ease of use (PEOU) as antecedents of individual's intention to adopt new technology. In recent times there has been a growing chorus among IS researchers to "open up the black box" of PU and PEOU and explain what makes a system useful or easy to use so as to provide action-able guidance for application design [6, 11, 27]. Furthermore, most

H. Chen et al. (Eds.): ICSH 2017, LNCS 10347, pp. 104–115, 2017.
https://doi.org/10.1007/978-3-319-67964-8_10

TAM studies have investigated individual adoption of office productivity systems or business information systems in an organizational setting [37]. Since a chronic illness creates a serious psychological and emotional burden on the patient, an individual's technology adoption behavior is likely to be influenced by his/her strategy to cope with the illness.

This research report attempts to enhance our understanding of individual adoption of mobile technologies in chronic care management. In particular we study individual's intention to adopt mobile technologies for diabetes self-care. We draw on two critical streams of research (1) technology affordance theory and (2) illness representations to explain this phenomenon. Our study makes several contributions. First, it is one of the earliest studies that empirically investigate the adoption of mobile technologies in chronic care management. Mobile technologies have tremendous potential to improving care delivery and lower healthcare cost. Thus, it is imperative to understand people's adoption behavior to promote technology adoption. Second, technology affordance, with its origin in ecological psychology, has been found to offer meaningful insight into technology use. Within IS, Volkoff and Strong [61] define affordances as "the potential for behaviors associated with achieving an immediate concrete outcome and arising from the relation between an object (e.g., an IT artifact) and a goal-oriented actor or actors." Our study follow this definition to develop an instrument to measure affordances of mobile technologies for diabetes self-management (AMTDSM) and validate it within a nomological network.

The remainder of the report is presented as follows. We articulate the theoretical underpinnings of the study and present the research model explicating its key constructs and relationships. The research plan to measure and validate technology affordance and its antecedents is then presented. The research findings are discussed and the paper is concluded with a presentation of implications of the findings and directions for future research.

2 Theoretical Background and Research Model (Nomological Net)

To understand the role of technology affordances in the larger context of technology adoption for diabetes management, we position the construct within a nomological network as shown in Fig. 1. This model draws on two streams of research, namely affordance theory and illness representation. We provide brief introductions to these research streams before presenting the arguments for the research model.

2.1 Technology Affordance

Theory of affordance has its roots in perceptual and ecological psychology [13, 25]. Affordances arise in the context of an actor-object system where the object affords possibilities for action based on the actor's capabilities and goals [54, 61]. Consider for example, a large rock on the ground. This rock affords a weary traveler an opportunity for resting whereas to a small burrowing animal, the same rock affords shelter. Thus,

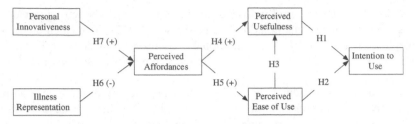

Fig. 1. Theoretical model

affordance is a relational concept [13, 33]. The fundamental premise of the theory is that affordances stimulate action. However, presence of affordance in an actor-object system does not imply that the activity will occur [28, 56]. Perceived affordance is a precursor to action.

Recently, IS researchers have adopted the concept of affordance to explain IT use behavior of individuals within the organizational context. Affordance theory has been used to study the role of social media in facilitating customer engagement [10], change in work routines [38], organizational changes driven by IT implementation and use [61], Electronic Health Record (EHR) implementation [55], media choice by knowledge workers [34], information quality and system quality [26], and smartphone adoption and use [57]. In summary, three key aspects emerge from the literature on technology affordance: (1) technology affordance is unique to the technology and specific to the context; (2) affordance influences technology use leading to IT driven organizational change; (3) individual or organization-al goals and capabilities influence technology affordance. The significance of technology affordance is evident from the growing body of affordance related research in IS. However, the discourse on affordance so far has been primarily at the conceptual level, and there is a paucity of instrumentation to measure affordance. A primary goal of this research is to develop and validate an instrument to measure technology affordance.

2.2 Illness Representation

Individuals experiencing chronic illness are under severe physical and psychological duress. In order to study the technology use behavior of chronically ill patients, it is imperative to understand their coping strategies. The common sense model of self-regulation [39], with its origin in health behavior research, is widely used to understand the coping behavior of patients experiencing chronic conditions. According to this model, individuals build cognitive and emotional representations of their illness when they are faced with health threats, and these illness representations drive their response strategies to cope with the threats [40, 41, 48].

Illness representations consist of five cognitive dimensions: identity, cause, timeline, consequences, and cure/control. Identity refers to the signs and symptoms that the individual ascribes to their health condition. Consequences are the patient's perception of physical, social, and economic impact or outcome on the individual's life and the emotional feelings due to the disease. Causes refer to the individual's perceptions about the origin of their health condition. Timeline refers to the perceived duration (e.g., acute, chronic, cyclical) of the illness and how long it might take to cure the illness. Finally, cure/control refers to the individual believes that the illness can be either cured or controlled by a treatment process [36, 41]. To these five dimensions of cognitive illness representation, Moss-Morris et al. [45] added coherence and emotional representations. Coherence refers to patient's understanding or comprehension about their illness [42]. Emotional representations include elements such as anger, anxiety, fear, and depression. Based on these dimensions a chronically ill patient's illness representation may fall in one of two categories: positive or negative. Those with positive illness representations believe that they are in control of the situation and don't feel the need to seek external help to cope with their chronic conditions. On the other hand, patients with negative illness representations look for external resource to manage their conditions. Obviously, this has significant implications for technology adoption and use in the context of individuals experiencing chronic conditions.

2.3   Hypotheses Development

Originated from the theory of reasoned action (TRA) [3, 21] and its extension, the theory of planned behavior (TPB), TAM has become a well-established model in the IS literature in predicting an individual's behavioral intention to adopt a new information technology. There is a substantial body of work [32, 43] on TAM and several empirical studies have clearly demonstrated the positive effect of perceived usefulness and perceived ease of use on an individual's behavioral intentions of using technology. Drawing from the extant TAM literature, we propose:

H1:   *Perception of usefulness of mobile technologies for diabetes management has a*
        positive effect on the patient's behavioral intention to use the technology.
H2:   *Perception of ease of use of mobile technologies for diabetes management has a*
        positive effect on the patient's behavioral intention to use the technology.
H3:   *Perception of ease of use of mobile technologies for diabetes management has a*
        positive effect on the patient's perception of usefulness of the technology.

Impact of Affordances on Perceived Usefulness and Perceived Ease of Use
Perception of affordance influences action or behavior. Literature shows that before one takes action, such as using technology, one must perceive its usefulness and/or ease of use. Temporally, whether the technology would be useful or easy to use depends on what the technology affords. In other words, technology affordances have an effect on usefulness and ease of use.

Technology affordance beliefs of smartphone design has been shown to positively influence perception of usefulness and ease of use in using smartphones [57]. Technology affordances are crucial for diabetes patients in managing their illness. For instance, eating a healthy and balanced diet in right proportions at right frequencies is vital in maintaining one's blood glucose level. Technology that can help a patient choose right kind and proportion of food has the potential to influence his/her belief on the usefulness of the technology. To reduce risks of side effects from diabetes, it might be necessary to periodically share blood glucose or other measurements with a healthcare provider. If the user has to save the data in a different tool and then transmit it to their provider, it might be cumbersome to use the technology. On the other hand, if the technology affords measurement and transmission of blood glucose levels, it would be easy for the patient to use the technology. Perceived affordances of mobile technologies for diabetes self-management is expected to positively affect usefulness and ease of use beliefs. Thus, we hypothesize:

H4:   *Perceived affordance of mobile technologies for diabetes management has a positive effect on the patient's perception of usefulness of the technology.*

H5:   *Perceived affordance of mobile technologies for diabetes management has a positive effect on the patient's perception of ease of use of the technology.*

Antecedents of Technology Affordances

Affordances of the technology and abilities of the individual are closely related to each other to make a particular behavior possible [28, 56]. An individual must have a need and capability to perceive affordances in the objects [54, 61].

In diabetes management, a blood glucose-measuring device may afford patients the opportunity to transmit blood glucose measurements to their health care provider, but the patient may not perceive this affordance unless he/she has a need and/or capability of engaging in such an action. According to the self-regulation model, patient's illness perceptions, which represent the patient's belief about health status and/or control, form their needs that drive coping behavior. Patient's need for managing health condition and leading a better life can influence perception of whether or not the technology can facilitate them in their coping process. Research has demonstrated that the patient's belief and estimate of his health severity have consistently predicted their compliance with treatment recommendations [20]. This illustrates that individuals with negative illness perceptions find a need to do something about it and will look for resources for help in getting their health under control. Similarly, patients who think their health status is good and are in control of their health, do not look for any help. Those who have positive illness perceptions may not believe that technology or external gadgets will afford anything for them to manage their illness. We theorize that individuals with positive illness representations are less likely to perceive affordances of the technology compared to those who with negative illness perceptions. Thus,

H6:   *Positive illness representations will have a negative effect on the perception of affordances of mobile technologies for diabetes management.*

Affordances of the object depend on individual abilities [13]. Personal innovativeness in the field of information technology is conceptualized as an individual's willingness to try out different things with a new technology [1]. According to Rogers [53], "innovators are active information-seekers about new ideas" (p. 22). While discussing innovativeness and adopter categories, he refers innovativeness as the degree to which an individual is quick in adopting new ideas compared to others who are less innovative. Personal innovativeness, conceptualized as an individual's characteristic, is likely to influence their discovering and realizing new affordances of the technology. For example, consider a spreadsheet like software that affords several possibilities for performing statistical and mathematical operations. An individual who is eager to explore is likely to notice affordances of this software more than those who are less innovative. We posit that an individual with greater personal innovativeness, considered as a proxy to an individual's capability in this study, is more likely to perceive new affordances of the technology compared to an individual who is less capable. Thus,

H7:   Personal innovativeness will have a positive effect on perception of affordances of mobile technologies for diabetes management.

3   Instrument Development

3.1   Affordances of Mobile Technologies for Diabetes Self-management

A four-stage process, based on the guidelines available in the literature [14, 18, 44], was used to develop the instrument for measuring affordances of mobile technologies for diabetes self-management (AMTDSM). The domain is specified and constructs are defined in Stage 1. Items for each scale are developed in Stage 2. Items are refined through sorting and pretesting in Stage 3. Finally, the instrument is validated in Stage 4.

Clearly specifying the domain helps develop relevant items for each scale and ensures content validity. Chronic illness self-management involves managing various complex tasks such as monitoring symptoms, conditions, and vital signs; tracking food intake, medication dosages; actively engaging in physical exercises to keep themselves active; and complying with treatment regimen [15, 31]. To help diabetics in managing their illness and experience a good quality of life, the American Association of Diabetes Educators (AADE7™) has developed an evidence-based framework comprising of seven key self-care behaviors [4]: (1) healthy eating, (2) being active, (3) monitoring, (4) taking medications, (5) problem solving, (6) healthy coping, and (7) reducing risks. Research shows that healthcare interventions that improve these seven self-care behavioral objectives have a positive effect on one's health [8]. Mobile technologies that are designed for diabetes self-management will be more effective when these technologies afford patients to accomplish the AADE7 self-care objectives. These seven behavioral objectives formed the basis of developing our instrument.

A list of items for each self-care behavior was developed based on the review of literature on diabetes self-management, extensive discussions with healthcare practitioners engaged in diabetes management, and experts in the College of Nursing in a major university. Experts were given the definition for the overall construct, descriptions for various scales/dimensions, and asked to describe the actions that mobile apps and devices can/should afford to the patients in order for them to accomplish the self-care objectives. An initial list of 52 items was created after rewording, rephrasing, and simplifying the descriptions. Six judges with expertise and/or experience in diabetes management reviewed this initial list to assess if the items accurately described various affordances offered by mobile apps and devices.

The instrument was refined by placing items into appropriate categories through sorting followed by pretesting to improve construct validity [44]. A total of nine individuals with experience and/or expertise in diabetes management categorized the items according to how closely they were related to each dimension/scale of the construct. Ambiguous items were eliminated in this step resulting in a list of 37 items (73% of the original list of 52). This list was pre-tested by conducting an online web-based survey with a group of 25 individuals. In addition to filling out the survey, the respondents were also requested to provide feedback on various aspects of the survey instrument, such as clarity of items and time taken to complete the survey. The survey instrument was further refined based on their feedback. The resulting instrument contained 27 items.

Finally, the instrument is validated in stage 4. The final instrument resulted in 26 items with five dimensions. We then tested the instrument for convergent, discriminant, and nomological validity by performing confirmatory factor analysis using the data collected through a final survey of over 208 diabetes patients.

3.2 Other Constructs

Items for measuring intention to adopt were adapted from Venkatesh et al. [59]. Perceptions of usefulness and ease of use were assessed by adapting items from Venkatesh and Davis [58] and Venkatesh et al. [59]. We used a brief illness perception questionnaire (Brief IPQ) [9] to measure illness representation. To assess an individual's willingness to try out new mobile technologies, we adapted personal innovativeness items from Agarwal and Prasad [1]. All the items were measured using a five-point Likert scale, ranging from strongly disagree (1) to strongly agree (5) with the exception of items for illness representation, which were measured on an eleven-point scale.

4 Methodology

The unit of analysis for the study is an individual, the diabetes patient. To empirically test the hypothesized relationships in the research model, we collected data anonymously in a cross-sectional study using an online web-based survey methodology. Participants comprise of diabetes patients who do not currently use any technology for managing their conditions, but they knew about those technologies. We collected data anonymously using an online survey questionnaire through a third party data collection agency from diabetes patients who are over 18 years of age and live within the United States of America. A total of 208 completed and useful responses were returned from the survey. Among the total respondents, 56.3% of the respondents are female and 43.8% are male.

5   Results

The partial least squares (PLS) approach to structural equation modeling (SEM) technique was used for evaluating the measurement of latent variables and testing relationships between them. To test the hypothesized relationships and establish nomological validity, we used the SmartPLS [52] software. In the model, intention to use, perceived usefulness, perceived ease of use, and personal innovativeness are measured as first-order reflective constructs. Illness representation is measured as second-order formative and first-order reflective constructs. Perceived technology affordances are measured as second-order reflective-reflective construct. In the model assessment, internal consistency is evaluated using both Cronbach's alpha and composite reliability. Indicator reliability is assessed using factor loadings. Average variance extracted (AVE) is used to evaluate convergent validity. Discriminant validity is assessed using item cross loadings and Fornell-Larcker criterion.

5.1   Measurement Model

Cronbach's alpha, with an acceptable value of 0.70, is usually evaluated as a means of measuring internal consistency [47]. Composite reliability, with a value of over 0.70 is considered satisfactory, and is another means of evaluating internal consistency. In the measurement model (not shown due to space constraints), composite reliability and Cronbach's alpha of all constructs were over 0.7, thus establishing internal consistency of all the variables in both models.

The outer loadings of the indicators along with the average variance extracted (AVE) are used in assessing convergent validity of the variables. A minimum value of 0.5 for AVE is considered acceptable [22]. The outer loadings of all the indicators were above the acceptable level of 0.708 [29], thus establishing convergent validity. Cross loadings of the indicators and the comparison of average variance extracted for each construct against inter-construct correlations are used to evaluate discriminant validity [22]. We checked the cross-loadings of the items and found all the items to load well with respect to their constructs indicating that they measured what they were intended to measure. Item cross-loadings and inter-construct correlations illustrated sufficient discriminant validity. Due to the limitation of article size, we are unable to show the outer loadings, item cross-loadings, reliability and validity test results in this article.

5.2   Structural Model

This study guaranteed respondent anonymity and also performed pretest to refine questionnaire items to help reduce common method bias [50]. In addition to this, we also ran Harman's Single Factor test [49]. The first general factor explained 33.82% and 33.49% of the total variance in the non-user and user models respectively indicating that common method bias is not likely to cause an issue with our results. The path coefficients and the proportion of variance in the dependent variable explained by the independent variables are presented in Fig. 2. Survey respondents' demographic

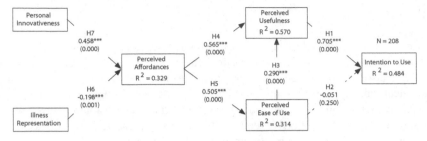

Fig. 2. Structural model

characteristics were used as controls to eliminate any confounding of results. None of the controls were significant.

It is evident from the PLS results that data provide strong support for hypotheses, essentially drawn from TAM [16], H1 and H2. The finding that hypothesis H3 was not supported is consistent with that obtained by Davis et al. [17]. Hypotheses H4 and H5 were strongly supported indicating that Perceived Affordances significantly impact Perceived Usefulness (H4) and Perceived Ease of Use (H5). Likewise, Illness Representation and Personal Innovativeness have significant effects on Perceived Affordances (H6 and H7). In addition to the models tested above, we examined whether there is a full mediation of the effects of Affordances on Intention. To perform this, we added the direct effect of Perceived Affordance on Intention to Use in the model. The effect was insignificant ($\beta = 0.034$, $p = 0.319$).

6 Discussion and Conclusion

In this research we developed an instrument to measure perceived affordances of mobile technologies in diabetes self-management and validated it within a nomological network in the context of technology adoption. The results clearly demonstrate the influence of technology affordances as the antecedent of PU and PEOU.

Our research makes several contributions to theory. Since perceived affordance is a relational construct between the IT artifact and the user, understanding technology affordance can lead to specific recommendations to improve IT artifact design. Thus, at a theoretical level, our research fulfills the recent calls to action to "open the black box" and explain what leads to perceived usefulness and perceived ease of use. Technology affordance, as a construct, has wider implication for IS research beyond technology adoption. This is evident from the small but growing body of literature on technology affordance (as cited earlier in this report) that investigate diverse IS phenomena. Most of these studies use technology affordance at a conceptual level. Thus, by developing and validating an instrument to measure technology affordance, our research makes a significant methodological contribution to advancing research in this area. Mobile technologies hold the potential to improve the quality of life and lower care delivery cost of chronically ill patients. In order to ensure rapid adoption and use of such technologies we need to understand adoption behavior of patients experiencing chronic conditions, which is very different from the adoption behavior of technology users in organizations. Drawing on the extant research in health behavior we adapted and used illness representation as a construct in our model to explain mobile technology adoption by chronically ill patients.

Our study also has implications for practice. Technology designers must assess the affordances from the user's perspective in order to design and deliver technologies that will have wider adoption. Considering the criticality of perceived affordance in technology adoption it is also imperative to enhance perception of affordance through training and promotions to ensure wider adoption.

References

1. Agarwal, R., Prasad, J.: A conceptual and operational definition of personal innovativeness in the domain of information technology. Inform. Syst. Res. **9**, 204–215 (1998)
2. Aitken, M., Lyle, J.: Patient Adoption of mHealth: Use, Evidence and Remaining Barriers to Mainstream Acceptance. IMS Institute for Healthcare Informatics, New York (2015)
3. Ajzen, I., Fishbein, M.: Understanding attitudes and predicting social behaviour. Prentice-Hall, Englewood Cliffs (1980)
4. American Association of Diabetes Educators: AADE7^{TM} - Self-Care Behaviors (2010). www.diabeteseducator.org, https://www.diabeteseducator.org/patient-resources/aade7-self-care-behaviors. Accessed 6 Feb 2016
5. Barlow, J., Wright, C., Sheasby, J., Turner, A.: Self-management approaches for people with chronic conditions: a review. Patient Educ. Couns. **48**, 177–187 (2002)
6. Benbasat, I., Barki, H.: Quo vadis TAM? J. Assoc. Inform. Syst. **8**, 211–218 (2007)
7. Bodenheimer, T., Lorig, K., Holman, H., Grumbach, K.: Patient self-management of chronic disease in primary care. J. Am. Med. Assoc. **288**, 2469–2475 (2002). doi:10.1001/jama.288.19.2469
8. Boren, S.A.: AADE7^{TM} self-care behaviors: systematic reviews. Diab. Educ. **33**, 866–871 (2007)
9. Broadbent, E., Petrie, K.J., Main, J., Weinman, J.A.: The brief illness perception questionnaire. J. Psychosom. Res. **60**, 631–637 (2006)
10. Cabiddu, F., De Carlo, M., Piccoli, G.: Social media affordances: enabling customer engagement. Ann. Tourism Res. **48**, 175–192 (2014). doi:10.1016/j.annals.2014.06.003
11. Carter, M., Grover, V.: Me, My Self, and I(T) - conceptualizing information technology identity and its implications. MIS Q. **39**, 931–957 (2015)
12. Centers for Disease Control and Prevention: Chronic Disease Overview (2015). http://www.cdc.gov/chronicdisease/overview/index.htm. Accessed 23 Apr 2016
13. Chemero, A.: An outline of a theory of affordances **15**, 181–195 (2003). doi:10.1207/S15326969ECO1502_5
14. Chu, A.M.Y., Chau, P.Y.K.: Development and validation of instruments of information security deviant behavior. Decis. Support Syst. **66**, 93–101 (2014). doi:10.1016/j.dss.2014.06.008
15. Clark, N.M., Becker, M.H., Janz, N.K., Lorig, K.: Self-management of chronic disease by older adults a review and questions for research. J. Aging Health **3**, 3–27 (1991)
16. Davis, F.D.: Perceived usefulness, perceived ease of use, and user acceptance of information technology. MIS Q., 319–340 (1989)

17. Davis, F.D., Bagozzi, R.P., Warshaw, P.R.: User acceptance of computer technology: a comparison of two theoretical models. Manage. Sci. **35**, 982–1003 (1989)
18. DeVellis, R.F.: Scale Development: Theory and Applications. Sage Publications, Newbury Park (2012)
19. El-Gayar, O., Timsina, P., Nawar, N., Eid, W.: A systematic review of IT for diabetes self-management: are we there yet? Int. J. Med. Informatics **82**, 637–652 (2013)
20. Feuerstein, M., Elise, L.E., Andrzej, K.R.: Health Psychology: A Psychobiological Perspective. Plenum Press, New York (1986)
21. Fishbein, M., Ajzen, I.: Belief, Attitude, Intention and Behavior: An Introduction to Theory and Research. Addison-Wesley, Reading (1975)
22. Fornell, C., Larcker, D.F.: Evaluating structural equation models with unobservable variables and measurement error. J. Mark. Res. **18**, 39–50 (1981)
23. Free, C., Phillips, G., Galli, L., Watson, L., Felix, L., Edwards, P., Patel, V., Haines, A.: The effectiveness of mobile-health technology-based health behaviour change or disease management interventions for health care consumers: a systematic review. PLoS Med. **10**, 1–45 (2013). doi:10.1371/journal.pmed.1001362
24. Funnell, M.M., Anderson, R.M.: Empowerment and self-management of diabetes. Clin. Diab. **22**, 123–127 (2004). doi:10.2337/diaclin.22.3.123
25. Gibson, J.J.: The Ecological Approach to Visual Perception. Lawrence Erlbaum Associates, Hillsdale (1986)
26. Grgecic, D., Holten, R., Rosenkranz, C.: The Impact of functional affordances and symbolic expressions on the formation of beliefs. J. Assoc. Inform. Syst. **16**, 580–607 (2015)
27. Grover, V., Lyytinen, K.: New state of play in information systems research: the push to the edges. MIS Q. **39**, 275–296 (2015)
28. Greeno, J.G.: Gibson's affordances. Psychol. Rev. **101**, 336–342 (1994)
29. Hair Jr., J.F., Hult, T.M., Ringle, C., Sarstedt, M.: A Primer on Partial Least Squares Structural Equation Modeling (PLS-SEM). SAGE Publications, Thousand Oaks (2014)
30. Hartz, J., Yingling, L., Powell-Wiley, T.M.: Use of mobile health technology in the prevention and management of diabetes mellitus. Curr. Cardiol. Rep., 1–11 (2016). doi:10.1007/s11886-016-0796-8
31. Hill-Briggs, F.: Problem solving in diabetes self-management: a model of chronic illness self-management behavior. Ann. Behav. Med. **25**, 182–193 (2003)
32. Holden, R.J., Karsh, B.-T.: The technology acceptance model: Its past and its future in health care. J. Biomed. Inform. **43**, 159–172 (2010)
33. Hutchby, I.: Technologies, texts and affordances. Sociology **35**, 441–456 (2001)
34. Jung, Y., Lyytinen, K.: Towards an ecological account of media choice: a case study on pluralistic reasoning while choosing email. Info Syst. J. **24**, 271–293 (2013)
35. Kass-Bartelmes, B.: Preventing disability in the elderly with chronic disease. Res. Action, 1–8 (2002)
36. Lau, R.R., Hartman, K.A.: Common sense representations of common illnesses. Health Psychol. **2**, 167–185 (1983)
37. Lee, Y., Kozar, K.A., Larsen, K.R.T.: The technology acceptance model: past, present, and future. Commun. Assoc. Inform. Syst. **12**, 1–31 (2013)
38. Leonardi, P.M.: When flexible routines meet flexible technologies: affordance, constraint, and the imbrication of human and material agencies. MIS Q. **35**, 147–167 (2011)
39. Leventhal, H., Nerenz, D.R., Steel, D.J.: Illness representations and coping with health threats. In: Baum, A., Taylor, S.E., Singer, J.E. (eds.) Social Psychological Aspects of Health, pp. 219–252. Lawrence Erlbaum Associates, Hillsdale (1984)

40. Leventhal, H., Benyamini, Y., Brownlee, S., Diefenbach, M., Leventhal, E.A., Patrick-Miller, L., Robitaille, C.: Illness representations: theoretical foundations. In: Petrie, K.J., Weinman, J.A. (eds.) Perceptions of Health and Illness: Current Research and Applications, pp. 19–46. Harwood Amsterdam, Amsterdam (1997)
41. Leventhal, H., Brissette, I., Leventhal, E.A.: The common-sense model of self-regulation of health and illness. In: Cameron, L.D., Leventhal, H. (eds.) The Self-Regulation of Health and Illness Behavior, pp. 42–65. Routledge, New York, NY (2003)
42. Leventhal, H., Weinman, J.A., Leventhal, E.A., Phillips, L.A.: Health Psychology: The Search for Pathways between Behavior and Health. Annu. Rev. Psychol. **59**, 477–505 (2008)
43. Marangunić, N., Granić, A.: Technology acceptance model: a literature review from 1986 to 2013. Univ. Access Inf. Soc. **14**, 81–95 (2014)
44. Moore, G.C., Benbasat, I.: Development of an instrument to measure the perceptions of adopting an information technology innovation. Inform. Syst. Res. **2**, 192–222 (1991)
45. Moss-Morris, R., Weinman, J., Petrie, K., Horne, R.: The revised illness perception questionnaire (IPQ-R). Psychol. Health **17**, 1–16 (2002)
46. National Institutes of Health. NIH Fact Sheets - Self-management 1–2 (2010). Report.nih.gov
47. Nunnally, J.C., Bernstein, I.H.: Psychometric Theory, 3rd edn. McGraw-Hill, New York (1994)
48. Petrie, K.J., Weinman, J.A.: Perceptions of Health and Illness: Current Research and Applications, pp. 1467–1480 (1997)
49. Podsakoff, P.M., Organ, D.W.: Self-reports in organizational research: problems and prospects. J. Manag. **12**, 531–544 (1986). doi:10.1177/014920638601200408
50. Podsakoff, P.M., MacKenzie, S.B., Lee, J.-Y., Podsakoff, N.P.: Common method biases in behavioral research: a critical review of the literature and recommended remedies. J. Appl. Psychol. **88**, 879–903 (2003). doi:10.1037/0021-9010.88.5.879
51. Powers, M.A., Bardsley, J., Cypress, M., Duker, P., Funnell, M.M., Fischl, A.H., Maryniuk, M.D., Siminerio, L., Vivian, E.: Diabetes self-management education and support in type 2 diabetes. Diab. Educ. **41**, 417–430 (2015). doi:10.1177/0145721715588904
52. Ringle, C.M., Wende, S., Will, A.: SmartPLS Software 3.2.3 (2015). http://www.smartpls.de. Accessed Apr 2016
53. Rogers, E.M.: Diffusion of Innovations, 5th edn. Free Press, New York (2003)
54. Stoffregen, T.A.: Affordances as properties of the animal-environment system. Ecol. Psychol. **15**, 115–134 (2003)
55. Strong, D.M., Volkoff, O., Johnson, S.A., Pelletier, L.R., Tulu, B., Bar-On, I., Trudel, J., Garber, L.: A theory of organization-EHR affordance actualization. J. Assoc. Inform. Syst. **15**, 53–85 (2014)
56. Thompson, W., Fleming, R., Creem-Regehr, S., Stefanucci, J.K.: Visual Perception from a Computer Graphics Perspective. CRC Press, Boca Raton (2011)
57. Tsai, J.-P., Ho, C.-F.: Does design matter? Affordance perspective on smartphone usage. Ind. Manage. Data Syst. **113**, 1248–1269 (2013). doi:10.1108/IMDS-04-2013-0168
58. Venkatesh, V., Davis, F.D.: A theoretical extension of the technology acceptance model: four longitudinal field studies. Manage. Sci. **46**, 186–204 (2000)
59. Venkatesh, V., Morris, M.G., Davis, G.B., Davis, F.D.: User acceptance of information technology: toward a unified view. MIS Q. **27**, 425–478 (2003)
60. Venkatesh, V., Davis, F.D., Moris, M.G.: Dead or alive? The development, trajectory and future of technology adoption research. J. Assoc. Inform. Syst. **8**, 267–286 (2007)
61. Volkoff, O., Strong, D.M.: Critical realism and affordances: theorizing IT-associated organizational change processes. MIS Q. **37**, 819–834 (2013)

Analyzing mHeath Usage Using the mPower Data

Jiexun Li[1(✉)] and Xiaohui Chang[2]

[1] Western Washington University, Bellingham, WA, USA
Jiexun.Li@wwu.edu
[2] Oregon State University, Corvallis, OR, USA
Xiaohui.Chang@oregonstate.edu

Abstract. The emergence of mHealth products has created capability of monitoring and managing health of patients with chronic disease. In this paper, we analyze the participants' usage of a mobile app named mPower, developed for Parkinson disease. We identify the demographic/usage difference between different groups of participants, which provides insights into better design and marketing of mHealth products.

Keywords: mHealth · mPower · Parkinson disease (PD) · Data analysis

1 Introduction

In recent years, the rapid growth of mobile devices, wearables and smart sensors have enabled the adoption of Internet of Things (IoT) technologies into healthcare (i.e., mobile health or mHealth). These mHeath products have creates unprecedented capacity of monitoring and managing healthcare, particularly for patients with chronic diseases that are in need for smarter approaches beyond traditional clinical settings. The mHealth products have demonstrated some initial success in chronic disease management, including improvement of glycemic control for diabetes patients [1] and measurements in obese patients with hypertension [2]. However, the adoption of mHealth products and their effectiveness in health management are still in early stage and requires in-depth investigation.

The major challenges that inhibit the effectiveness of mHealth solutions are the following: (1) failure to take the demographic and socio-economic information of user population, such as age and digital literacy, into consideration, and (2) inability to account for different disease progressive subtypes of patients. Therefore, for mHealth products to establish themselves in healthcare industry and to provide essential information to both healthcare providers and patients, it is important for researchers to include user demographic and disease information into the analysis.

In this work, we seek to tackle the challenges with empirical analysis using the data collected from mPower mobile Parkinson Disease (PD) study [3]. The mPower project is a mobile-app-based study that interrogates various aspects of this movement disorder using surveys and sensor-based recordings from both the diseased ones and the

H. Chen et al. (Eds.): ICSH 2017, LNCS 10347, pp. 116–122, 2017.
https://doi.org/10.1007/978-3-319-67964-8_11

controls. With a large longitudinal cohort of volunteers, the mPower data serves as a good benchmark for studying the demographics and progression of PD patients.

Our study is aimed at analyzing the mPower data and answering the following research questions:

- *What the demographic characteristics of participants in the mPower study? Which activity app is generating the most/least data?*
- *What are the subtypes of participants in the mPower data?*
- *What are the key factors that affect the usage of the mPower application?*

2 The mPower Data

PD patients suffer a movement disorder, whose manifestations can include tremor, changes in gait, slowness (bradykinesia) and rigidity. Patients may demonstrate significant variation of these symptoms. Typically, a PD patient needs to visit a physician every 4–6 months. This, however, does not allow monitoring the day-to-day variability of symptoms or the effects of medications on these symptoms. If we can quantitatively assess PD patients in a much more frequent fashion, this could help better understand the disease heterogeneity and reveal opportunities for interventions that might improve quality of life for those with PD.

Sage Bionetworks is a non-profit research organization with funding from the Robert Wood Johnson Foundation. It proposed a new approach to monitor health in PD using a mobile app, named mPower. This mobile app is developed to monitor key indicators of PD symptoms with quantitative metrics gleaned from sensor-rich mobile devices [3]. mPower has provided an alternative to traditional approach of visits, which makes it possible to measure and track PD symptoms in a frequent, scalable, inexpensive, and non-invasive fashion [4]. The mPower project has survey a large cohort of volunteers with PD and those without to participate as controls. The current release of data encompasses the first six months of data donation (03/09/2015–09/09/2015).

Table 1 summarizes the basics of this dataset. The mPower datas contains three survey datasets (i.e., demographics, MDS-UPDRS, and PDQ8) and four activity datasets (memory, tapping, voice, and walking):

Table 1. A summary of the mPower data

Task name	Type of task and schedule	Unique participants	Unique tasks
Demographics	Survey - once	6,805	6,805
MDS-UPDRS	Survey - monthly	2,024	2,305
PDQ8	Survey - monthly	1,334	1,641
Memory	Activity	968	8,569
Tapping	Activity	8,003	78,887
Voice	Activity	5,826	65,022
Walking	Activity	3,101	35,410

(1) *Demographics*: a survey about general demographic topics and health history.
(2) *MDS-UPDRS*: a survey of selected questions from the Movement Disorder Society's Unified Parkinson's Disease Rating Scale.
(3) *PDQ-8*: a survey of the Parkinson's Disease Questionnaire short form.
(4) *Memory*: participants complete a short visuospatial game related to the Corsi block tapping test. This app was released three months later than the other three.
(5) *Tapping*: participants repeatedly tap their phone's screen.
(6) *Voice*: participants record themselves saying "aaah" for 10 s.
(7) *Walking*: participants walk back and forth for 20–30 s with their smartphone. They are then asked to stand still for another 20–30 s.

3   mPower Data Analysis

3.1   Exploratory Data Analysis

We conducted a series of exploratory data analysis on the mPower data using a popular data visual analytics tool named Tableau. Such exploratory visual analysis provides a better understanding of the demographic distributions of participants and their activities in the mPower study.

In the Demographics survey data, attribute "Professional diagnosis" indicates whether a participant has been diagnosed with Parkinson disease. As shown in Fig. 1:

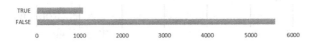

Fig. 1. Distribution of participants with vs. without PD

the majority of participants are not diagnosed with PD.

Furthermore, we looked at other dimensions in the demographic survey data, including age, gender, and smartphone use ("*How easy is it for you to use your smartphone?*"). As shown in Fig. 2, (a) there are more young participants than old ones, which contradicts with the fact that PD is more common for elderly people; (b) there are more male than female participants; and (c) the majority of participants find smartphone easy or very easy to use and therefore should be confident in using the mPower app to complete tasks.

For the four activities implemented in the mPower app, Fig. 3 shows that tapping is the most popular, followed by voice, walking and memory. Tapping can be performed anywhere with the least physical effort. Voice requires a quiet environment. Walking requires the most time and physical effort. The lower usage of the memory app may be attributed to the fact that this app was released later than the other three.

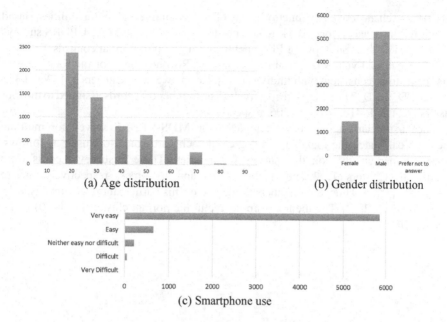

(a) Age distribution

(b) Gender distribution

(c) Smartphone use

Fig. 2. Distribution of participants in three demographic dimensions

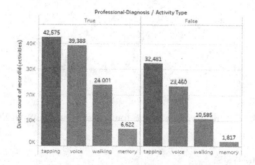

Fig. 3. The same order holds for both participants diagnosed with PD and those not.

3.2 Cluster Analysis

One of the standard surveys used for PD assessment is MDS-UPDRS. It was presented monthly throughout the course of the six-month study. Due to the length of the instrument, mPower only included a subset of questions from MDS-UPDRS focusing largely on the motor symptoms of PD. Out of the 2,024 unique participants in this MDS-UPDRS survey dataset, 1,871 completed the survey only once and there are only four participants who have completed the survey for seven times.

According to research by Wang et al. [5], there are three progressive subtypes for PD patients: (1) patients who have significant function decay of cognitive abilities but normal motor abilities; (2) those who have normal cognitive abilities but severe motor problems;

and (3) those characterized by function decay of both cognitive and motor abilities. Based on their findings, we performed a k-means cluster analysis on the MDS-UPDRS surveys with k = 4, i.e., three subtypes of PD patients plus a group of normal controls. Figure 4 shows the centroid values of variables (MDS-UPDRS questions) for the four clusters. This seems to be consistent with findings in [5]. Hence, we label Clusters 0, 1, 2 and 3 as Normal, PD_1, PD_2 and PD_3, respectively. The number of records assigned to the four clusters are 1,271, 418, 410 and 206, respectively.

Since a participant may have completed the MDS-UPDRS survey for multiple times, we calculated the membership degree of each participant to cluster as follows. Suppose a participant took this survey for n times. These n survey records were assigned to Clusters 1, 2 and 3 for n_1, n_2 and n_3 times, respectively, where $n_1 + n_2 + n_3 \leq n$. Thus, the membership degree of this participant to cluster i is: n_i/n, where i is in $\{1, 2, 3\}$. The membership degree to the normal cluster (cluster 0) is $(n-n_1-n_2-n_3)/n$.

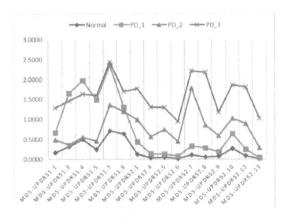

Fig. 4. Centroid values of the four clusters in MDS-UPDRS

3.3   Regression Analysis

The dependent variable is the total number of times a participant has performed a task. There are five different activity types: memory, tapping, voice, walking and all activities combined. The independent variables include age measured in years, gender, a dummy variable for professional diagnosis outcome (1 if a participant has been diagnosed by a medical professional with PD, and 0 otherwise), 5-factor level digital literacy represented by the answer to smartphone use (1 for complete digital illiteracy and 5 for full digital literacy), and membership degrees to the four clusters (Normal, PD_1, PD_2, and PD_3). Negative binomial regression models provide more suitable fit for the mPower data due to overdispersion that is evident in Poisson regression models for the data. The estimated activity counts are presented in Table 2. For example, for all activities, while controlling all other variables constant, a 1-year increase in age increases a participant's all activity count by 3% ($\times 1.03$); while controlling all other variables constant, a participant with PD is 2.46 times more likely to perform one of the four activities in the mPower app than one without PD.

In summary, professional diagnosis of PD is the key determinant factor for activity counts. Participants diagnosed with PD tend to be significantly ($\sim$2.3 times) more active than those without PD in using the mPower app and performing the activities. As evidenced by the coefficient of age, older participants tend to contribute more to the study. For participants in the PD_1 cluster, who have function decay of cognitive abilities but normal motor abilities, their activity counts are significantly lower (around 80%) than that in the Normal cluster except for memory. For those in PD_3, who have function decay of both cognitive and motor abilities, their activity counts are significantly lower (from 50% for memory to 77% for voice) compared to the Normal cluster except for walking. On the other hand, the activity counts of PD_2, who have function decay of motor abilities but normal cognitive abilities, are not statistically different from that of Normal.

Table 2. Estimated activity count ratios using negative binomial regression models. Estimates that are significant at the 5% significance level are highlighted. Significant estimates are marked by *** at 0% significance level, ** at 0.1% level and * at 1% level respectively. Female Normal participants are used as the baseline.

Independent variables	Dependent variable (activity count per participant)				
	memory	*tapping*	*voice*	*walking*	*all activities*
age	1.03***	1.03***	1.03***	1.04***	1.03***
gender	1.18	0.92	0.88*	1.00	0.96
professional diagnosis	2.39***	2.29***	2.30***	2.47***	2.46***
digital literacy	0.86	0.97	0.96	0.82**	0.96
PD_1	0.67	0.77***	0.81**	0.79*	0.78***
PD_2	0.70	0.86	0.89	0.99	0.86
PD_3	0.50**	0.76*	0.77*	0.75	0.73**

4 Conclusions

The mPower app provides a new way to measure and track PD symptoms in a scalable, inexpensive, and non-invasive fashion. In this paper, we analyzed the big data collected via mPower and discovered several interesting demographic and usage patterns between different groups of participants. These findings can potentially provide insights into better design and marketing of mHealth products and improve the capability of health management of patients with chronic disease.

References

1. Nundy, S., et al.: Mobile phone diabetes project led to improved glycemic control and net savings for Chicago plan participants. Health Aff. 33(2), 265–272 (2014)
2. Park, M.-J., Kim, H.-S., Kim, K.-S.: Cellular phone and Internet-based individual intervention on blood pressure and obesity in obese patients with hypertension. Int. J. Med. Inform. 78(10), 704–710 (2009)

3. Bot, B.M., et al.: The mPower study, Parkinson disease mobile data collected using ResearchKit. Scientific Data **3** (2016)
4. Wilbanks, J., Friend, S.H.: First, design for data sharing. Nature Biotechnol. (2016). doi:10. 1038/nbt.3516
5. Wang, F., Liang, J., Xiao, C.: Subtyping Parkinson's Disease with Deep Learning Models (2016). https://www.michaeljfox.org/foundation/grant-detail.php?grant_id=1518

Zen_Space: A Smartphone App for Individually Tailored Stress Management Support for College Students

Marguerite McDaniel and Mohd Anwar[⊠]

North Carolina Agricultural and Technical State University,
Greensboro, NC, USA
manwar@ncat.edu

Abstract. Alleviating stress reduces the risk of developing many chronic health problems. Though the effects of stress on the body may not always be immediately evident, exposure to chronic stress can lead to serious health problems and/or exacerbate existing medical conditions. This research study explores how a personal computing device such as a smartphone can be used to provide information regarding individually tailored stress management activities for college students. Since the use of smartphones is pervasive, one way to address this issue would be to develop a smartphone application in which a user can monitor stress as well as obtain various interventions for stress management. The proposed stress management application is based on information obtained from the user regarding stress type and intensity. An application that provides recommendations for stress-relieving activities can have a positive impact on a student's health and well-being.

Keywords: Stress management · Mobile health · Health behavior · Personalized health

1 Introduction

Mobile applications (apps) are emerging in the healthcare domain. With innovative technology, medical professionals can utilize mobile health apps to make better clinical decisions [1]. These apps can also help individuals monitor their health [1, 2].

The research study examines how a personal computing device such as a smartphone can be used to provide information regarding individually tailored stress management activities for college students. Zen_Space, a mobile health app that provides recommendations for stress-relieving activities, can have a positive impact on a student's health and well-being. The application would help reduce stress among college students.

Research shows that stress is a major issue for students at universities [3]. Stress is a mental as well as a physical response by the student's body to real or perceived changes and challenges [4]. Excessive demands and responsibilities as well as getting adjusted to a new environment can leave many students feeling fatigued and overwhelmed [4]. Stress-related problems that are not addressed may result in health issues

© Springer International Publishing AG 2017
H. Chen et al. (Eds.): ICSH 2017, LNCS 10347, pp. 123–133, 2017.
https://doi.org/10.1007/978-3-319-67964-8_12

for college students [4]. Though the effects of stress on the body may not always be immediately evident, exposure to chronic stress can lead to serious health issues and/or exacerbate existing medical conditions.

An excessive academic workload is one of the leading causes of stress for college students [4]. Students may feel overwhelmed from having too many challenging assignments, especially if they have to be completed in a short time span [4]. Classes that are difficult or hard to comprehend can leave students feeling frustrated [4]. Students may even feel the need to forgo sufficient sleep to meet their academic demands [4]. Insufficient sleep can contribute to a student's stress. Without proper coping strategies, stress can lead to various health problems. This includes depression, mood swings, and anxiety [4]. Stress can also lead to physical and mental exhaustion. Zen_Space helps reduce the risk of developing those health problems by providing stress management activities for a user's specific needs.

Zen_Space can assist college students greatly with their stress management needs. This app can provide insight as to what mechanisms are effective regarding alleviating stress among college students. Zen_Space can also provide health care professionals further information on the causes and impact of stress respecting students. This information could also be useful to health care providers at universities.

The remainder of the paper is as follows. Section 2 provides a discussion on similar mobile health apps that help individuals monitor and alleviate health issues. In Sect. 3, we provide in-depth background information regarding stress. In Sect. 4, we present the layout of Zen_Space to show the design and functionality of the app. The same section discusses the algorithms used to provide stress management recommendation(s) based on the evaluation of a user's stress type and intensity. Section 5 provides Zen_Space use case scenarios to show features of the app. Finally, Sect. 6 summarizes work completed on the app and future developments.

2 Related Work

There are similar health apps targeting college students. This includes StudentLife. Developed at Dartmouth, this app provides insight as to the effects of pressures that college students endure [5]. The app collects data through user-input as well as through phone sensors. The app assesses various items including workload, sleep, sociability, and mood. Similar to Zen_Space, StudentLife also uses stress scales (e.g., Perceived Stress Scale) and other types of resources to determine which type of user data should be collected. From the collection of data, StudentLife shows how a student's academic performance declines as he or she overlooks healthy habits while dealing with the pressures and demands of college [5]. In contrast, Zen_Space not only provides college students insight on health issues, but also provides personalized stress management recommendations.

Psychologist in a Pocket (PiaP) is a mobile health app that incorporates text analysis to help detect depression [6]. PiaP is geared towards young adults. Words that indicate signs of depression are categorized by sections, including the following: mood, psychomotor agitation, suicide, and anxiety [6]. Words used for the assessment are derived from various resources, including medical professionals, group studies, as well as depression scales. Similar to PiaP, we use scales, such as the Hassles and Uplifts Scale (HUS) to categorize different types of stressors college students typically endure. We also incorporate data analysis on user data. However, Zen_Space does not detect stress, but evaluates the user's stress type and intensity to provide personal recommendations. When college students use Zen_Space, they have a sense of their stressor (s). Moreover, Zen_Space is designed to prevent students from developing stress-related illnesses. The app seeks to assist students with developing positive health habits to alleviate stress.

Another similar app is PopTherapy. PopTherapy is an app that provides micro-interventions for users to help alleviate stress and develop appropriate strategies to deal with stress [7]. This app provides micro-interventions based on user-input, such as stress level and mood. The micro-interventions are categorized into four sections based on "most commonly used stress-management psychotherapy approaches." The actual techniques provided for users are popular web apps [7].

From a research study, authors found that participants preferred the Machine Learning aspect of the recommender system that provides interventions based on passed data performance. Though Zen_Space seeks similar goals in helping users alleviate stress, our audience and strategy are different. Zen_Space is customized for college students, since stress is a major health problem that they may endure. In terms of strategy, the interventions utilize more of the user's information to provide an individual with the appropriate recommendation. Another difference is that our interventions are not based on psychotherapy. Though we do use research from the medical field and other related areas in Zen_Space for developing strategies to address the user's condition, our strategy goes beyond relaxation techniques. In many cases, we help individuals resolve their stressor.

In addition to mobile health apps, there are also other tools used to help an individual alleviate stress. This includes using general stress scales, such as the College Undergraduate Stress Scale, in which students obtain insight regarding their stress levels [8]. In comparison to the Social Readjustment Ratings Scale, students are provided a rating scale and choose stressors (e.g., financial difficulties) applicable to them. When finished, students add up each rating value of the chosen stressor. Also, theories regarding coping with stress include Richard Lazarus's [9] appraisal theory or transactional theory of stress [10]. Lazarus's theory asserts that when individuals deal with situations, the situations themselves are neither negative nor positive. How one handles or reacts to the situation determines if the situation will negatively affect the individual.

3 Taxonomy of Stress

In the following section, we provide background information on stress as well as its effects on the body to further show how beneficial a stress management tool would be to college students.

Stress is the mental as well as physical reaction and adaptation of one's body to real or perceived change or challenges [4]. Common stressors among college students that increase the risk of health problems are typically forms of distress (negative stress). Distress is any type of event that leaves one in deliberate tension or strain. There are various types of distress, including the following: acute stress, episodic acute stress, and chronic stress [4].

Acute stress derives from either demands or pressure from the past or those anticipated in the future [4]. This type of stress typically has a short duration [4]. With regard to college students, an example includes anxiety over a class presentation. An overwhelming occurrences of acute stress on a daily basis is known as episodic acute stress, such as ceaseless worrying [11]. Though not immediately evident, chronic stress can have a severe impact on one's body. Chronic stress is an ongoing state of psychological arousal in reaction to various perceived threats. Effects of chronic stress include heart attack, suicide, and even cancer [11].

Often, the normal mode of an individual's biological system is in a homeostasis or balance state. When undergoing stress, the body becomes unbalanced, and takes an adaptive response to return it to normal. The process of returning to a balance state is known as the general adaptation syndrome (GAS) [4]. Developed by Hans Selye, GAS consists of three phases: alarm, resistance, and exhaustion [10]. In the alarm stage, when an individual initially experiences any type of stress (real or imaginary), that stress prevents the body from being stable. The part of the brain that processes the stressor (cerebral cortex) stimulates an automatic nervous system response, preparing the body to either fight or escape from a real or perceived threat [4]. An automatic nervous system response is an operation of the central nervous system that manages bodily functions that are not typically consciously controlled by an individual [4]. During the process of the automatic nervous system response, the body also releases several stress hormones. Specifically, this portion of the process is known as the sympathetic nervous system. Besides the release of stress hormones, the body also takes other actions. This includes the action of the hypothalamus: part of the brain that acts as the main controller of the automatic nervous system as well as determines the body's reaction to stressor(s). The hypothalamus gets signals that additional energy is needed to fight a stressor, and stimulates adrenal glands to release the epinephrine or adrenaline hormone. As a result of adrenaline, the heart in turn is stimulated to pump more blood, which consequently increases the intake of oxygen, the breathing rate, and the release of glucose to fuel muscular exertion [4].

In the resistance phase, the body has calmed down from the alarm stage, but still has not reached homeostasis [4]. Since an individual still perceives some sort of stressor, bodily functions used to reduce stress will continue to operate.

In the exhaustion stage, the body is drained from trying to adapt to a stress response [4]. There is very little physical or emotional energy remaining to alleviate stress. Consequently, one's resistance falls below normal.

Especially when experiencing chronic stress, the body releases so much cortisol from the adrenal glands that it can lower immunocompetence [4]. The immune system is compromised of its ability to protect an individual from infectious diseases [4].

4 Zen_Space - Mobile App Based Stress Management Tool

Zen_Space acts as a stress management tool to provide stress relieving activities that addresses an individual's needs. In the following sections, we discuss the design layout of Zen_Space as well as the algorithms used for the mobile app.

4.1 Design of Application

Zen_Space is designed to be user-friendly and appealing to college students. Its colors and images are intended to create a calming visual environment for individuals throughout the use of the mobile app.

The layout of the app is as follows. Once the user opens Zen_Space and clicks start, the main menu appears. The main menu shows three types of stressors: academic, financial, and social (See Fig. 1). Each section has stressful situations and conditions that college students typically endure. These stressful conditions are based on related research, reports, and surveys of stress among college students [9, 12–20]. For instance, in the academic category, students can choose from the following (See Fig. 2): anxiety, grade performance, and exam stress (difficulty studying).

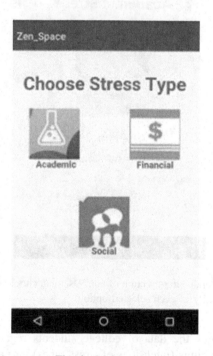

Fig. 1. Main menu.

For each category mentioned above, the user chooses a stressful condition that is most applicable and rates it. The rating scheme is also based on the HUS developed by Richard Lazarus, which we further discuss in the Algorithms section. If the student's stress level is low, the user should choose somewhat severe as the intensity level. For a medium stress level, the choice should be moderately severe. If the stressful condition is high, extremely severe should be chosen. Each level of severity also has an intensity score associated with it: somewhat severe (score 1), moderately severe (score 2), and extremely severe (score 3). Once a user rates all applicable stressful conditions and clicks finish, personal recommendations to help the college student relieve his or her stress are provided (See Fig. 3). Consequently, the personal recommendations or interventions are based on applicable stress type and intensity chosen by the student. For instance, if the user has an academic stressor and a social stressor, Zen_Space would take into consideration the intensity of each one separately and provide an intervention for both stressors. This would assist college students with mental stress management by helping them find more effective ways to address stress-related problems.

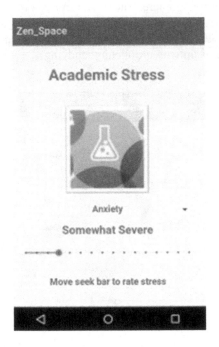

Fig. 2. Figure shows academic stress section of app. User can choose from options of academic stressors and rate the intensity of each selected option.

Zen_Space also stores the data of college students regarding stress conditions (stress types) and their ratings (intensities of stress types) into a secure database using aspects of Structured Query Language (SQL). When a user reopens the app, the previous stress level rate (overall) is shown (See Fig. 4). After seven-days of app usage, Zen_Space would give a history of a college student's stressful condition(s). Through graphs, the report will display stress types (e.g., academic) and the average of their intensities over seven-days of app usage. The report is beneficial to college students because it provides them insight as to what conditions cause them the most stress. With various stressful situations that many college students endure on a daily basis, the report is especially intended to make users more aware and cautious about their stress and its impact on their health.

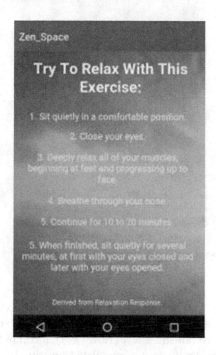

Fig. 3. Recommendation for user based on previous figure of stress type and intensity.

4.2 Algorithms

Algorithms used in Zen_Space to assess stress-related issues among college students are primarily based on the HUS, a self-assessment tool that helps individuals evaluate their stress [12]. The scale is divided into two sections: daily hassles and uplifts. Daily hassles consist of items that reflect "experiences and conditions of daily living that have been appraised as salient and harmful to the [individual's] well-being." This might include borrowing money or not having enough time for family relationships [12]. Uplifts also consist of items, but reflect "experiences and conditions of daily living that have been appraised as salient and positive or favorable to the [individual's] well-being" [12]. Examples of uplifts include socializing and exercising. Among other resources, our recommendations of stress-relieving activities are based on the uplifts section. In Zen_Space, stressors from HUS that are common to college students were incorporated in the mobile app. As mentioned, from the rating scheme of HUS, we can calculate the frequency, cumulated severity, as well as intensity of stressors among college students [12].

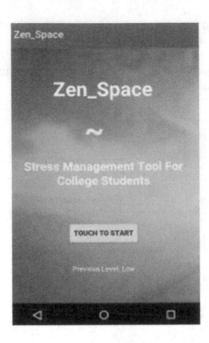

Fig. 4. Start View. After first time of use, the user will see previous stress level(s) when opening Zen_Space again.

In Zen_Space, users choose applicable items that are common stressors (e.g., managing money) and rate their intensity (e.g., somewhat severe). Once finished, the mobile app provides an overall stress level (low (1–3), medium (4–6), and high (7–9)) for each section. We consider this as the cumulated severity. In general, the cumulated severity for HUS is the sum of all the "3-point severity ratings" of stressors applicable to an individual. We sought to obtain the cumulated severity for each section to accurately capture the stressor and thus provide appropriate recommendations for the user. There are some exceptions, including when a user chooses only extremely severe. Though the overall score is three, the mobile app would consider the condition as extreme and thus categorize it as high. Once the user has completed the section, stress-relieving activities based on each applicable stress type and its overall intensity are shown. The overall stress level for each section is also stored in the database, where the average is calculated after seven-days of app usage.

5   Use Case Scenarios of Zen_Space

In this section, we will discuss scenarios of how Zen_Space can be used to help college students alleviate stress.

Our first scenario involves a student experiencing academic stress. Student Ava has a heavy course load this semester. Besides computer science courses, she has Calculus II and Physics II. Consequently, due to numerous demands during the semester, she begins to experience anxiety. If this continues, Ava's anxiety can worsen and lead to serious health problems.

Ava decides to use the stress management tool Zen_Space. Once in the main menu, she chooses her stress type - academic. Among the various options, Ava chooses one most applicable to her health needs. Once Ava chooses a stressor from a particular category, she can now rate the severity of that stress type. As mentioned, the intensity of stress type includes the following: somewhat severe (low level), moderately severe (medium level), and extremely severe (high level). Since Ava is just beginning to experience anxiety, she chooses somewhat severe as the stress intensity.

After choosing stress type and its intensity, the app provides a recommendation for Ava. The intervention is a proactive relaxation technique to help Ava reduce her anxiety (Fig. 3). Derived from the Relaxation Response made popular by Dr. Herbert Benson of the Harvard Medical School, the technique acts as a "mentally active process" that relaxes the body [21, 22]. The intervention results in Ava successfully lowering her stress level. By engaging in this relaxation technique, Ava becomes more aware of how important it is to address her stress-related issues.

In our second scenario, Brandon's stress deals with financial matters. One of the most stressful aspects of college life is dealing with financial issues. Research shows that over 70% of college students deal with stress related to their personal finances [20]. This includes student loans and debt [20]. Brandon's stressor mainly deals with managing loans. Due to limited family and scholarship funding, he had to obtain a loan to pay for his tuition. Brandon chooses a stress type (managing loans (payment budgeting)) and stressor applicable to him. His intensity level is moderately severe. Based on stress type and intensity, Zen_Space suggests that Brandon create a structured budget plan, in which he may assess his monetary needs and spending habits [4].

6 Conclusion

Zen_Space is a stress management tool for college students. It provides personalized stress interventions based on an individual's stress type and intensity. Research shows that daily stress-related hassles can have a major impact on one's health. We hope that students using Zen_Space will become more cognizant of stress and its impact on their health.

Further research is needed regarding Zen_Space. Specifically, experiments involving Zen_Space users can provide information on how to modify the app so that it is more beneficial to college students. We plan to conduct a human-subject study at our college campus to assess the impact of Zen_Space in alleviating stress among college students. We will recruit college students to use the app over a one month period. After the month usage, we will ask students to answer the following evaluation questions:

1. How likely are you to use Zen_Space if the app is available on your device?
2. How easy is it to use Zen_Space on a regular basis?
3. How easy is it to find information that you are looking for in Zen_Space?
4. How likely are you to recommend Zen_Space to other people?
5. What changes do you believe would improve Zen_Space?

There also needs to be collaboration with other professionals in the health domain so that Zen_Space can become more efficacious. We also want to incorporate more data analysis in the app. We hope to use data derived from the seven day report provided by Zen_Space users. This information will allow us to modify and refactor Zen_Space's recommendation system so that even more recommendations can be provided for college students through the app.

Acknowledgment. We thank Amari Vaughn for his contribution to the app. This research is partly funded by the North Carolina-Louis Stokes Alliances for Minority Participation.

References

1. Mobile Health Apps | Knowledge Hub | athenahealth. In: Athena Health. http://www.athenahealth.com/knowledge-hub/mobile-health-technology/apps. Accessed 1 Apr 2017
2. Husain, M.D.I., Misra, M.D.S: The best medical apps released in 2015 for iPhone & Android. In: iMedicalApps (2016)
3. Written by A. Holterman | Published on August 25, 2016 Mental Health Problems for College Students Are Increasing. In: Healthline (2016). http://www.healthline.com/health-news/mental-health-problems-for-college-students-are-increasing-071715#1. Accessed 17 Jan 2017
4. Donatelle, R.J.: Health: The Basics, 11th edn. Pearson, Boston (2015)
5. Wang, R., Chen, F., Chen, Z., Li, T., Harari, G., Tignor, S., Zhou, X., Ben-Zeev, D., Campbell, A.T.: StudentLife: assessing mental health, academic performance and behavioral trends of college students using smartphones. In: 2014 ACM International Joint Conference on Pervasive and Ubiquitous Computing, pp. 3–14. ACM, New York (2014)
6. Cheng, P.G.F., Ramos, R.M., Bitsch, J.Á., Jonas, S.M., Ix, T., See, P.L.Q., Wehrle, K.: Psychologist in a pocket: lexicon development and content validation of a mobile-based app for depression screening. JMIR mHealth and uHealth (2016). doi:10.2196/mhealth.5284
7. Parede, P., Gilad-Bachrach, R., Czerwinski, M., Roseway, A., Rowan, K., Hernandez, J.: PopTherapy: Coping with History Stress through Pop – Culture
8. College Undergraduate Stress Scale
9. Cooper, C.L., Dewe, P.: Stress: A Brief History, p. 10. Blackwell, Malden (2005)
10. Richard Lazarus's Theory of Stress Appraisal - Video & Lesson Transcript. In: Study.com. http://study.com/academy/lesson/richard-lazaruss-theory-of-stress-appraisal.html. Accessed 1 Apr 2017
11. Miller, L.H., Smith, A.D.: Stress: The different kinds of stress. In: Pardon Our Interruption. http://www.apa.org/helpcenter/stress-kinds.aspx. Accessed 1 Apr 2017, Adapted from The Stress Solution
12. Kanner, A.D., Coyne, J.C., Schaefer, C., Lazarus, R.S.: Comparison of two modes of stress measurement: Daily hassles and uplifts versus major life events. J. Behav. Med. **4**, 1–39 (1981)
13. Bulo, J.G., Sanchez, M.G.: Sources of stress among college students. CVCITC Res. J. **1**(1), 16–25 (2014)
14. Trombitas, K.: Financial Stress: An Everyday Reality for College Students (2012)
15. Stress. Wellness Center at Boston University
16. American College Health Association. American College Health Association-National College Health Assessment II: Reference Group Executive Summary Spring 2015. Hanover, MD: American College Health Association (2015)

17. Moninger, J.: 10 Relaxation Techniques That Zap Stress Fast. In: WebMD. http://www.webmd.com/balance/guide/blissing-out-10-relaxation-techniques-reduce-stress-spot#1. Accessed 1 Apr 2017
18. Causes of Stress. In: WebMD. http://www.webmd.com/balance/guide/causes-of-stress#1. Accessed 1 Apr 2017
19. Iida, M., Shrout, P.E., Laurenceau, J.-P., Bolger, N.: Using Diary Methods In Psychological Research (2012)
20. National Student Financial Wellness Study, cfw.osu.edu/posts/documents/nsfws-key-findings-report-2.pdf
21. Steps to Elicit the Relaxation Response. In: Steps to Elicit the Relaxation Response. http://www.relaxationresponse.org/steps/. Accessed 1 Apr 2017
22. YOU REALLY NEED TO RELAX: Effective Methods http://www.med.umich.edu/painresearch/patients/Relaxation.pdf
23. Atlanta Metropolitan State College. In: Atlanta Metropolitan College. http://www.atlm.edu/. Accessed 1 Apr 2017
24. 3kW System - Platinum - System Summary. In: solarhub. http://monitoring.solarhub.net.au/solar-panel-systems/3kw-system-lg-sma. Accessed 1 Apr 2017
25. Social Media Agency Birmingham & London. In: Ricemedia. https://www.ricemedia.co.uk/social-media-marketing/. Accessed 1 Apr 2017
26. RelaxIn: Flickr (2016). https://www.flickr.com/photos/icemanphotos/31023305921. Accessed 1 Apr 2017

Segmentation of Human Motion Capture Data Based on Laplasse Eigenmaps

Xiaodong Xie, Rui Liu, Dongsheng Zhou$^{(\boxtimes)}$, Xiaopeng Wei,
and Qiang Zhang$^{(\boxtimes)}$

Key Laboratory of Advanced Design and Intelligent Computing,
Ministry of Education, Dalian University, Dalian 116622, China
{zhoudongsheng, zhangq}@dlu.edu.cn

Abstract. The segmentation of motion capture data is to separate the different types of human motion data contains long movement sequence into motion clips with independent semantics in order to facilitate the storage in the database as well as medical analysis. This paper proposed a method for human motion capture data segmentation based on Laplacian Eigenmaps (LE) algorithm. Firstly, the LE algorithm is used to reduce the dimension of original data by realizing the mapping from the high dimensional data to the low dimensional space. And then a specified window was drawn in the low dimensional space which was used to calculate the space distance from frames in the specified window to each frame in the former fragment. Finally we detected the similarity to get the final segmentation points, thus obtained motion clips with independent semantics. The validity of the segmentation method is verified by experiment.

Keywords: Motion capture · Segmentation · LE

1 Introduction

Motion capture technology has been widely used in the field of medical correction analysis. The motion capture data can be used to analyze 3D space trajectory of human bones and joints, as well as data curve of rotational motion. Compared with the motion curve of normal people, the patient can be treated more effectively and quickly. In healthcare, such as gait analysis and rehabilitation training, the independent motion clips are usually needed. Although, the independent motion clips can be captured separately, as the long motion sequences are more comfortable for patients to perform and contain more natural transitions from one motion to the next, the independent motion clips are usually extracted from a long motion sequence by the method of motion segmentation. On the other hand, capture a long motion sequence is more efficient than capturing short motion clips one by one. So the motion segmentation is significant for healthcare. However, the captured motion sequence is complex and variable and always consists of multiple movements which is inconvenient for data analysis and storage. To solve this problem, we need to segment the long motion sequence which contains different types of human motion into short motion fragments which have independent meanings to make the motion data to be convenient for storing in the database and analysis in medical correction.

© Springer International Publishing AG 2017
H. Chen et al. (Eds.): ICSH 2017, LNCS 10347, pp. 134–145, 2017.
https://doi.org/10.1007/978-3-319-67964-8_13

The most original motion segmentation method is manual segmentation. Manual segmentation can get relatively better segmentation results, but it is very complicated and time-consuming. Therefore, there is a need to have a highly efficient and accurate automatic segmentation method to replace the manual work. At present, many scholars have done a lot of research in the field of motion segmentation, and made a series of theoretical and practical results. The current motion segmentation method can be divided into three main categories:

(1) Method based on the dimension reduction

J. Barbic et al. [1] proposed human motion segmentation methods based on principal component analysis (PCA) [2], probabilistic principal component analysis (PPCA) and Gaussian Mixture Model (GMM). The first two methods are online, that is, to achieve segmentation in the process of motion sequence capture. Segmentation method based on Gauss mixture model is a batch process using the expectation maximization algorithm to estimate a mixed Gauss model. The segmentation is processed according to the different elements of continuous frame sequence belongs to this model. Liu et al. [3] proposed a motion capture data segmentation method based on PCA and Mahalanobis distance. Xiao [4] proposed a segmentation method for 3D human motion capture data based on ISOMAP [5]. Dimension is reduced by using ISOMAP in nonlinear space. Then K-means clustering algorithm is adopted to realize the automatic segmentation between different motions. But, the method is not strong, and it is not accurate when motions have many different gestures. Peng et al. [6] reduced the number of dimensions through extracting the center distance feature of 12 dimensions including distances from three joints of limbs respectively to root joint. And then they through the use of low pass filter to reduce the noise of human motion capture data to obtain behavior segmentation points. Experiments show that this method is poor when it is used on the long motion sequence contains many complex types of motion.

(2) Method based on models

Method based on models mainly uses some existing mathematical models in the segmentation of human activities. The two typical models are Hidden Markov Model (HMM) [7] and Gaussian Mixture Model (GMM) [8]. Reference [9] proposes an approach for online, automated segmentation and identification of movement segments from continuous time-series data of human movement, obtained from body-mounted inertial measurement units or from motion capture data. This approach uses a two-stage identification and recognition process, based on velocity features and stochastic modeling of each motion to be identified. Barbic [1] and others believe that motions have different types of semantics belong to different clusters, and all the cluster obey Gauss distribution. Then they put forward that if a coherent frame belong to two different GMM models at the same time while using GMM on different types of motion sequence clustering, it is the segmentation point of these two types of behavior motions. But the limitation of this method is that the user needs to determine the number of types of movement in advance. Lu et al. [10] proposed double threshold segmentation algorithm based on multi dimension by decomposing the complex human motion capture data into a simple sequence of dynamic linear model. But this method is only applicable to human motion capture data which has cyclic behavior. Wang et al. [11] applied Kernel Dynamic Texture (KDT) [12] to human motion behavior segmentation. Firstly, the reference sequence and the subsequence segment were selected as the similarity comparison. And then the KDT models were built. Finally they measured the similarity through Mahalanobis distance between each KDT model to determine the different motion segmentation point. However, this method had a low efficiency of calculation in dealing with long motion sequence.

(3) Method based on the classifier

The classifier has been widely used in human motion capture data segmentation. The hierarchical clustering method is used to divide the action data into different classes in the literature [13] and each class corresponds to a segment. Arikan et al. [14] segmented motion capture data by using Support Vector Machine (SVM) [15]. SVM trained by manual labeled training data set can realize automatic segmentation of the original long motion sequence. Zhou et al. [16] transform the human behavior segmentation into energy minimization problem by using Aligned Cluster Analysis (ACA). They measured the similarity of motion sequence fragments have different lengths by using core k-mean [17] to complete the classification of human motion behavior. On this basis, the dynamic programming was used to obtain the behavioral segmentation point of the split. But the users need to determine the number of cluster while the time sequence is reduced and the number of sequence types. After that, Zhou et al. [18] proposed a segmentation method based on hierarchical clustering analysis on this basis. The method has higher segmentation accuracy compared with the basic behavior method. But it has a high computational complexity. Yang Yuedong et al. [19] proposed a motion segmentation method based on "motion string". Motion data formed "motion string" by spectral clustering, timing recovery and maximum filtering and then used the "motion string" into motion segmentation. But this method can't handle the motions of human body which have big difference in the postures. Xiao et al. [20] proposed an automatic segmentation algorithm. Firstly, the original data is mapped to the low dimension space by using nonlinear dimensionality reduction technique, and then the clustering technique is used to separate the different types of motion. Hu Xiaoyan et al. [21] proposed a regular motion data segmentation algorithm based on spectral clustering. The motion capture data is decomposed into motion data segments with identical lengths. And then they calculated the similarity between these small fragments based on principal component analysis to obtain the similarity matrix of motion data. After that they convert the similarity matrix into corresponding Laplacian matrix by using the spectral clustering algorithm. Finally the k-means algorithm was used to obtain the clustering result, and then the final segmentation point was got.

In summary, the dimension reduction technique has been widely used in the segmentation algorithm, and manifold learning is an important method for nonlinear dimension reduction. LE algorithm is one of the most important methods in manifold learning, and it has a better robustness. It is relatively simple in selection of the weight. We can directly set the weights and do not need to solve a linear equation. Therefore, this paper proposes a motion sequence segmentation method based on LE algorithm which is used to reduce the dimension of the original data to obtain the accurate segmentation results.

2   Proposed Approach

This paper presents a method of human motion capture data segmentation based on LE algorithm. Firstly, the original data dimension was reduced by using LE algorithm to realize the mapping of high dimensional data to the low dimensional space. And then draw a specified window in the low dimensional space to calculate space distance from frames in the specified window to each frame in the former fragment. Finally we detected the similarity to get the final segmentation points, thus obtained motion clips with independent semantics. The flow chart of the algorithm is shown in Fig. 1.

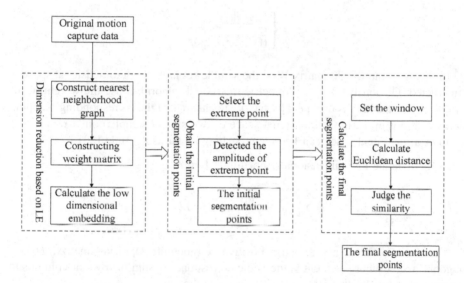

Fig. 1. Motion segmentation process based on LE algorithm

2.1   Dimension Reduction Based on LE

LE is a high computational efficiency algorithm proposed by Mikhail Belkin and Partha Niyogi in 2003. It is a nonlinear dimensionality reduction method in manifold learning, the purpose of which is to find the low dimensional manifold structure embedded in high dimensional data space and give an effective low dimensional representation method [22]. The basic idea of this algorithm is that the sample points which have closer distances in the high dimensional space are neighboring after they are projected into the low dimensional target space. LE algorithm constructs local neighborhood relationship between sample points based on the concept of Laplacian spectrum and maps the local neighborhood relationship into low dimensional space to recover the relationship in the low dimensional space.

Given a set of sample data sets $X = (x_1, x_2, \cdots, x_N)$, $x_i \in R^D$, there is the mapping:

$$f : R^D \to R^d \quad (d \ll D)$$

The mapping data set on the low dimensional embedding space R^d is $Y = (y_1, y_2, \cdots, y_N)$, $y_i \in R^d$, $d \ll D$. LE algorithm's procedure is as follows:

(1) Construct nearest neighborhood graph. Calculate the Euclidean distance $d_E(x_i, x_j)$ between each sample points x_i and other sample points. We use the k-nearest neighbor method to find out k nearest neighbor sample points of the sample points x_i and establish edge according to the KNN adjacent criterion. And then construct the local neighborhood relationship $N_i(x_{ij}|j = 1, 2, \cdots, k)$ between sample points.

(2) Constructing weight matrix. After the nearest neighborhood graph was constructed, each edge needs to be given the corresponding weight value w_{ij}:

$$w_{ij} = \begin{cases} e^{\frac{\|x_i - x_{ij}\|^2}{t}} & x_{ij} \in N_i \\ 0 & x_{ij} \notin N_i \end{cases}$$

In this way, the weight matrix W of the sample set in the high dimensional space is constructed. Obviously, W is a symmetric matrix. LE algorithm use the weight w_{ij} of sample points x_i and x_j as the "penalty factor" to ensure that the corresponding mapping points y_i and y_j in the low dimensional space of two similar sample points x_i and x_j in the high dimensional space can keep approaching as far as possible [23].

(3) Calculate the low dimensional embedding. For Y:

$$\frac{1}{2} \sum_{ij} \|y_i - y_j\|^2 w_{ij} = tr(YLY^T)$$

The $L = D - W$ is a symmetric positive semidefinite laplacian matrix, D is a diagonal matrix whose element value is the corresponding sum of rows or columns to the weight matrix W, that is:

$$D_{ij} = \sum_j w_{ij}$$

By adding constraints on $YDY^T = I$ to eliminate the effects of scale factors [24], LE algorithm is transformed into the optimization problem:

$$\begin{cases} \arg \min tr(Y^T L Y) \\ s.t. Y^T D Y \end{cases}$$

Finally it can be transformed into the solving of generalized eigenvalue:

$$Lf = \lambda Df$$

Assume that the $d+1$ minimum eigenvalue are $0 = \lambda_0 \leq \lambda_1 \leq \cdots \leq \lambda_d$ and the corresponding feature vector are $f_0, f_1, \cdots, f_d$, so we can see that the low dimensional embedding Y are the $d+1$ minimum feature vectors $f_0, f_1, \cdots, f_d$ corresponding to the $d+1$ minimum eigenvalues in matrix L, that is:

$$Y = [f_0, f_1, \cdots, f_d]^T$$

LE algorithm retains the manifold local neighbor information which can reflect the intrinsic geometric information embedded in the low dimensional manifold of data set and can be used for data clustering. The characteristic of the algorithm is to transform the problem into the solution of eigenvalue problem which does not need to use iterative algorithm and the process is simple and fast.

2.2   The Segmentation of the Motion Sequences

After the dimension of the motion sequence was reduced by LE algorithm, we can obtain the characteristic curve. Then we processed smoothing, filtering and denoising on the curve to get a smooth characteristic curve for accurate data segmentation.

First of all, we detected the amplitude of the obtained characteristic curve to gain the initial segmentation points, which mainly include the following steps:

(1) Calculate the maximum and minimum points of the curve. The extreme point of the characteristic curve represents a relatively larger change of the human motion gesture. Therefore, we first selected all the extreme points of the curve as the initial segmentation point.

(2) Detect the difference of amplitude between each maximum (minimum) point and its neighboring minimum (maximum) point of both sides. If the smaller one is $\lambda(0 < \lambda < 1)$ times smaller than the larger one, the extreme point is the initial segmentation points. That is because a larger amplitude variation may represent a turning in different semantic movements, so extreme points which meet this condition were retained as the initial segmentation point.

(3) In order to ensure that the segmentation points were not too dense. Here we set threshold T = 150 and detect whether the length between the two adjacent points is larger than it. If so, the two frames are both used as the initial segmentation points, otherwise remove the larger frame. Terminate the judgment when reach the final frame.

Through the above three steps, we got the initial segmentation points. Afterwards, we confirmed the initial segmentation points further to obtain accurate segmentation points by the following steps:

(1) Set $m = 2$.

(2) Set a window with a length of $2\alpha + 1$ around the m-th point F_m, they are the frames $[F_m - \alpha, F_m + \alpha]$. Calculate the frame distance $D(F_p, F_q)$ from each frame

in the window to each frame to the previous cluster $[F_{m-1} : F_m - \alpha]$. Here we selected Euclidean distance as the frame distance which is defined as follows:

$$D(F_p, F_q) = \sqrt{(p_1 - q_1)^2 + (p_2 - q_2)^2 + \cdots + (p_n - q_n)^2} \qquad n = 93$$

(3) Judge the similarity of the frames. We put the frame distance into the matrix D and set $\beta = 5 \min(D)$ as the threshold. If the frame distance $D(F_p, F_q)$ is less than the threshold, it is indicated that this frame belongs to the former cluster and mark 1 in the corresponding window; otherwise it belongs to the latter one and mark 0.

(3) Judge whether the current frame is the last frame. If so, switch to step (4), otherwise, $m = m + 1$ and switch to step (2).

(4) Count the number of frames marked with 1 and record as N, the precise point of the segmentation is set as $F_m - \alpha + N$.

3   Experiments and Analysis

In this paper, the method is verified by experiments and compared with the different segmentation algorithms. The efficiency of the algorithm is proved strictly through the comparison of the error rate of the segmentation. The input motion capture data is from the motion capture database of Carnegie Mellon University (CMU). The motion sequences are captured by the marker based motion capture equipment Vicon MX-40. The data format is BVH and the sampling frequency is 120 frames per second. We selected two groups of motion sequences with different semantic and complexity in the experiments and compared the method with the existing algorithms.

Experiment 1: segmentation of simple motion sequence.

Select a simple sequence of motion with 824 frames. The semantic is "go forward, pick up items, put down items" which is shown in Figs. 2, 3 and 4.

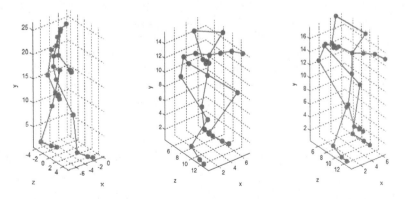

Fig. 2. The motion "move forward", "pick up items", "put down items"

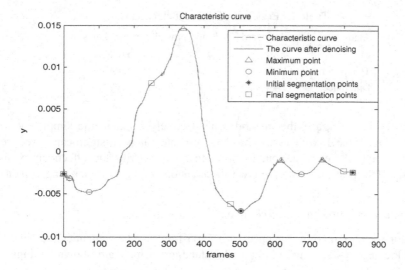

Fig. 3. Motion characteristic curve and its annotation

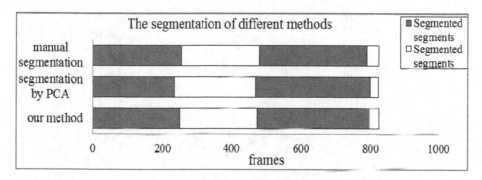

Fig. 4. The segmentation of different methods

In order to ensure the accuracy of manual segmentation, the result of manual segmentation is from multiple people. To verify the effectiveness of this method, this paper takes the manual segmentation results as a reference and used the error rate(ER) [25] to measure the effectiveness of the algorithm which is defined as follows:

$$ER = \frac{N_{miss} + N_{extra}}{N} \times 100\%$$

N_{miss} means the missed frames of semantic segmentation fragments, N_{extra} means the number of extra frames in the segmentation segment, N expresses the length of segmentation segment by manual segmentation. The error rates of motion segmentation by different algorithms are shown in Table 1:

Table 1. Error rate of different algorithms

Algorithms	Move forward	Pick up items	Put down items
PCA	4.3%	7.5%	5.4%
This paper	1.9%	4.4%	3.8%
Difference	2.4%	3.1%	1.6%

As shown in the figure, the method can effectively segment the simple motion sequence. From Table 1, we can see that the error rate has been significantly reduced compared with PCA segmentation. In order to further verify the effectiveness and universality of the proposed algorithm, we choose another more complex long sequence to test.

Experiment 2: segmentation of complex motion sequence.

Select a complex motion sequence with 2465 frames. The semantics are "jump", "twist", "kicking", "squatting", "jogging", "standing" which are shown in Figs. 5, 6 and 7.

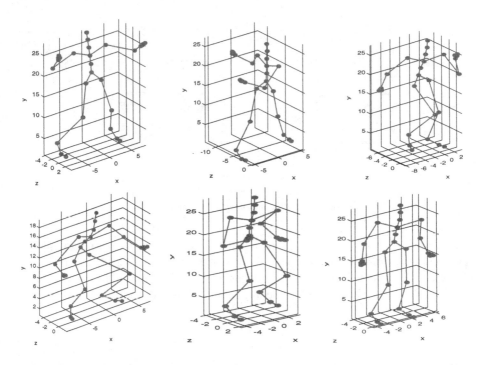

Fig. 5. The motion "jumping", "twisting", "kicking", "squatting", "jogging", "standing"

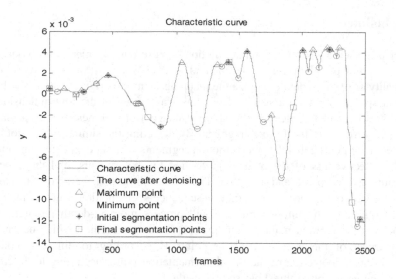

Fig. 6. Motion characteristic curve and its annotation

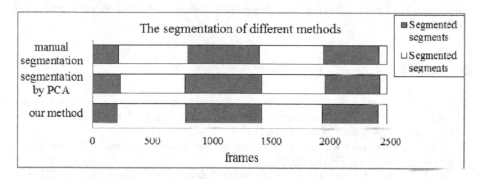

Fig. 7. The segmentation of different methods

The error rate of motion segmentation by different algorithms are shown in Table 2:

Table 2. Error rate of different algorithms

Methods	Jumping	Twisting	Kicking	Squatting	Jogging	Standing
PCA	7.5%	6.2%	7.2%	6.5%	5.7%	13.3%
This paper	4.5%	4.4%	5.4%	4.6%	2%	6.1%
Difference	3%	1.8%	1.8%	1.9%	3.7%	7.2%

By comparison, we can find that the method can effectively segment the motion capture data precisely in semantic and the method is also suitable for complex motion sequences. As can be seen from Table 2, the error rate of this algorithm is greatly reduced compared with the PCA algorithm, which can be used to realize the segmentation of motion sequence.

4 Conclusions

This paper proposed a method of human motion capture data segmentation based on Laplacian Eigenmaps algorithm. The method uses LE algorithm to reduce the dimensionality of original data to realize the mapping from the original data to the low dimensional space. And then a specified window was drawn in the low dimensional space which was used to calculate the space distance from frames in the specified window to each frame in the former fragment. By detecting the similarity, we got the final segmentation points; thereby obtain motion segments with independent semantics. Finally, the effectiveness of the method is verified by experiments, and the experimental results are compared and analyzed. The results show that the algorithm has a great improvement on the accuracy of motion sequence segmentation. But this method is still inadequate. In the future work, we will process more in-depth research and improvement of the method mainly including: (1) Finding a method which has automatic adjustment of the nearest neighbor points K according to different motion sequence. (2) In the detection of the initial segmentation point, according to different motion, finding an adaptive threshold setting method.

Acknowledgement. This work is supported by the National Natural Science Foundation of China (No. 61370141, 61300015), the Program for Dalian High-level Talent's Innovation (2015R088).

References

1. Barbic, J., Safonova, A., Pan, J.Y., et al.: Segmenting motion capture data into distinct behaviors. In: Proceedings of Graphics Interface, pp. 185–194. Canadian Human-Computer Communications Society, Canada (2004)
2. Wold, S., Esbensen, K., Geladi, P.: Principal component analysis. Chemom. Intell. Laboatory Syst. **2**(1), 37–52 (1987)
3. Liu, X.P., Lu, J.T., Xia, X.Y.: Motion captured data segmentation based on PCA and mahalanobis distance. J. Hefei Univ. Technol. (Natural Science) **37**(5), 563–566 (2014)
4. Xiao, J., Zhuang, Y.T., Wu, F.: Getting distinct movements from motion capture data. In: 19th Proceeding of the International Conference on Computer Animation and Social Agents, pp. 33–42 (2006)
5. Tenenbaum, J.B., De, S.V., Langford, J.C.: A global geometric framework for nonlinear dimensionality reduction. J. Sci. **290**(5500), 2319 (2000)
6. Peng, S.J.: Motion segmentation using central distance features and low-pass filter. In: International Conference on Computational Intelligence and Security, pp. 223–226 (2010)
7. Baum, L.E., Petrie, T.: Statistical inference for probabilistic functions of finite state Markov chains. Annal. Math. Stat. **37**(6), 1554–1563 (2012)
8. Reynolds, D.A., Rose, R.C.: Robust text-independent speaker identification using Gaussian mixture speaker models. IEEE Trans. Speech Audio Process. **3**(1), 72–83 (1995)
9. Lin, F.S., Kulić, D.: Online segmentation of human motion for automated rehabilitation exercise analysis. IEEE Trans. Neural Syst. Rehabil. Eng. **22**(1), 168 (2014). A Publication of the IEEE Engineering in Medicine & Biology Society
10. Lu, C.M., Ferrier, N.J.: Repetitive motion analysis: segmentation and event classification. IEEE Trans. Pattern Anal. Mach. Intell. **26**(2), 258–263 (2004)

11. Wang, M.J., Wang, W., Li, Y., et al.: Motion capture data segmentation using kernel dynamic texture. In: International Conference on Audio Language and Image Processing, pp. 592–596. IEEE (2010)
12. Doretto, G., Chiuso, A., Wu, Y.N., et al.: Dynamic textures. Int. J. Comput. Vis. **51**(2), 91–109 (2003)
13. Yang, Y., Chen, J.F., Liu, Z.Z., et al.: Low level segmentation of motion capture data based on hierarchical clustering with cosine distance. Int. J. Database Theory Appl. **8**(4), 231–240 (2015)
14. Arikan, O., Forsyth, D.A., O'Brien, J.F.: Motion synthesis from annotations. In: ACM Siggeraph, pp. 402–408 (2003)
15. Cortes, C., Vapnik, V.: Support-vector networks. J. Mach. Learn. **20**(3), 273–297 (1995)
16. Zhou, F., Torre, F., Hodgins, J.K.: Aligned cluster analysis for temporal segmentation of human motion. In: 8th IEEE International Conference: Automatic Face and Gesture Recognition, pp. 1–7. IEEE (2008)
17. Mavroeidis, D., Marchiori, E.: Feature selection for k-means clustering stability: theoretical analysis and an algorithm. J. Data Mining Knowl. Discov. **28**(4), 918–960 (2014)
18. Zhou, F., De, l.T.F., Hodgins, J.K.: Hierarchical aligned cluster analysis for temporal clustering of human motion. IEEE Trans. Pattern Anal. Mach. Intell. **35**(3), 582–596 (2013)
19. Yang, Y.D., Wang, L.L., Hao, A.M.: Motion String: a motion capture data representation for behavior segmentation. J. Comput. Res. Dev. **45**(3), 527–534 (2008)
20. Xiao, J.: Feature visualization and interactive segmentation of 3D human motion. J. Softw. **19**(8), 1995–2003 (2008)
21. Hu, X.Y., Sun, B., Zhu, X.M., et al.: Motion capture data segmentation based on spectral clustering. J. Comput.-Aided Des. Comput. Graph. **28**(08), 1306–1315 (2016)
22. Jin, C.B., Cui, R.Y., Jin, X.F.: Improvement of Laplacian eigenmaps for human action recognition. J. Appl. Res. Comput. **31**(12), 3613–3616 (2014)
23. Liu, H.H., Zhou, C.H.: Semi-supervised Laplacian Eigenmap. J. Comput. Eng. Design. **33**(2), 601–605 (2012)
24. Zhou, M., Liu, B.H.: Classifier design based on Laplacian Eigenmap. J. Comput. Eng. **35**(16), 178–180 (2009)
25. Peng, S.J.: Double-feature combination based approach to motion capture data behavior segmentation. J. Comput. Sci. **40**(8), 303–308 (2013)

Online Community

The Effects of the Externality of Public Goods on Doctor's Private Benefit: Evidence from Online Health Community

Min Zhang, Tianshi Wu[✉], Xitong Guo, Xiaoxiao Liu,
and Weiwei Sun

School of Management, eHealth Research Institute,
Harbin Institute of Technology, Harbin, China
minzhang233@gmail.com, xiaoxiaoliuhit@gmail.com,
{wutianshi,xitongguo}@hit.edu.cn, sunweiwei45@126.com

Abstract. In order to explore the effects of the externality of public goods in the online healthcare domain, we investigate the relationship between the contributions to Q&A (public goods) and the private benefits of family doctors based on the theory of public goods and externality. We analyze a panel dataset of 1,323 doctors from an online healthcare community, and our results show that participation in public goods will significantly increase the private benefits of family doctors. Moreover, we also find that the physician's ranking has a moderating effect on this relationship.

Keywords: Externality · Public goods · Online healthcare community

1 Introduction

One of the most prominent problems in the world of the medical industry is the shortage of medical resources. In recent years, a substantial increase in China's medical costs indicates that the public demand for medical and health services is increasing. For a long period, China has experienced a serious shortage, and imbalanced allocation of medical resources. With the rapid development and numerous innovations in Internet technology, Internet medicine has become a new direction for healthcare services. At the same time, a variety of social networking sites have become popular, and the growth of the online health community has become more dynamic.

The Internet has changed people's relationships with health information, while the use of the Internet has enabled patients to access search engines, online symptom checkers, and health information sites to contribute to positive health outcomes for themselves. Humans have information needs, which lead people to perform certain behaviors in order to meet such needs [2]. Social networking sites (SNSs), including Facebook and Twitter, have been widely adopted for online communication, and many people rely on SNSs to seek information [3], a behavior referred to as social questioning and answering (social Q&A). In social Q&A (SQA) sites, where users ask question, seek answers, and rate content, while interacting around it, queries are matched against an index of existing documents, and simultaneously become new

© Springer International Publishing AG 2017
H. Chen et al. (Eds.): ICSH 2017, LNCS 10347, pp. 149–160, 2017.
https://doi.org/10.1007/978-3-319-67964-8_14

documents themselves [4]. There is a representative platform known as Baidu Knows. In online health care portals, the Question and Answer (Q&A) platform of the xywy. com portal also belongs to this category. Few researchers have focused on such types of public questioning and answering and its effects on private benefits.

In 2004, the website xywy.com launched the first domestic medical platform, known as the Q&A to enable doctors and patients to communicate with each other. The doctors can provide free questioning and answering services. In 2014, the website launched the Family Doctor platform. On this platform, doctors can freely fix a fee, and patients can consult the doctors in their spare time. There are two types of services that the doctors can provide: free services (e.g. Q&A) and paid services (e.g. Family Doctor). The information produced in the Q&A platform has the attributes of public goods, which are non-rivalrous and nonexclusive. A public good problem arises naturally in situations characterized by positive externalities or negative externalities [5].

The focus of this paper is on whether doctors' participation in the free contribution of public goods will produce externality, that is, will it affect their private benefits on the Family Doctor platform. Therefore, we will attempt to answer the following research questions through panel data regression and the analysis of the results:

- Is there any externality of contributions to public goods in the online health community?
- Is this externality positive or negative?
- How do the externality effects vary across doctors of different rankings?

2 Literature Review and Hypotheses

2.1 Online Public Goods

2.1.1 Public Goods

In the field of economics, a public good is a one that is both non-excludable and non-rivalrous. Individuals cannot be effectively excluded from its use and moreover, use by one individual does not reduce its availability to others [6].

A non-rivalrous attribute is one where some individuals' consumption of a product will not affect others' consumption of this product; and when some people benefit from this product, this will not prevent other people from benefiting from it also. There is no conflict of interest between the beneficiaries. A non-exclusive good or service is one for which the costs of preventing nonpayers from enjoying its benefits are prohibitive.

A public good is a typical resource that is generated and sustained by volunteerism, while private products are produced for profit.

2.1.2 Online Public Goods

Online public goods can be viewed as extensions of public goods. We can also refer to them as digital public goods [7] or public goods on the Internet, and so on. Examples include the open source software communities (Linux, Apache), open content outputs (Wikipedia, OpenCourseWare), content sharing networks (Flickr, YouTube), and so on [8].

Using the description of the characteristics of online public goods in [7], we will define the question and answer information generated by the Q&A community as an online public product. The main points are as follows:

Non-rivalrous goods. A non-rivalrous good is the most basic feature of public goods. It is one for which the consumption of goods will not be reduced or exhausted [9]. Paul Samuelson [10] first examined the non-rivalrous nature of public goods. The information on products and services generated through a network are non-rivalrous because a person using these products and services does not cause a reduction in the product and does not affect the use of the product by others. In this paper, information generated by the Q&A community has such a characteristic. All the site users and visitors can search for and view the relevant questions and answers, and a person's behavior does not affect its use by other people.

Non-exclusive. The non-exclusive feature is also related to public goods [11]. Non-excludability refers to any product or service that is impossible to provide without its being available for many people to enjoy. The production of public goods results in positive externalities for which producers do not receive full payment. Consumers can take advantage of public goods without paying for them. The information of Q&A is also non-exclusive, in other words, a user's behavior does not prevent others from viewing and using useful information, and users who do not contribute to the community can also benefit from the relevant information.

Online features. An online feature is one in which the information generated is accessed by all participants who may enter the site, and there are different ways in which the online community can restrict participants from accessing and using the information products. For example, in an online community, the site can limit the number of users entering and using some of the information by making them pay and using a password to log in. In some sites, only certain members can create and send content. There is a similar situation in the case of a Q&A community, i.e. only registered users can post questions, and registered doctors can answer questions. But there is no restriction on the reading and use of information.

Participation in the online community is voluntary, and everyone can choose whether or not to participate. The users make personal choices on how to participate, for example, to decide on whether to ask questions, continuously ask questions, make comments, and so on, while the content of the questions and the extent of the information accessed is also a personal choice.

Currently, the establishment and continuity of many online public goods is totally dependent on the users' free contributions, and hence the motivations of the behavior relating to free contributions are the focus of many researchers [12, 13]. In some study models, a contributor receives not only utility from total provision of the public good, but also a rather selfish, private benefit or warm glow, such as moral satisfaction and joy of giving [8]. In fact, some researchers have used open source software as topics for examining the motivations behind contributions to online public goods [8]. In a study [14] of the open source software platform, Krishnamurthy and Tripathy posited that the external motivation for public product contribution behavior is derived from external incentives, such as material rewards, job promotion opportunities, signaling quality and so on. Zhang X et al. in their study [1] examined the relationship between the size of a group and the motivations of contribution behavior in this study, and the results of this study have shown that social impacts do control the "free ride" motivation, indicating the importance of social impacts in the supply of public goods.

2.2   The Externality Theory

The externality theory was created by Marshall in his "Principles of Economics" in 1890 [15]. Externality is the cost or benefit that affects a party who did not choose to incur that cost or benefit [16]. Based on different effects, externality can be divided into positive externalities and negative externalities. The beneficial objects of externality in this article are the contributors themselves, and if this externality exists, this externality does not need to be controlled.

In general, public goods are a manifestation of externalities. Externality will enable some third parties who are not investors or contributors to gain from benefits or the sharing of costs. Here, we include three categories of doctors involved in the Q&A, i.e., the experts, the family doctors and other certified doctors. The two platforms, i.e., the Q&A and Family Doctor, can be linked by the free questioning and answering functions (see Fig. 3). What we want to determine is whether the contributions to public goods generate externality. This article seeks to explore whether the family doctors' participation in the Q&A community will impact the private benefit of the family doctors personally, in other words, whether the doctors' contributions to the Q&A will produce externality, so that the participants can gain the benefits; and also whether the externalities of participation in the contribution of public goods are positive or negative.

Franc in his study [17] suggested that volunteer contributors can be divided into two categories: investors who expect benefits from contribution behavior, and donors who do not demand returns. Some studies [1, 14, 18] explore the potential benefits of providing public goods to providers from the perspective of contributing behavioral motivations. This shows that the contribution of public goods does provide benefits for the contributors personally. Here, we focus on the monetary benefits (e.g. earnings in the Family Doctor portal) of family doctors' contributions to the Q&A platform (public goods). Combining the characteristics of externality, this paper explores whether a contributor's contribution to public goods will affect his/her private benefits at the Family Doctor website at the individual level and assumes that its effects are positive.

Based on the preceding arguments we present the following hypotheses.

Thus, we hypothesize that:

H1:   **Contributions to public goods have a significant positive impact on the private benefits of family doctors.**

H2:   **The higher the quality of public goods contributed by the family doctor, the better would be his/her private benefits.**

2.3 Doctors' Titles

There are two categories of doctors' titles in China: physician's ranking and academic titles. Every doctor has a physician's ranking, but many doctors do not have an academic title [19]. Furthermore, patients are more concerned about a doctor's physician's ranking than an academic title. Thus, a doctor's title in this study focuses on a physician's ranking.

The family doctor is purchased as a product, and thus the physician's ranking is seen as a product characteristics. Some researchers have examined the moderating of product characteristics, such as product popularity [20], product category [21] and so on. Liu et al. in their study [22] concerning online doctors' reputations indicated that a physician's ranking has a moderating effect on the relationship of a doctor's efforts and performance. Thus, we hypothesize that physician's ranking has moderating effect (Fig. 1).

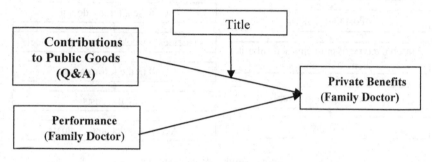

Fig. 1. The research model

H3: **The higher the doctor's title, the greater would be the impacts of the contributions of public goods on the private benefits of the family doctor.**

3 Empirical Analyses

3.1 The Research Context

Our research focuses on the xywy.com website, which was established in 2004 and is a trusted one-stop Internet medical service platform in China. In addition, it is one of the platforms for exploring and practicing online medical services in the early stages of the Internet. Since 2016, the website has gathered more than 120 million registered users, more than 22 million independent visitors, and more than 320 million independent visitors monthly, thus giving it a first ranking in the health care industry.

Next, we briefly describe the functions of the two platforms. The Q&A platform is the basic forum that has existed since the website was developed. It is a Q&A platform for all users (doctors and patients), which gathers together Q&A content on other platforms of the site. The forum can quickly retrieve previous similar problems or the replies of related questions for the doctors and the users based on the patients' questions. Moreover, if there are no existing similar problems, a doctor is available to provide a timely answer for the users' questions. The Family Doctor platform provides convenient advisory services for the majority of users who have health needs. This kind of service is provided by doctors belonging to Third-Level Referral Hospitals or Second-Level Referral Hospitals. The service provides one-to-one telephone counseling, and once a person has signed on, the whole family can use the service. Using the platform, family doctors will help users in analyzing health records, and understanding a patient's medical history and physical conditions, thus providing advice and health guidance. The specific behavioral patterns of the doctors and patients is shown in Fig. 2.

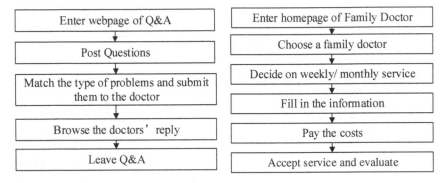

Fig. 2. Doctors' service process in xywy.com

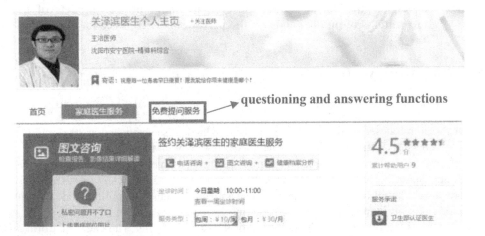

Fig. 3. The web page of the family doctor platform

There exists a link between the two platforms. The family doctor platform gives access to a free service for users to post questions, and the contents of questions and answers between a patient and the family doctor in this 'free question' forum will be collected in the Q&A platform (Fig. 4).

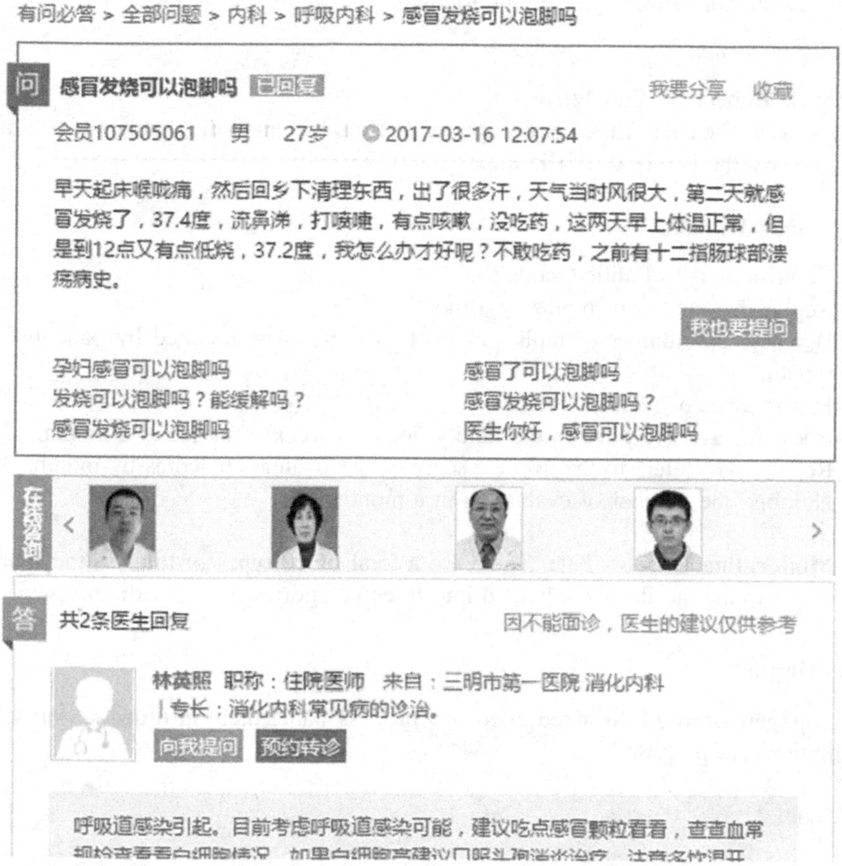

有问必答 > 全部问题 > 内科 > 呼吸内科 > 感冒发烧可以泡脚吗

问 **感冒发烧可以泡脚吗** 已回复   我要分享 收藏

会员107505061 │ 男 │ 27岁 │ ◎ 2017-03-16 12:07:54

早天起床喉咙痛，然后回乡下清理东西，出了很多汗，天气当时风很大，第二天就感冒发烧了，37.4度，流鼻涕，打喷嚏，有点咳嗽，没吃药，这两天早上体温正常，但是到12点又有点低烧，37.2度，我怎么办才好呢？不敢吃药，之前有十二指肠球部溃疡病史。

我也要提问

孕妇感冒可以泡脚吗   感冒了可以泡脚吗
发烧可以泡脚吗？能缓解吗？   感冒发烧可以泡脚吗？
感冒发烧可以泡脚吗   医生你好，感冒可以泡脚吗

在线咨询 <   >

答 **共2条医生回复**   因不能面诊，医生的建议仅供参考

林英照 职称：住院医师 来自：三明市第一医院 消化内科
│专长：消化内科常见病的诊治。
向我提问 预约转诊

呼吸道感染引起。目前考虑呼吸道感染可能，建议吃点感冒颗粒看看，查查血常规检查看看白细胞情况，如果白细胞高建议门服头孢当水治疗，注意多休渴工

Fig. 4. Questions and Answers platform (Q&A)

3.2   The Data

The main sources of data for this study are the data of the Family Doctor platform and the Q&A platform in the website. In the Family Doctor platform, we collect the basic personal information of family doctors, their evaluations and purchase records. In the Q&A platform, as the amount of data in this platform proved to be too large, it has been difficult to crawl all the questions and answers. Therefore, only 477,242 questions related to diabetes and their responses were collected, involving 16,215 doctors, and including 744 family doctors' questions and answers.

The data studied in this paper included the records of family doctors, ranging from August 2014 to October 2016.

Variables.
In this paper we focused on whether the inclusion of contributions to public goods was external, that is, whether the activities of the Q&A forum would impact the connected Family Doctor platform. We used the following variables.

Dependent Variables

Private Benefits of Family Doctor
Purchase: The data of the Family Doctor platform refers to the number of contracts signed by the family doctor in a month.

Independent Variables

(a) Contributions to Public Goods
Reply: the number of replies in a month
B_reply: the number of replies of doctors' who were adopted by patients in a month.
(b) Performance of Family Doctor
Price: the average price of the family doctor's weekly service in a month.
Reputation: Refers to the average score of the evaluation scores by month.
Number: the number of evaluation in a month.

The Moderating Effects. Title: There are a total of 10 types of titles in the Family Doctor platform, and they are divided into three categories (high, medium, low).

3.3 Method

In this paper, we used the fixed effects to process panel data, in order to verify the assumptions we proposed.

Model 1:

$$Purchase_{it} = Price_{it} + Reputation_{it} + Reply_{it} + Reply_{it}^2 + B_{reply_{it}} + Number_{it} + \varepsilon_{it} \quad (1)$$

Model 2:

$$Purchase_{it} = Price_{it} + Reputation_{it} + Reply_{it} + Reply_{it}^2 + Title2 \times Reply_{it} + Title3$$
$$\times Reply_{it} + + B\_reply_{it} + Number_{it} + \varepsilon_{it}$$

$$(2)$$

4 Results

We present the summary statistics of our major variables in Table 1 and the correlations between variables in Table 2. Table 3 presents the main estimated results of this paper.

By observing the regression results of Model 1, it is perceived that the contribution of public goods has a positive, significant effect on the contributor's private benefits (purchases). This result is consistent with our assumptions about the externalities of the Q&A, and thus H1 is supported. However, the optimal response number of the doctor

Table 1. Summary statistics of variables

Variable	Obs	Mean	Std. Dev.	Min	Max
Reputation	36423	0.6380455	1.636251	0	5.333333
Number	36423	1.24866	6.264256	0	291
B_reply	36423	0.025698	0.3104333	0	15
Reply	36423	0.4963896	4.621918	0	250
Price	36423	6.419409	60.47767	0	3000

Table 2. Correlations

	1	2	3	4	5	6	7
Reputation	1						
Number	0.462	1					
B_reply	−0.005	0.001	1				
Reply	0.010	0.000	0.604	1			
Price_week	0.082	0.041	0.007	0.007	1		
Price_month	0.043	0.028	0.002	0.002	0.487	1	
Purchase	0.089	0.054	0.015	0.022	0.043	0.030	1

Table 3. Regression coefficients and model summary

Independent variables	Model 1	Model 2
Ln(Reputation)	0.1385517***	0.1390141***
Ln(Reply)	0.1597685***	0.1033189***
Ln(Reply)^2	−0.0292761***	−0.0259094***
Ln(Price_week)	0.2285782***	0.2285544***
Ln(B_reply)	0.0094241	−0.0174405
Ln(Number)	−0.0228516**	−0.0226486**
Ln(Reply) × Title2		0.1257936***
Ln(Reply) × Title3		−0.0533086**
R-square	0.15028	0.15078
Adjusted R-square	0.11747	0.11794
F-test	1033.69***	778.248***

* indicates p < 0.1 ** indicates p < 0.05 ***indicates p < 0.01

has no significant effect on the website of the family doctor (Ln (B_reply) regression coefficient = 0.0094, p > 0.1), and thus H2 is not supported.

Next, we analyze the moderating role of the doctor's title on the significant effects. First, the doctor's title is defined as a dummy variable in this article. Title1 represents 1, and that indicates that the doctor's title is a low rating; Title 2 represents 2, and that indicates that the doctor's title is an intermediate rating; Title 3 represents 3, and indicates that the doctor's title is that for a senior doctor. As can be seen in the regression results of Model 2, the moderating effects of the title do not affect the main effects of the amount of responses on the number of sales, and it remains a positive, significant impact ((Ln (Reply) regression coefficient = 0.1033189, p < 0.01)). The number of best replies has no significant impact. Model 2 also shows the results of the interactions between Title 2 and the replies which is positive and statistically significant, indicating that when a physician has a higher rating, the impacts of doctor's reply on physicians' private benefit will be more influential. The interactions between Title 3 and the replies is negative and statistically significant, indicating that the purchase of a doctor with a high rating will be less than a doctor with a low rating if that doctor does contribute to public goods. Moreover, the results show that the title is a pure moderator, indicating that the relationship between a reply and a purchase is contingent upon a doctor's title. ((Ln (Reply) × Title 2 regression coefficient = 0.1257936, p < 0.01); (Ln (Reply) × Title 3 the regression coefficient = −0.0553086, p < 0.05)). The preliminary results reveal that the purchase of a family doctor's service with a medium rating will be more than that of a doctor with a low rating if the family doctor makes more contributions to public goods. More research is needed to test the moderating effects (Table 4).

Table 4. Summary hypotheses

Hypotheses	Supported?
H1: Contributions to public goods have a significant positive impact on the private benefits of family doctors	Yes
H2: The higher the quality of public goods contributed by the family doctor, the better would be the private benefits of the family doctor	No
H3: The higher the doctor's title, the greater would be the impacts of the contributions of public goods to the private benefits of the family doctor	Partially

5   Discussion

In this paper, we examine the impacts of public product contributions on the private benefit of family doctors. Specifically, it is from the doctor's personal level that one can test the effects of both the number of replies and best replies of doctors in the Q&A forum on the number of family doctors' contracts. At the same time, the moderating effects of doctors' titles is tested. By regressing the panel data of family doctors, we find that the contributions to the public goods of family doctors in the Q&A forum does have a significant effect on the private benefit of the family doctor and it is seen to be positive. However, only the number of replies has a significant effect, and the best numbers of replies in the two models do not have any significant impact. Our study employs physician's ranking as a moderating variable. Doctors with a low rating have the potential to overcome the shortage of doctors with low ratings to increase their number of patients in a short time if they pay attention to the contribution of public goods. More research is needed to test the moderating effects. Generally, our results suggest that doctors who have a low ratings benefit in a short period when they make contributions to the Q&A platform.

There are some limitations of this paper: (1) There are many diseases for doctors provide answers to in the online healthcare community, and we only chose the questions on diabetes to test the model. (2) The value of R-square in the model is low, indicating that we may have missed some variables, and further research is needed.

Doctors treating different diseases may have different choices in answering the questions. The many different diseases may influence doctors' motivation to contribute. Therefore, in future research, we can use different diseases to test the model and compare results.

6 Conclusion

This paper provides an empirical analysis that investigates whether contributions to public goods indicate externalities on private benefits. Our setting focuses on the two platforms of the xywy.com website: the Q&A and Family Doctor platform. There is a link between the two platforms. Users can sign on with any family doctor, while they can also view the doctors' contributions to the Q&A forum. We show first, that if family doctors make contributions to the Q&A forum, their private benefit in the Family Doctor platform will show an improvement, and the title of the doctor can moderate this effect. As we have mentioned previously, our research indicates that online public goods generate externality, and hence the externality is positive. Physician's rankings can enhance the effect of contributions to public goods on private benefits.

Our most insightful finding concerns the externalities generated by contributions to public goods which reflect on private benefits. When a doctor makes contributions to the Q&A forum, that doctor will be granted a better benefit in the Family Doctor platform, thus generating a positive externality. The results regarding the moderation of physician's ranking can indicate that doctors with a lower ranking need to contribute more to public goods.

References

1. Zhang, X., Wang, C.: Network positions and contributions to online public goods: the case of Chinese wikipedia. J. Manag. Inf. Syst. 29(2), 11–40 (2012)
2. Given, L.M., Mai, J.E., Case, D.O.: Looking for Information: A Survey of Research on Information Seeking, Needs, and Behavior. Emerald Group Publishing, Bingley (2016)
3. Liu, Z., Jansen, B.J.: Analysis of question and answering behavior in question routing services, pp. 72–85 (2015)

4. Gazan, R.: Social Q&A. J. Am. Soc. Inf. Sci. Technol. **62**(12), 2301–2312 (2011)
5. Dybvig, P.H., Spatt, C.S.: Adoption externalities as public goods. J. Public Econ. **20**(2), 231–247 (1983)
6. Varian, H.R.: Microeconomic analysis. Nort. Co., New York (1992)
7. Wasko, M.M., Teigland, R., Faraj, S.: The provision of online public goods: examining social structure in an electronic network of practice. Decis. Support Syst. **47**(3), 254–265 (2009)
8. Zhang, X., Zhu, F.: Group size and incentives to contribute: a natural experiment at Chinese Wikipedia. Am. Econ. Rev. **101**(4), 1601–1615 (2011)
9. Shmanske, S.: Public Goods. Mixed Goods and Monopolistic Competition. Texas A&M University Press, College Station (1991)
10. Samuelson, P.A.: The pure theory of public expenditure. Rev. Econ. Stat. **36**(4), 387 (1954)
11. Head, J.G.: Public goods and public policy. In: Readings in Industrial Economics, pp. 66–87. Macmillan Education UK, London (1972)
12. Lerner, J., Tirole, J.: Some simple economics of open source. J. Ind. Econ. **50**(2), 197–234 (2003)
13. Lakhani, K.R., von Hippel, E.: How open source software works: 'free' user-to-user assistance. Res. Policy **32**(6), 923–943 (2003)
14. Krishnamurthy, S., Tripathi, A.K.: Monetary donations to an open source software platform. Res. Policy **38**(2), 404–414 (2009)
15. Wang, H., Shao, S.: Study on the eco-tourism environment protection based on the external theory. Asian Soc. Sci. **5**(1), 13 (2009)
16. Buchanan, J.M., Stubblebine, W.C.: "Externality," in Classic Papers in Natural Resource Economics, pp. 138–154. Palgrave Macmillan UK, London (1962)
17. Franck, E., Jungwirth, C.: Reconciling rent-seekers and donators – the governance structure of open source. J. Manag. Gov. **7**(4), 401–421 (2003)
18. Bramoullé, Y., Kranton, R.: Public goods in networks. J. Econ. Theory **135**(1), 478–494 (2007)
19. Yang, H., Guo, X., Wu, T.: Exploring the influence of the online physician service delivery process on patient satisfaction. Decis. Support Syst. **78**, 113–121 (2015)
20. Zhu, F., (Michael) Zhang, X.: Impact of online consumer reviews on sales: the moderating role of product and consumer characteristics. J. Mark. **74**(2), 133–148 (2010)
21. Kushwaha, T., Shankar, V.: Are multichannel customers really more valuable? The moderating role of product category characteristics. J. Mark. **77**(4), 67–85 (2013)
22. Liu, X., Guo, X., Wu, H., Vogel, D.: Doctor's Effort Influence on Online Reputation and Popularity, pp. 111–126 (2014)

Do Online Reviews of Physicians Reflect Healthcare Outcomes?

Danish H. Saifee, Indranil Bardhan, and Zhiqiang (Eric) Zheng[✉]

Jindal School of Management, University of Texas at Dallas,
Richardson, TX 75080, USA
{danish.saifee,bardhan,ericz}@utdallas.edu

Abstract. Patients are increasingly using online reviews to choose physicians. However, it is not known whether online reviews accurately capture the true quality of care provided by physicians. This research addresses this issue by empirically examining the link between online reviews of a physician and the actual clinical outcomes of patients treated by the physician. Specifically, this study uses online reviews from Vitals.com, and combines that data with patient health outcomes data collected from Dallas-Fort Worth Hospital Council. Our econometric analyses show that there is no clear relationship between online reviews of physicians and their patients' health outcomes, such as readmission and ER visit rates. Our results imply that online reviews may not be as helpful in the context of healthcare as they are for other experience goods such as books, movies, or hotels. Our findings have important implications for healthcare providers, healthcare review websites, and healthcare consumers.

Keywords: Online reviews · Healthcare · Clinical outcomes · Topic modeling · Sentiment analysis · Chronic obstructive pulmonary disease (COPD)

1 Introduction

Online reviews of physicians have the potential to reduce information asymmetry between healthcare providers and patients, empowering patients to make better decisions. A pertinent question, then, is *whether, and to what extent, patients benefit from online reviews of physicians.*

Ascertaining this efficacy is important because of the greater role that online reviews play in patients' decisions about which physicians to see and which ones to avoid (Hanauer et al. 2014). In fact, many physicians monitor their reviews and ratings closely and try to boost their ratings on review sites such as Yelp, Vitals, and RateMDs.[1] There are even numerous instances in which physicians have filed defamation lawsuits over negative patient reviews.[2] Evidently, patients are increasingly using online reviews to select physicians as well as other healthcare providers,

---

[1] https://www.washingtonpost.com/news/to-your-health/wp/2016/05/27/docs-fire-back-at-bad-yelp-reviews-and-reveal-patients-information-online, last accessed 03/31/2017.
[2] http://www.oregonlive.com/today/index.ssf/2015/11/doctor_sues_patient_over_negat.html and http://blog.ericgoldman.org/archives/2015/01/another-failed-doctor-lawsuit-against-a-patient-for-online-reviews-brandner-v-molonguet.htm, last accessed on 03/31/2017.

© Springer International Publishing AG 2017
H. Chen et al. (Eds.): ICSH 2017, LNCS 10347, pp. 161–168, 2017.
https://doi.org/10.1007/978-3-319-67964-8_15

prompting providers to take these reviews rather seriously. Despite the increasing importance of online reviews in healthcare, it is not at all clear that these reviews are actually leading to better patient choices. Put differently, the relationship between physician reviews and quality of physician care remains largely unexplored. A major challenge lies in the difficulty of accurately measuring the quality of care provided by physicians. Some researchers have used surveys to assess patients' perceptions of physicians to construct a proxy for physician quality (Doyle et al. 2013). However, patient perception may not be the same as reality.

To address this challenge, we obtained research data for this study from two sources. The first dataset (spanning from 2006 to 2015) was obtained from Dallas Fort Worth Hospital Council's (DFWHC) Research Foundation database on COPD patients. This dataset consists of approximately 630,000 inpatient admission-discharge records, 10,200 attending physicians, and 330,000 patients. The second dataset of about 14,500 physicians in North Texas (spanning from 2007 to 2015) was collected from Vitals.-com. This dataset provides data on physician characteristics and online reviews, including textual reviews, review ratings, and years of physician practice. We integrated the data from these two data sets, using physician names, to create a unique dataset that provides patient health outcomes for physicians who are also rated and reviewed by their patients and examine whether online reviews of physicians are reliable predictors of their patients' clinical outcomes. In other words, if a physician receives very positive online reviews, does that also mean that her patients also exhibit good health outcomes?

Our results show that patients under the care of physicians with better online reviews may not necessarily experience better clinical outcomes, compared to patients receiving care from physicians with worse review ratings. Our results have broader implications for healthcare providers and consumers.

2 Literature Review

A few recent studies in the information systems area examine online ratings and reviews of care providers. For example, Bardach et al. (2013) suggest that reviewers on Yelp may possess knowledge on important aspects of care. Gao et al. (2015) find that physicians who are rated lower in quality (by the patient population) in offline surveys are less likely to be rated online and online ratings are positively correlated with patient reviews, and that online ratings tend to be exaggerated at the upper end of the quality spectrum. They construct their quality measure using patient surveys conducted by Consumers' Checkbook using the instrument and procedure designed by the U.S. Agency for Healthcare Research and Quality. Gray et al. (2015) don't find a clear evidence of association between physician website ratings and traditional quality measures such as blood pressure or low-density lipoprotein controlled. Although these papers shed much needed light on patient perception of providers, they either (1) rely on limited care quality measures such as offline patient satisfaction surveys or (2) are mostly limited to aggregated numeric ratings of physicians as a surrogate for patient perception and often do not consider the rich sentiments expressed in textual reviews.

Studies in medical journals examining the relationship between patient experience and clinical outcomes, such as the mortality rate, 30-day readmission rate, and clinical safety, are also relevant (e.g., Glickman et al. 2010; Boulding et al. 2011). A comprehensive review, conducted by Doyle et al. (2013), summarizes prior research that examined the relationship between patient experience and clinical outcomes. Majority of these studies find positive connection between patient satisfaction and clinical outcomes. Although these findings provide important insights, a bulk of the studies in this literature stream rely on offline surveys to solicit patient experience, which do not allow significant parsing of the textual content through sentiment-mining and topic-modeling techniques as can be done with online reviews. These prior studies have also often relied on cross-sectional hospital- or clinic-level data, limiting the extent to which their findings can be extrapolated to the context of patient experience at the physician level. Finally, the use of these survey findings by patients is not nearly as widespread as is that of websites containing reviews of physicians.

The stream of research on online consumer reviews has generally found that online reviews of products, such as books, and services, and hospitality, enable consumers to make more informed decisions by providing them information on other consumers' perspectives (e.g., Vermeulen and Seegers 2009; Chevalier and Mayzlin 2006). However, it is not clear whether the findings in prior research relating to the efficacy and usefulness of reviews automatically are applicable to a healthcare context. That is, the true quality of healthcare services could be significantly more difficult to assess when compared to the context of hotels, restaurants, or other similar services.

3 Research Question

Online reviews of physicians can contain rich information and often provide significantly more information than numeric (star) ratings. For example, they can help users gather information about the experience of past patients of a physician including, but not limited to, bedside manners of the physician, whether she spends sufficient time with her patients, follows up after the visit, and the thoroughness of explanations (of diagnoses and procedures) provided by her or her staffs. Some aspects of online reviews, such as detailed accounts of procedures and clinical steps performed by a physician, may even provide useful cues about the clinical aspects of care. Moreover, online reviews can influence patients' choices. Based on a survey of patients, Hanauer et al. (2014) report that 35% of the respondents selected physicians with good ratings, while 37% avoided those with bad ones. Thus, it suggests that prospective patients expect physicians who receive largely positive online reviews to deliver better clinical outcomes. However, to the best of our knowledge, *there is no data-driven evidence that this is indeed the case.*

There ought to be a concern about the reliability of online reviews of a physician in predicting the quality of service delivered by the physician because a patient, who typically lacks a comprehensive medical training, may not be well equipped to ascertain the clinical proficiency of a physician.[3] Also, an online review of a physician may not necessarily provide information on the clinical characteristics of that physician's care delivery and could easily overemphasize factors such as flexibility in scheduling appointments, promptness and courteousness of the staff, receptiveness and of the medical team, etc. These factors are not necessarily indicative of the level of clinical care provided by the physician. This leads us to our central research question:

Are physicians who receive better online reviews more likely to deliver better clinical outcomes for their patients?

4   Research Framework

4.1   Variables

The two clinical outcome measures used in our study, *Future30DayReadm* and *FutureERVisit*, are constructed from the DFWHC dataset. *Future30DayReadm* is the proportion of future patient admissions within thirty days of the previous discharge date, for a given physician at a given point in time (quarter), due to the same principal diagnosis (i.e. COPD). We construct a binary variable that equals 1 for a patient visit only if that patient's next admission date is within 30 days of his current discharge date. Then, for each attending physician, we calculate the rolling average of this dummy variable, beginning from the chronologically last (most recent) inpatient admission record to obtain *Future30DayReadm*. *FutureERVisit* is the proportion of future patient admissions involving a visit to an emergency room, with construction similar to *Future30DayReadm*.

The key explanatory variables with regard to online reviews are *OverallRating* and *SentimentScore*. *OverallRating* is the average of the overall star ratings of a physician at a given time, and *SentimentScore* is the average of the sentiment score (up to a time-point) derived from textual reviews in vitals.com. The sentiment analysis technique that we applied classifies the sentiment of each word in a review into four sentiment categories: very positive, positive, very negative, and negative (based on the vocabulary provided by Nielsen 2011). Then, aggregation across all sentiment words within a review yields an overall sentiment score, *SentScorePerReview,* for the review.[4] To control for variations in clinical outcomes arising from variations in the patient-mix handled by physicians, we create several controls. (Note that these controls as well as the key explanatory variables are backward-looking, as opposed to the forward-looking outcome variables *Future30DayReadm* and *FutureERVisit*.) We also control for sentiment variance, and *latent topics* underlying the textual content of online reviews.

We, next, conduct a fine-grained textual analyses of the online reviews by deploying latent Dirichlet allocation (LDA) (Blei et al. 2003) to derive latent topics

---

[3] Source: http://health.usnews.com/health-news/patient-advice/articles/2014/12/19/are-online-physician-ratings-any-good%20, last accessed on 03/31/2017.

[4] $SentScorePerReview = 2 \times number\ of\ very\ positive\ words + 1 \times number\ of\ positive\ words$
$- 1 \times number\ of\ negative\ words - 2 \times number\ of\ very\ negative\ words.$

underlying the textual content in online reviews. Figure 1 plots the distribution of the sentiment category (positive, neutral, or negative) across these four latent topics.[5] Reviews under the latent topic "Overall Care" tend to be rated more positively, as opposed to reviews for the other three latent topics, while reviews for the latent topic "Promptness" tend to be more negative, compared to the rest. This provides some insights into how the types of underlying themes might be driving sentiments expressed in online reviews.

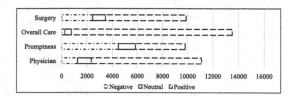

Fig. 1. Frequency of sentiments by latent topics

4.2   Estimation Model and Results

To account for potential physician-time-level fixed effects and omitted variable biases, we consider a two-stage two-way fixed-effects panel regression with instrument variables. The physician fixed effects account for time-invariant physician attributes that are not captured in our data. The use of forward-looking measures for the outcome variables helps us mitigate possible biases in coefficient estimates of our key explanatory variables, which can arise from simultaneity between these explanatory variables and clinical outcomes. We construct two instrument variables (IV), which represent the average sentiment score of online reviews and average score of online ratings received by the focal attending physician's peer physician group in the same hospital system, over the previous two and a half years (10 quarters). A physician's reviews (online perception) can be reliably predicted using the online perception of other physicians in the same hospital system, aggregated over time. But, this time-aggregated online perception of her peer group need not systematically determine clinical outcomes of her (i.e. focal physician's) patients. The first stage regression results indicate that these IVs are strong. Table 1 presents the second-stage regression estimation results.

The coefficient estimates of our key explanatory variable—*SentimentScore* and *OverallRating*—in Table 1 demonstrate that physicians who receive better online reviews or higher online star ratings, compared to their peers, do not necessarily exhibit better health outcomes as measured by the future 30-day readmission or ER visit rates of their patients. In fact, higher overall ratings are associated with a higher frequency of future ER visits, casting additional doubts on the efficacy of online reviews and ratings.

---

[5] If *SentScorePerReview* is greater than zero, we label the review "positive;" if it is less than zero, we label it "negative," and "neutral" if it is zero.

Table 1. Two-stage Two-way fixed effects IV estimation results (second-stage)

| | Future30DayReadm | | FutureERVisit | |
	(1)	(2)	(3)	(4)
SentimentScore	−0.013 (0.037)	−	0.129$^+$ (0.067)	−
OverallRating		0.151$^+$ (0.081)		**0.515** (0.188)**
SentimentVariance	0.134 (0.257)	−0.111 (0.086)	−0.857 (0.471)	−0.478* (0.200)
ReviewWordsNum	0.000 (0.000)	0.000 (0.000)	−0.001 (0.000)	0.001* (0.000)
TopicSurgery	−0.049 (0.078)	0.036 (0.032)	0.284* (0.135)	0.221** (0.074)
TopicPhysician	−0.035 (0.037)	0.026 (0.027)	0.181** (0.068)	0.224** (0.064)
TopicPromptness	−0.069 (0.137)	0.234 (0.136)	0.536* (0.254)	0.929** (0.322)
Experience	−0.002 (0.004)	0.003 (0.005)	0.026* (0.011)	0.043** (0.014)
ERVisit	−0.011 (0.024)	−0.016 (0.021)	−	−
30DayReadm	−	−	0.659*** (0.171)	0.375** (0.143)
VisitsNum	0.000 (0.000)	0.000 (0.000)	0.000 (0.000)	0.000* (0.000)
LOS	0.011** (0.004)	0.010** (0.004)	−0.021* (0.009)	−0.017 (0.009)
Expired	−0.518* (0.262)	−0.738* (0.316)	−1.895** (0.643)	−2.609*** (0.706)
PtAge	0.002 (0.002)	−0.001 (0.001)	−0.012*** (0.003)	−0.015*** (0.003)
Female	0.030 (0.035)	0.009 (0.028)	−0.32** (0.113)	−0.203** (0.075)
SevMajExt	0.030 (0.052)	0.069 (0.046)	−0.238* (0.101)	−0.200 (0.112)
MortMajExt	−0.260*** (0.058)	−0.205*** (0.051)	0.340** (0.115)	0.405** (0.128)
SwitchHospSys	−0.030 (0.034)	−0.044 (0.028)	−0.129 (0.075)	−0.308*** (0.067)
SwitchHosp	0.064* (0.031)	0.082** (0.028)	0.118 (0.072)	0.298*** (0.066)
EthnHisp	0.123* (0.050)	0.182*** (0.051)	0.124 (0.148)	0.095 (0.128)
RaceWhite	−0.047 (0.027)	−0.012 (0.028)	0.098 (0.075)	0.114 (0.073)

$p < 0.10^+$, $p < 0.05*$, $p < 0.01**$, $p < 0.001***$, standard error in parenthesis

Hence, our results suggest that *neither sentiments expressed in reviews nor numeric ratings are accurate predictors of actual clinical outcomes.*

5 Robustness Checks

An endogeneity concern could arise from potential self-selection by patients, i.e. patients with poor health may choose to go to physicians perceived to be of high quality. When that happens, physicians who deliver better clinical outcomes could end up receiving relatively poor reviews. To deal with possible self-selection, we apply the two-stage Heckman selection method. The results from the Heckman method do not lend any evidence to the possibility that patient self-selection is indeed driving our main finding that reviews and ratings are not as useful in predicting clinical outcomes, as commonly believed. These results are omitted due to space constraints.

Next, we consider the possibility that physicians whose patients experience poor clinical outcomes (high readmission or ER visit rates) may be involved in of review manipulation. To examine this, we divided our physicians into two groups: those whose patients have experienced below-average readmission rates (*AvgFut30DayReadm = 0*), and those whose patients have experienced above-average readmission rates (*AvgFut30DayReadm = 1*). We repeat this for ER visit rates and again create two groups for *AvgFutERVisit* = 0 and *AvgFutERVisit* = 1, respectively. We, next scrape the numbers of "recommended" and "not-recommended" reviews for physicians from Yelp. Reviews not recommended are potentially suspicious due to potential for manipulation. Thus, if we find that physicians whose patients have experienced relatively poorer clinical outcomes have a disproportionately larger number (or fraction) of such reviews, we can suspect some manipulation on Yelp, and perhaps other web sites as well. None of the t-tests' results in Table 2 suggest that physicians who deliver above-average readmission or ER visit rates receive a higher number (or fraction) of "not-recommended" reviews, compared to physicians who deliver below-average readmission or ER visit rates, not providing any evidence that physicians are engaging in active manipulation of online reviews.

Table 2. Comparison of number and percent of not-recommended yelp reviews

	Number of Not-Reco reviews				Percent of Not-Reco reviews			
	AvgFut30DayReadm		AvgFutERVisit		AvgFut30DayReadm		AvgFutERVisit	
	0	1	0	1	0	1	0	1
Mean	0.653	0.268	0.762	0.310	37.382	37.734	37.785	37.557
(Std Dev)	(4.394)	(0.917)	(5.250)	(1.550)	(39.244)	(39.659)	(39.672)	(39.266)
No. of obs.	623	370	399	490	198	93	132	122
t	2.12		1.66		−0.07		0.05	
p	0.035		0.097		0.944		0.963	

6   Contributions and Implications

In summary, our paper contributes to and builds on prior research in the following four ways: (1) it attempts to study the relationship between online reviews of a physician and actual clinical outcomes of the physician's patients, (2) it measures clinical outcomes *objectively* based on the readmission rate and ER visit rate at the patient-admission level, (3) it analyzes the fine-grained textual content of reviews, rather than relying only on aggregated numeric ratings, in examining patients' opinions, and (4) it applies text mining techniques as well as econometric methods, including a series of robustness checks, to investigate whether the textual content in reviews of physicians is indeed a reliable predictor of clinical outcomes. To the best of our knowledge, there is no prior research that has addressed all of the above dimensions in a unified framework, as we have proposed in this paper.

Our study has several managerial and healthcare policy implications. First, healthcare consumers need to be cautious, when using online reviews and ratings to form opinions about physician quality. Physicians who receive better online reviews, may not necessarily exhibit better quality as measured by their patients' health outcomes. Second, our results suggest that online reviews require further scrutiny than what is currently done to decipher physician quality. Our study lends support to the concerns raised in the popular press about over-reliance on online reviews of physicians to assess actual physician quality particularly in the context of chronic conditions.

Third, hospitals and clinics should be careful about relying on online reviews of physicians for evaluating physician performance, since they do not serve as accurate predictors of future patient health outcomes.

References

Bardach, N.S., Asteria-Penaloza, R., Boscardin, W.J., Dudley, R.A.: The relationship between commercial website ratings and traditional hospital performance measures in the USA. BMJ Qual. Saf. **22**(3), 194–202 (2013)

Blei, D.M., Ng, A.Y., Jordan, M.I.: Latent Dirichlet Allocation. J. Mach. Learn. Res. **3**, 993–1022 (2003)

Boulding, W., Glickman, S.W., Manary, M., Schulman, K.A., Staelin, R.: Relationship between patient satisfaction with inpatient care and hospital readmission within 30 days. Am. J. Managed Care **17**(1), 41–48 (2011)

Chevalier, J.A., Mayzlin, D.: The effect of word of mouth on sales: online book reviews. J. Mark. Res. **43**(3), 345–354 (2006)

Doyle, C., Lennox, L., Bell, D.: A systematic review of evidence on the links between patient satisfaction and clinical safety and effectiveness. BMJ Open **3**(1), 1–18 (2013)

Gao, G.G., Greenwood, B.N., Agarwal, R., McCullough, J.S.: Vocal minority and silent majority: how do online ratings reflect population perceptions of quality? MIS Q. **39**(3), 565–589 (2015)

Glickman, S.W., Boulding, W., Manary, M., Staelin, R., Roe, M.T., Wolosin, R.J., Ohman, E. M., Peterson, E.D., Schulman, K.A.: Patient satisfaction and its relationship with clinical quality and inpatient mortality in acute myocardial infarction. Circ. Cardiovasc. Qual. Outcomes **3**(2), 188–195 (2010)

Gray, B., Vandergrift, J.L., Gao, G.G., McCullough, J.S., Lipner, R.S.: Website ratings of physicians and their true quality of care. JAMA Internal Med. **175**(2), 291–293 (2015)

Hanauer, D.A., Zheng, K., Singer, D.C., Gebremariam, A., Davis, M.M.: Public awareness, perception, and use of online physician rating sites. J. Am. Med. Assoc. **311**(7), 734–735 (2014)

Nielsen, F.Å.: A new ANEW: evaluation of a word list for sentiment analysis in microblogs. In: Proceedings of the ESWC2011 Workshop on 'Making Sense of Microposts': Big Things Come in Small Package, CEUR Workshop Proceedings, no. 718, pp. 93–98 (2011)

Vermeulen, I.E., Seegers, D.: Tried and tested: the impact of online hotel reviews on online hotel reviews on consumer consideration. Tour. Manag. **30**(1), 123–127 (2009)

Social Support and User Roles in a Chinese Online Health Community: A LDA Based Text Mining Study

Jiang Wu[⊠], Shaoxin Hou, and Mengmeng Jin

School of Information Management,
Wuhan University, Wuhan 430072, Hubei, China
jiangw@whu.edu.cn

Abstract. Online health communities (OHCs) have become increasingly popular for people with health issues in China, which have been regarded as one of the major sources of social support. In this study, we designed a Chinese content analysis process to understand social support and user engagement in OHCs. Based on the social support theory, the process used Chinese text mining and machine learning techniques. Using a case study of an OHC among diabetics, we first divided users' posts and replies into different types of social support. Then, we aggregated each user's texts of different social support types. At last, we revealed the roles of the users by clustering. Considering the high dimensions of Vector Space Model (VSM) transformed from user texts, we proposed a new method to extract features based on LDA. In order to improve the effect of user clustering, we optimized the clustering algorithm with the principle of Maximum Distance and Elbow Method. Results showed that the process performed well in classification and clustering.

Keywords: OHCs · LDA · Feature extraction · Text classification · User clustering · K-means

1 Introduction

Online health communities (OHCs) refer to the internet platforms that allow participants to exchange and share information without the limitation of time and space. OHCs are of great significance for integrating medical resources, improving medical services and user's health awareness [1, 2].

Previous studies have shown that OHCs can provide effective social supports for participants [2–4] and have a positive impact on the health behavior of users [5]. Literatures on social support suggest that OHCs mainly feature three types of social support: information support, emotional support, and companionship [6, 7]. Does a user's involvement to different categories of social support affect his/her engagement in an OHC? To answer the question, Kang et al. used machine learning techniques to reveal the types of social support embedded in text from an OHC among breast cancer survivors [3]. By examining the user generated content, Kang et al. extracted various types of features for classifiers: basic features, lexical features, sentiment features, and

© Springer International Publishing AG 2017
H. Chen et al. (Eds.): ICSH 2017, LNCS 10347, pp. 169–176, 2017.
https://doi.org/10.1007/978-3-319-67964-8_16

topic features. This kind of feature extraction method not only retains text information, but also reduces the number of data dimension and the number of human annotated data.

However, most studies took English OHCs as their research objects, while few focused on Chinese OHCs. It is universally acknowledged that some methods used in English text mining process cannot be perfectly adapted to the text analysis of Chinese content. The reason lies in the nature of Chinese. It is a semantic language which focuses on the meaning rather than form. Furthermore, the ambiguities of Chinese characters, grammar, semantics and other aspects is very outstanding [8]. At the same time, Chinese text mining needs abundant basic resources, such as lexical dictionary, professional dictionary, semantic and grammar rule base and commonsense knowledge base [9]. Compared to English, Chinese text processing resources are not complete and entirely available.

Based on the characteristics of Chinese text analysis, in order to understand the social support and user engagement in OHCs, we use "Sweet Home (http://bbs.tnbz.com/)", a popular diabetes OHC in China, as a case study. In this research, we have addressed three research gaps: (1) The paper uses the LDA to extract topic features from analysis corpus to improve the traditional text vector space representation. (2) Based on the Binary Classification method, we test different classification algorithms for each type of social support and select the best one to build classifiers to improve the performance of classification. (3) We optimize the clustering algorithms by using the principle of Maximum Distance to select the cluster centers and utilizing Elbow Method to determine the optimal number of clusters.

2   Research Design

Figure 1 illustrates the proposed social support classification and user clustering process. The major components including data acquisition and preprocessing, features extraction, user text classification, and user clustering will be discussed in detail in the following subsections, respectively.

2.1   Data Collection and Process

First, we used a web crawler to collect data from "Sweet Home", a popular diabetes OHC in China. The original dataset consists of all the public posts and replies of users in the community. Then the experiment dataset derived from the original dataset after data cleaning and selection. Kang et al. [3] indicated some basic features of the text are important in social support classification. For instance, the texts including URL is more likely to provide information support. The basic features of each text include: the text length, whether the text is a post or a reply, whether the text contains URLs, whether the text contains "!", and whether the text contains "?". Finally, the experiment dataset was split into four datasets: training set, test set, forecast set, and LDA training set.

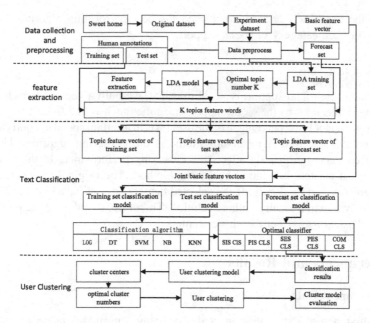

Fig. 1. Social support classification and user clustering process.

2.2 Feature Extraction Based on LDA

Then, we used LDA to extract topic features from the data set. LDA (Latent Dirichlet Allocation), namely a three-tier Bayesian probability model, is a document topic generation model, containing the three-tier structure of words, topics, and documents [10]. We referenced the research of Blei [10], which uses the perplexity as a criterion to determine the best number K of topics. After training the LDA model, we extracted more special and exclusive words from each topic as topic features. Finally, we obtained the feature libraries of K topics.

2.3 User Text Classification

After features extraction, we used the topic feature libraries to form the three k-dimensions topic feature vector. The classification model was built by combining the topic feature vector and basic feature vector. According to the social support theory [6, 7], the OHCs user text can be classified as the following five types: seeking informational support (SIS), providing informational support (PIS), seeking emotional support (SES), providing emotional support (PES), and companionship (COM). Adopting the principle of binary classification, we built a classifier for each category of social support. In order to build the best classification model, various classification algorithms, such as Logistic, Decision Tree, Naive Bayes, KNN, and SVM algorithm with different kernel function, were applied to each category of social support. Then, each model was trained 10 times with the 90% training data randomly selected from training set. At last, using the average accuracy and the average F1 (F-measure when α = 1) as the evaluation criteria, we picked the best performing algorithm to build classifiers for each category of social support.

2.4   User Clustering

After revealing the social support types of user text, we built a vector for each user by aggregating his/her texts by the social support categories such as (0.2,0.3,0.1,0.4,0). Each element in the vector is the percentage of the user texts in a certain social support category.

Furthermore, we used K-means algorithm as the clustering algorithm [11]. The number of clusters significantly affects the clustering performance. In this study, the best number of clusters is inferred by Elbow Method. The original cluster centers of K-means are selected randomly. If the selected centers are not far away, the K-means algorithm may trap in a locally optimal solution. Therefore, we adopted the principle of Maximum Distance to select the cluster centers.

3   Experiments and Results

3.1   Experiment Data

After the first step of data collecting and processing, the final datasets are shown in Table 1.

Table 1. Dataset descriptions

	Post	Reply	Total
Training set	1349	953	2302
Test set	319	141	460
Predict set	1323655	30000	1353655
Total	1325323	31094	1356417

The training set and test set need to be labeled manually. It's important to note that a text could belong to more than one of social support categories. For instance, the text, "饮食 运动 主要是运动, 你的情况和正常人一样, 要是吃了不动, 以后可真的悲催了, 少吃糖, 没事的", both belongs to the categories of PIS and PES. The results of human annotations of training set are shown in Table 2.

3.2   Feature Extraction Results

To choose the best number of topics, we calculated the perplexity with various k values (from 10 to 80). The perplexity-topic number curve is shown in Fig. 2. With the increasing of number of topics, the perplexity decreases. When the number of topics outnumbers 50, the ratio of the perplexity-topic number curve decreases significantly, which shows that the perplexity tends to be stable. Therefore, the best number of topics is determined to be 50 in this paper. Using the data set to train the LDA model, we selected 300 words that can mostly represent the topic characteristics from each topic [13]. Finally, we obtained 50 topic feature libraries.

Table 2. The number of human annotations of training set

Social support category	Number
Seeking Informational Support (SIS)	599
Providing Informational Support (PIS)	671
Seeking Emotional Support (SES)	380
Providing Emotional Support (PES)	294
Companionship(COM)	897
Total	2841

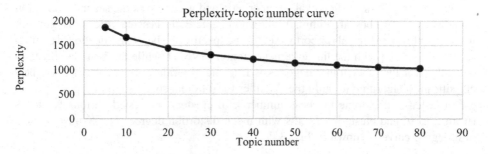

Fig. 2. The perplexity-topic number curve

3.3 User Text Classification

The performance of these algorithms on each type is shown in Table 3. In the table, the kernel functions of SVM1, SVM2, SVM3, SVM4 are the linear function, the polynomial function, the Radial Bayesian Function (RBF), and the Sigmoid function, respectively.

Table 3. Algorithm evaluation

Algorithms	Evaluation criteria	SIS	PIS	SES	PES	COM
Logistic	Accuracy	0.8711	**0.7781**	**0.9811**	**0.9611**	**0.7004**
	F1	0.7625	**0.7195**	**0.7698**	**0.7948**	**0.7934**
SVM1	Accuracy	**0.8753**	0.7768	0.9826	0.9579	0.7004
	F1	**0.7679**	0.7145	0.7648	0.7878	0.7933
SVM2	Accuracy	0.7818	0.7152	0.9826	0.9579	0.5414
	F1	0.4713	0.5440	0.6635	0.7259	0.6895
SVM3	Accuracy	0.8505	0.7690	0.9826	0.9579	0.7124
	F1	0.7487	0.6769	0.7414	0.7730	0.7918
SVM4	Accuracy	0.8497	0.7469	0.9826	0.9579	0.7078
	F1	0.7443	0.6399	0.7195	0.7593	0.7831

(*continued*)

Table 3. (*continued*)

Algorithms	Evaluation criteria	SIS	PIS	SES	PES	COM
KNN	Accuracy	0.8247	0.7321	0.9833	0.9590	0.6622
	F1	0.6789	0.6738	0.7384	0.7722	0.7898
Bayes	Accuracy	0.8666	0.7753	0.9805	0.9525	0.6961
	F1	0.7384	0.7174	0.7661	0.7939	0.7950
Decision Tree	Accuracy	0.8228	0.7026	0.9599	0.9236	0.7000
	F1	0.7399	0.7144	0.7635	0.7862	0.7777

We use the F1 as the first evaluation criteria and accuracy as the second evaluation criteria to select the best algorithm. As shown in Table 3, the best classification algorithm for different types of social support varies. To be specific, the best classification algorithm for "SIS" is SVM with the linear kernel function (SVM1), while the best classification algorithm for the other four categories is Logistic algorithm. Then, we used the best classification algorithm to build the classifier for different social support types.

In order to determine the best number k of clusters, we tested various K values (from 2 to 9) and clustering results with mean distortion degree. The K-mean distortion degree curve is shown in Fig. 3.

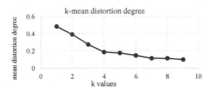

Fig. 3. K-mean distortion degree

As shown in Fig. 3, we can see that the point (4, 0.1859) is the inflection point of the curve. According to the Elbow Method, k = 4, the elbow of the curve, is the best number of clusters we need. The clustering centers are selected by the Maximization Distance principle The results of user clustering are shown in Table 4. The columns 2 to 6 separately show the proportion of each type text in each cluster. The "Total" represents the number of users in the corresponding cluster. As you can see, the proportion of "SIS" category in Cluster1 is much bigger than others, which indicates the majority of users in Cluster1 post to seek information support. According to this feature, such users can be summarized as "information demanders". In Cluster3, the proportion of "PIS" category is 92.55%, which indicates the majority of users in Cluster3 post to provide information support and can be summarized as "information sharers". Almost 96% user texts in Cluster2 belong to the "COM" category. Different from information-driven users, the users in Cluster2, whose results show that they prefer to share their life, chat with others, and make friends in the community, can be summarized as "community companions". The ratio of each category in Cluster4 is more balanced than other clusters. However, the ratio of emotional categories "SES" and "PES" is significantly higher than the first three clusters, while the ratio of informational categories of "SIS" and "PIS" is balanced distributed. The users in Cluster4 engage the community activities without a clear purpose, and can be summarized as "community walkers".

Table 4. Results of user clustering

	SIS	PIS	SES	PES	COM	Total
Cluster1	**0.7874**	0.0577	0.0008	0.0018	0.152	6447
Cluster2	0.0155	0.019	0.0032	0.0062	**0.9558**	15250
Cluster3	0.0163	**0.9255**	0.0004	0.0037	0.0538	4153
Cluster4	0.2226	0.2624	0.0669	0.0872	0.3606	13825

4 Conclusions

In this study, using Chinese text mining and machine learning techniques, we designed a Chinese text analysis process to understand social support and user engagement in OHCs. Based on a case study of an OHC among diabetics in China, we firstly classified user's texts into different social support types. Then, we found that the users in the OHC play different roles. The results showed these methods can significantly reduce the amount of human annotated data required and perform well in classification and clustering. The results can help deepen understanding of user behavior and engagement to OHCs. We believe our work has certain reference significance to analyze the user behavior of OHCs and provides instructions of user's precision management for OHCs.

However, we discovered that the amount of data about emotional support in the OHC is much smaller than other social support types.The unbalanced data distribution can further affect the accuracy of prediction and performance of clustering. In the future research, we would like to consider the effect of unbalanced data distribution and eliminate the effect by adding the data about emotional support to make the training data distribution of each social support categories to be balanced.

References

1. Eijk, M.V.D., Faber, M.J., Aarts, J.W., Kremer, J.A., Munneke, M., Bloem, B.R.: Using online health communities to deliver patient-centered care to people with chronic conditions. J. Med. Internet Res. **15**, e115 (2013)
2. Wang, X., Zuo, Z., Zhao, K.: The evolution of user roles in online health communities – a social support perspective (2015)
3. Wang, X., Zhao, K., Street, N.: Social support and user engagement in online health communities. In: Zheng, X., Zeng, D., Chen, H., Zhang, Y., Xing, C., Neill, D.B. (eds.) ICSH 2014. LNCS, vol. 8549, pp. 97–110. Springer, Cham (2014). doi:10.1007/978-3-319-08416-9_10
4. Beaudoin, C.E., Tao, C.C.: The impact of online cancer resources on the supporters of cancer patients. New Media Soc. **10**, 321–344 (2008)

5. Ba, S., Wang, L.: Digital health communities: the effect of their motivation mechanisms. Decis. Support Syst. **55**, 941–947 (2013)
6. Keating, D.M.: Spirituality and support: a descriptive analysis of online social support for depression. J. Relig. Health **52**, 1014–1028 (2013)
7. Bambina, A.: Online Social Support: The Interplay of Social Networks and Computer-Mediated Communication. Cambria Press, Youngstown (2008)
8. Lu, C.: The Parataxis Network of Chinese Grammer. The Business Publisher, Beijing (2001). (in Chinese)
9. Chen, Z., Zhang, G.: Study on the text mining and chinese text mining framework. Inform. Sci. **25**, 1046–1051 (2007). (in Chinese)
10. Blei, D.M., Ng, A.Y., Jordan, M.I., Lafferty, J.: Latent Dirichlet allocation. J. Mach. Learn. Res. **3**, 993–1022 (2003)
11. Jain, A.K., Dubes, R.C.: Algorithms for Clustering Data. Prentice-Hall, Inc. (1988)
12. Rousseeuw, P.J.: Silhouettes: a graphical aid to the interpretation and validation of cluster analysis. J. Comput. Appl. Math. **20**, 53–65 (1987)
13. Sievert, C., Shirley, K.E.: LDAvis: a method for visualizing and interpreting topics. In: The Workshop on Interactive Language Learning, Visualization, and Interfaces at the Association for Computational Linguistics (2014)

Mining User Intents in Online Interactions: Applying to Discussions About Medical Event on SinaWeibo Platform

Chenxi Cui[1,2(✉)], Wenji Mao[1,2], Xiaolong Zheng[1], and Daniel Zeng[1,2]

[1] State Key Laboratory of Management and Control for Complex Systems, Institute of Automation, Chinese Academy of Sciences, Beijing, China
{cuichenxi2014,wenji.mao,xiaolong.zheng,dajun.zeng}@ia.ac.cn
[2] School of Computer and Control Engineering, University of Chinese Academy of Sciences, Beijing, China

Abstract. Mining user intents in online interactive behavior from social media data can effectively identify users' motives behind communication and provide valuable information to aid medical decision-making and improve services. However, it is a challenging task due to the ambiguous semantic, irregular expressions and obscure intention classification categories. In this paper, we first define user intent categories based on speech act theory. On the basis of this, we develop a novel method to further classify users' utterances according to their pragmatic functions. First, we design topic independent features by regularizing the utterance and categorizing the textual features. Then, we build a hierarchical model based on Hidden Markov Model (HMM) [1] to mine user intents in context sequence at both sentence and microblog level. Finally, we construct a dataset of microblogs about hot topics related to the medical event by a semi-automatic method. Experimental study shows the effectiveness of our method.

Keywords: User intention recognition · Speech act theory · Online communication · Markov multinomial model · Medical event

1 Introduction

Social media provides the major platform for people to discuss various issues through online interactions. Topics about medical events, and especially medical disputes, often provoke hot discussions. Mining communicative purposes from online discussions of medical events can help effectively identify users' motives and intents providing valuable information to improve services, ease doctor-patient relationship, and facilitate medical decision-making according to public demands.

Different from topic detection concerned with affairs and sentiment analysis concerned with polarities, mining user intents in online interactions pays more attention to current actions and future results. For example, in a microblog "Black-hearted hospital should publish video evidence!" topic detection concerns the subject "video evidence"; sentiment analysis concerns the negative feeling expressed with "black-hearted". Differently, intention mining focuses on the action "should publish". By mining directive

H. Chen et al. (Eds.): ICSH 2017, LNCS 10347, pp. 177–183, 2017.
https://doi.org/10.1007/978-3-319-67964-8_17

intent from the microblog, the hospital can quickly notice this public demand and adjust strategy to fulfill it.

Although recently, recognizing user intents in online interactions has been studied, it is usually confined to the particular application domain and corpus. Existing research on mining user intents in online communication has focused on two specific domains, search query [2, 3] and commercial purchase [4, 5]. Recent work [6, 7] applies user intention recognition from social media data, using domain-dependent intent classification scheme. Different from the previous research, our work aims to recognize users' communicative intents in online interactions by proposing a computational method and apply it to the medical related domain which has abundant online data resources.

However, recognizing user intents from online communication in social media platform is challenging due to the ambiguous semantic, irregular expressions and obscure categories. To deal with the challenges, in this paper, we identify user intent categories in online interactions based on speech act theory and propose a method to mine user intents. Firstly, we design features and employ a filtering process to characterize topic independent features. Then, we build a hierarchical model based on HMM that captures user intent types at both sentence level and microblog level. We apply this model to a microblog dataset about a medical event in China. The training data is generated by a semi-automatic label method and experimental study shows the effectiveness of our proposed method.

2   Related Works

2.1   Speech Acts and Chinese Sentence Patterns

Speech act theory is a subfield of pragmatics concerned with the ways in which words can be used not only to present information but also to carry out actions [8]. Founded by Austin [8] and further developed by Searle [9], speech acts are traditionally classified into five broad categories [9]: directive, commissive, expressive, representative, and declarative.

The speech act coding schemes can help identifying the speaker's intent in an utterance. According to Wu [10], the function of sentences is the intention of speech act. He reasons out 8 functional categories of Chinese sentences, including declarative, statement, directive, interrogative, expressive, provocative, commissive, and cooperative. Inspired by this, in our work, we define user intents based on this classification scheme and classify users' utterances according to their pragmatic functions.

2.2   Intention Recognition

Intention recognition is an essential component of text mining applications. It has been widely studied in AI field to detect agent's behavior in relatively close-systems, typically with predefined plan libraries. With the rapid development of social media platforms and online communication, recognizing user intents in online interactions has become an important research issue in text mining research and applications.

Current work on user intention mining in online communication and social media analytics is carried out in limited domains. Query intention mining focuses on expanding query characteristics and recovering semantics because data in search engine log usually lacks complete utterance. External knowledge is taken into consideration, such as Q&A websites [2] and users' feedback [3]. Purchase intention mining focuses on recognizing product entity [4] and judging users' consumption intents by means of natural language processing (NLP) methods [5].

Recent work applies user intention recognition to more general social media domain, but the definition of the intent classification scheme is still dependent on the specific domain. Wang et al. [6] propose a method to recognize six daily life intents from intent twitter, like "I want/plan to". Another work on Twitter identifies two specific intents "seeking" and "offering" help for crisis rescue application [7]. Different from aforementioned research, our work aims to recognize users' communicative intents in online interactions according to the pragmatic functions, which are more general.

3   User Intent Categories in Online Interactions

According to the speech act theory [8], speech is a kind of action with certain intent. On this view, we associate users' communicative intents with speech acts and define the categories of user intents exhibited in online texts. We examine the taxonomy of speech acts manifested in online texts by reviewing a large number of microblogs and divide user intents into nine broad categories. Besides, we also identify subcategories within each broad one. The categories are described as following (Table 1):

Table 1. Description of user intent categories in online interactions.

Intent categories	Description
Directive (D_1)	Want the others (not) to do something, including subcategories: general directive and moral directive. The moral directive force others to act through moral power
Question (Q)	Ask for information, including subcategories: yes-or-no question, alternative question, and specific questions
Statement (S)	Narrate events, describes something or explains relations, including subcategories: narration, description, and explanation
Comment (C_1)	Evaluate the possibility or necessity of something by subjective judgment, including subcategories: assertion, speculation, and prediction
Desire (D_2)	Describe one's desire/wish or plan of doing something
Commissive (C_2)	Promise (not) to do something in the future
Expressive (E_1)	Express his/her feelings or attitudes with polarity about something, including subcategories: sentiment and evaluation
Provocative (P)	Inspire certain emotions in others, including subcategories: blame and manners
Declarative (D_3)	Announce objective information

4   Features Representation

We use a filtering process to remove redundancy and characterize topic independent features. Inspired by the previous filtering work [11], we first regularize the utterance into grammatical skeletons as subject, object, predicate, attributive and tone.

Considering semantics, grammar and pragmatics, we then represent terms/phrases features in each skeletons with different attributes using external knowledge sources, including LIWC (Linguistic Inquiry and Word Count) dictionary [13] and HowNet [14]. We design feature classes according to the following attributes: personal pronoun (first/second/third), tense (past/present/future), modality (dynamic/deontic/epistemic), sentimental polarity (evaluation/emotion/positive/negative), objective degree and other special attributes like interrogative, temporal, positional, etc.

In terms of the corpus statistical property, we find the objective class contains more entity nouns (such as dates, organizations, and places) but fewer sentiment adjectives. So, we calculate the objective degree as (1) and characterize it as an objective person if the score is above a certain threshold.

$$S_{obj} = (C_e - C_s)/(C_w) \tag{1}$$

Where S_{obj} denotes the score of objective degree, C_e, C_s and C_w denote the count of entity nouns, sentiment adjectives and words, respectively.

We also distinguish performative verbs [12], modal particles, punctuations, manner words and dirty words since non-illocutionary meanings, intonations and idioms are important in intention recognition. Finally, we represent each feature with a three-tuple (feature class, grammatical class, position in syntax tree).

5   Hierarchical Model for User Intention Mining

HMM is a statistical model which describes the system using a Markov process with hidden states [1]. Since intents are not observable but can be inferred from linguistic characters, HMM is very suitable to describe our problem. In detail, we describe inter-active intents implied in each sentence from a document as hidden states and the utterances represented with features as observable states. Moreover, as a sequence learning model, HMM can represent both the sentences of context in a single microblog and the microblogs in a whole dialog with a sequence of states.

On the basis of this, we build a Hierarchical Model based on HMM. The model consists of two layers (see Fig. 1). The upper layer HMM aims to recognize user intent categories in each microblog. Each hidden state in upper layer represents an intent category in one microblog, which we called intent. The lower layer HMM aims to recognize user intent categories in each sentence. Each hidden state in lower layer represents an intent category in one sentence, which we called sub-intent. Since one microblog consists of several sentences, each hidden state in upper layer is naturally coupled with one Markov process of hidden states in lower layer. Each observable state is a sentence utterance represented with features we design.

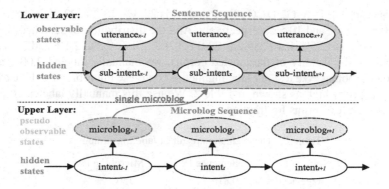

Fig. 1. Hierarchical model for user intention mining.

In general, the model describes a physical process of intention comprehension and expression: When user expresses an intent with a microblog in dialog, the audience first observes utterances composed of words. Then, audience captures a sequence of sub-intents by reading the microblog sentence by sentence. Finally, the audience understands the main intent in the whole microblog by summarizing the sub-intents. To continue the dialog, the audience can express another intent and start a new round. The task of intention mining corresponds to the decoding process [1] of hidden intent states according to observable utterance states. We can train model with the Baum-Welch algorithm and recognize user intents using decoding process with Viterbi algorithm [1].

6 Experiment

6.1 Datasets and Labeling Strategy

We crawl microblogs about a hot medical topic during 2016 from SinaWeibo, the most popular microblog platform in China. They cover a variety of discussions on medical events about "Maternal death in Peking University Third Hospital". After spam filtering and preprocessing, we get totally 35,128 microblogs for our analysis.

By reviewed a large number of microblogs and studied taxonomy, we annotate the microblogs with a semi-automatic method based on the intent classification scheme. Given a seed set of the intent markers in each category according to [10], for example, "you should", "I wonder", "In my opinion", we classify sentences into different intent categories. Then, we extract frequently co-occur phrases using sentence sets within each category. We examine the extracted phrases and regarded them as new intent markers for classifying. For instance, we extract phrase "by the report" using intent maker "Xinhua News reported" as they always appear together. This new phrase is kept as an intent marker of "declarative" by manual examination.

Through this iterative process, we extract many intent markers. Finally, we get a labeled corpus consisting of 81,097 sentences within 25,374 microblogs. Further, we use some simple priority rules to label intent categories for microblogs according to intent categories in sentences of microblog. The distribution of microblogs for each intent category D_1, Q, S, C_1, D_2, C_2, E_1, P and D_3 is 22.3%, 13.2%, 22.7%, 34.8%, 1.4%, 6.6%, 10.6%, 6.4% and 10.5%, respectively. And the distribution of sentences for each intent category is 12.5%, 8.4%, 39.2%, 22.0%, 0.4%, 2.1%, 9.8%, 2.1% and 3.5%.

To verify the validity of the labeled corpus, we manually labeled 2,000 random sampled microblogs. We test our labeling method on these microblogs and the average accuracy is pretty high as shown in Table 2. We use this manually labeled corpus for testing and the rest corpus for training.

Table 2. The evaluation result of labeling strategy.

Level	Sentence level	Microblog level
Average accuracy	0.819	0.750

6.2 Evaluation

With F1 value as performance metric, we compare our method with other classifiers (Logistic Regression, Decision Tree, and SVM) on both sentence and microblog level (Table 3).

Table 3. Performance Comparison with Other Methods (in terms of F1 value).

Intent categories	Sentence level				Microblog level			
	LR	DT	SVM	Our method	LR	DT	SVM	Our method
Directive (D_1)	0.685	0.692	0.734	**0.742**	0.673	0.670	**0.674**	0.654
Question (Q)	0.663	0.733	0.773	**0.790**	0.622	0.602	0.655	**0.731**
Statement (S)	0.614	0.583	0.595	**0.691**	0.604	0.561	0.590	**0.651**
Comment (C_1)	0.561	0.595	0.581	**0.683**	0.545	0.582	0.552	**0.673**
Desire (D_2)	0.613	0.640	0.591	**0.641**	0.613	**0.640**	0.593	0.530
Commissive (C_2)	0.665	**0.705**	0.635	0.667	0.665	**0.706**	0.635	0.679
Expressive (E_1)	0.667	0.614	**0.701**	0.690	0.666	0.621	**0.695**	0.661
Provocative (P)	0.734	0.740	**0.800**	0.784	0.678	0.720	0.642	**0.794**
Declarative (D_3)	0.832	0.832	0.832	**0.835**	0.832	0.831	0.832	**0.838**
Macro-average	0.670	0.682	0.694	**0.725**	0.655	0.659	0.652	**0.690**

We note that the performance on sentence level is better than microblog level since the features in one sentence are more concise and the training dataset on sentence level is more precise. We also find "desire", "commissive" and "expressive" categories don't achieve better results. It is worth noting that "directive" performs better at sentence level but weaker at microblog level. But "provocative" is the opposite.

The results provide several insights of user intention mining in medical events. First, users express self-related intents (desire/commissive/expressive) through clear expressions without being affected by context. Second, "directive" intent is implied in rich context but independent of dialogue sequence. Third, "provocative" intent has a strong correlation with dialogue sequence. And from the intent category distribution, we note that users express "statement" and "comment" intents to share their knowledge, experiences and opinions in most of the time. Moreover, "directive" and "question" takes a large proportion which need someone to solve and answer. So, we can infer that medical organizations can avoid negative attitudes of users by guiding the conversation online, such as providing the solution, answering the question and responding with politeness.

7 Conclusions and Future Work

In this paper, we explore user intents in online interactions based on speech act theory and propose a method to mine user intent categories. We first use a filtering process to represent features according to grammatical and semantic factors. Then, we propose a hierarchical model to mine user intents at sentence and microblog levels. Finally, we apply the model to a microblog dataset about an influential medical event on SinaWeibo platform. The experimental study demonstrates the effectiveness of our method. One limitation of our method we have presented is that the labeling method still requires a lot of manual examination of key terms. Going forward, we hope to address the limitation to automatically generate key terms suitable for different domains.

References

1. Rabiner, L., Juang, B.: An introduction to hidden Markov models. ASSP Mag. IEEE **3**(1), 4–16 (1986)
2. Tsur, G., Pinter, Y., Szpektor, I., Carmel, D.: Identifying web queries with question intent. In: International Conference on World Wide Web, pp. 783–793 (2016)
3. Yang, Y., Tang, J.: Beyond query: interactive user intention understanding. In: IEEE International Conference on Data Mining, pp. 519–528 (2015)
4. Fu, B., Liu, T.: Identifying consumption target in microblog based on cross social media search. J. Front. Comput. Sci. Technol. **9**, 1247–1255 (2015)
5. Gupta, V., Varshney, D., Jhamtani, H., et al.: Identifying purchase intent from social posts. In: International Conference on Weblogs and Social Media, pp. 180–186 (2014)
6. Wang, J., Cong, G., Zhao, X.W., Li, X.: Mining user intents in twitter: a semi-supervised approach to inferring intent categories for microblog. In: 29th AAAI Conference on Artificial Intelligence, pp. 318–324 (2015)
7. Purohit, H., Dong, G., Shalin, V.L., Thirunarayan, K., Sheth, A.P.: Intent classification of short-text on social media. In: 2015 IEEE International Conference on Smart City/SocialCom/SustainCom (SmartCity), pp. 222–228 (2015)
8. Austin, J.L.: How to do Things with Words. Oxford University Press, London (1975)
9. Searle, J.R., Kiefer, F., Bierwisch, M.: Speech Act Theory and Pragmatics, vol. 10. Springer, Dordrecht (1980). doi:10.1007/978-94-009-8964-1. Synthese language library
10. Wu, J.: Speech acts and Chinese sentence patterns, Doctoral dissertation, East China Normal University (2006)
11. Han, X., Zhao, T.: Two-fold filtering for Chinese subcategorization acquisition with diathesis alternations used as heuristic information. Inst. Comput. Linguist. **11**(2), 101–114 (2006)
12. Vanderveken, D., MacQueen, K.: Semantic analysis of English performative verbs. In: Meaning and Speech Acts, vol. 1, pp. 166–219 (1990)
13. Huang, C.L., Chung, C.K., Hui, N., Lin, Y.C., Seih, Y.T., Chen, W.C., Pennebaker, J.W.: The development of the Chinese linguistic inquiry and word count dictionary. Chin. J. Psychol. **54**, 185–201 (2012)
14. Dong, Z., Dong, Q.: Introduction to HowNet (2002). http://www.keenage.com

Online Health Communities the Impact of Social Support on the Health State of People with Chronic Illness

Zachary Davis[✉], Qianzhou Du, G. Alan Wang, Christopher Zobel, and Lara Khansa

Department of Business Information Technology,
Pamplin College of Business Virginia Tech, Blacksburg, VA 24060, USA
zached1@vt.edu

Abstract. People with chronic illnesses are engaged in the lifelong management of their disease and with this management comes the need for emotional support, informational support, and companionship from others, particularly those who have the same disease and can relate to their situation. More often people are seeking this social support through online health communities. The concern is that online health communities may not have a positive impact on the health condition since anyone can be providing information and the information provided may not be valid. We utilize an objective measure of the health condition to determine the impact social support, given and received, in an online health community has on the user's health condition over time.

Keywords: Social support · Online health community · Chronic illness

1 Introduction

At some point, not too many years ago, people sought healthcare information primarily from their doctor, or from family and friends if they happened to have some knowledge or experience with the illness or disease. However, with the ready availability of information and support through the internet this practice is rapidly changing. Online health communities are now allowing people to reach out and "talk" to large quantities of people who have the same condition for advice on management and to seek support (Fan et al. 2014). Beyond being a bit like social media, online health communities have benefits to users including being a source of education, emotional support, and information specific to the focus of the community. Online health communities provide a place for people with the disease, caregivers, and healthcare providers to interact in a non-threatening environment (Yan and Tan 2014). An online health community provides users the ability to connect with others with similar struggles and interests regarding disease management and the ability to do so is changing how people approach their care. Previous research has examined the social support received in online health communities and our research seeks to extend this by examining the impact that the social support received from an online health community has on a user's health condition. With this information, healthcare providers can better inform and expand the resources available to patients with chronic illnesses regarding their need for social support.

© Springer International Publishing AG 2017
H. Chen et al. (Eds.): ICSH 2017, LNCS 10347, pp. 184–188, 2017.
https://doi.org/10.1007/978-3-319-67964-8_18

2   Literature Review

We conducted a search in the literature examining the use of text analytics in online health communities. The majority of previous studies have examined the trustworthiness of the information shared in online health communities, which is logical since many people seek health advice from these sources. Fan et al. (2014) examined how trust is established in online health communities. They utilized variance theories and devised a three-step process for how trust is established in this environment. In an online health community, trust is essential as people seek advice and support in managing their disease. Similarly, Chomphoosang et al. (2012) examined online health communities to develop a method that people could use to determine the trustworthiness of a post. Yan and Tan (2014) examined the effects of sharing in online health communities focused on mental health. They found that social support had a positive effect on a patient's overall health, including an improved mental status. Batenburg and Das (2011) examined the effect of the sharing of negative experiences in online health communities and found that although the emotional response increases during the sharing, it results in feelings of well-being in the end if a response is received, even if the response is not necessarily worded in the way we would traditionally think is acceptable.

Previous research regarding online health communities has primarily been qualitative in nature, utilizing survey responses for the analysis (Zhao et al. 2014; Johnston et al. 2013; Welbourne et al. 2013). Yan and Tan (2014) provide an example of a method that is more quantitative, utilizing Partially Observed Markov Decision Process to examine a user's posts. We seek to extend this research by examining a more objective measure of the health condition and comparing this to the social support received in the online health community.

3   Modeling Framework

As we seek to examine the impact social support received in an online health community has on the users' health condition we created a model to depict this (see Fig. 1).

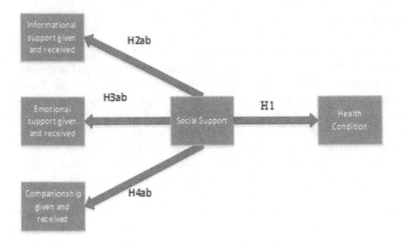

Fig. 1. Model

Following the model creation, we devise the following hypothesis:

Hypothesis 1: *Social support given and received in an online health community positively impacts a change in the user's health condition.*
Hypothesis 2: *Informational support given and received in an online health community
positively impacts the social support of the online health community.*
Hypothesis 3: *Emotional support given and received in an online health community
positively impacts the social support of the online health community.*
Hypothesis 4: *Companionship given and received in an online health community positively impacts the social support of the online health community.*

By examining the various aspects identified as social support and matching it to
participants in the online health community, we then examine the health condition and
compare these values to determine the change in the health condition, whether positive,
negative, or neutral and the extent to which the social support was impactful.

4 Methodology

In this paper we conduct our research on the online health community, http://www.diabe-
ticconnect.com/, which allows for the interaction of users allowing them to share information about the medical devices they use, diet plans, laboratory values and medications
as well as offer social support to one another. To obtain the data we utilized a web
crawling script that collected all fields and post data from every user on the health social
media site and extracted these data values to an excel CSV file. To analyze the model
we use RStudio Version 0.99.896 and structural equation modelling package sem. We
utilized a reflective causal structure whereby the latent variables of social support and
health condition flow to the indicator variables. The relationship between the indicator
variables and latent variables are presented in Table 1.

Table 1. Indicator variables

Indicator variable	Latent variable	Description
Emotional support received	Social support	The emotional support the user has received
Emotional support given	Social support	The emotional support the user has given
Informational support received	Social support	The informational support the user has received
Informational support given	Social support	The informational support the user has given
Companionship received	Social support	The companionship the user has received
Companionship given	Social support	The companionship the user has given
Healthy	Health condition	Binary variable: 1 = healthy value, 0 = unhealthy value
Lab value	Health condition	The last lab value the user posted
Delta lab value	Health condition	The change in overall lab values of the user since using the online community

5   Results

The results of the structural equation model analysis are presented in Table 2.

Table 2. SEM results

Hypothesis	Path	Estimate	Std error	Z value	Pr (>|z|)
1	Social support -> health condition	−0.088	0.051	−1.722	0.085
	Health condition -> lab value	1.663	0.107	15.583	<0.001
	Health condition -> delta lab value	1.337	0.177	7.537	<0.001
	Health condition -> healthy	−0.343	0.029	−11.744	<0.001
2a	Social support -> informational support received	35.751	1.553	23.014	<0.001
2b	Social support -> informational support given	8.706	1.057	8.240	<0.001
3a	Social support -> emotional support received	20.075	0.911	22.034	<0.001
3b	Social support -> emotional support given	4.232	0.496	8.538	<0.001
4a	Social support -> companionship received	22.106	0.878	25.169	<0.001
4b	Social support -> companionship given	6.392	0.778	8.24	<0.001

We can see from Table 2 that each of the paths of the indicator variables yields very significant results. The most interesting path we observed exists between the latent variables Social Support and Health Condition. We can see that at the 90% confidence level the users' health condition improves by about 0.08 with participation in the online health community.

6 Implications

Our study has many managerial implications for online health community providers, healthcare professionals, and patients with a chronic illness. First, providers can develop mechanisms to encourage social support behaviors, which lead to an improvement in the health condition for people managing a chronic illness. Second, our findings inform health professionals about the importance of community support and the relevance of receiving this support through participation in an online health community. Lastly, patients may respond differently to the support they receive in an online health community. Our research allows healthcare professionals to provide better education for patients so that they can respond to social support in a positive manner.

References

Batenburg, A., Das, E.: 'I Know How You Feel': Effects of Cognitive and Emotional Sharing of Negative Experiences in Online Support Groups. Etmaal van de Communicatiewetenschap (2011)

Chomphoosang, P., Durresi, A., Durresi, M., Barolli, L.: Trust management of social networks in health care. In: 15th International Conference on Network-Based Information Systems (NBiS), pp. 392–396. IEEE, November 2012

Fan, H., Lederman, R., Smith, S.P., Chang, S.: How trust is formed in online health communities: a process perspective. Commun. Assoc. Inf. Syst. 34(1), 28 (2014)

Johnston, A.C., Worrell, J.L., Di Gangi, P.M., Wasko, M.: Online health communities: an assessment of the influence of participation on patient empowerment outcomes. Inf. Technol. People 26(2), 213–235 (2013)

Welbourne, J.L., Blanchard, A.L., Wadsworth, M.B.: Motivations in virtual health communities and their relationship to community, connectedness and stress. Comput. Hum. Behav. 29(1), 129–139 (2013)

Yan, L., Tan, Y.: Feeling blue? Go online: an empirical study of social support among patients. Inf. Syst. Res. 25(4), 690–709 (2014)

Zhao, K., Yen, J., Greer, G., Qiu, B., Mitra, P., Portier, K.: Finding influential users of online health communities: a new metric based on sentiment influence. J. Am. Med. Inform. Assoc. 21(e2), e212–e218 (2014)

Predictive Diagnosis

Deep Learning Through Two-Branch Convolutional Neuron Network for Glaucoma Diagnosis

Yidong Chai[1(✉)], Luo He[1], Qiuyan Mei[1], Hongyan Liu[1(✉)], and Liang Xu[2(✉)]

[1] School of Economics and Management, Tsinghua University, Beijing, China
chaiyd@yeah.net, hell6@mails.tsinghua.edu.cn, mei_qiuyan@qq.com,
liuhy@sem.tsinghua.edu.cn
[2] Tongren Hospital, Beijing, China
xlbio@yahoo.cn

Abstract. Glaucoma is a group of eye diseases that damage the optic nerves progressively and lead to deterioration in vision irreversibly. Diagnosing glaucoma based on retinal images automatically is meaningful both in practice and research area. While deep learning models have achieved superior performance in natural images recognition and have been also used for medical image diagnosis recently, the models usually rely on large dataset and expensive computing resources, thus limiting the wider use in medical areas. So how to train a deep learning model with relatively small amount of medical data is challenging. In this paper, we propose to incorporate domain knowledge to construct a two-branch Convolutional Neural Networks (CNN) to learn a classifier for glaucoma diagnosis based on the retinal image. Our two-branch CNN framework can analyze the whole image and pay special attention to discriminative local region of image at the same time. Experiments conducted on real medical dataset demonstrate the advantages of our method over traditional computer vision algorithm and classical CNN.

Keywords: Deep learning · Convolutional neuron networks · Domain knowledge · Glaucoma diagnosis · Medical image analysis

1 Introduction

Glaucoma is a group of complicated eye diseases that damage the optic nerve and affect peripheral vision [1]. It is the second biggest cause of blindness [2] and about 44.7 million people in the world were diagnosed with glaucoma in 2010 [3]. The figure is expected to rise to 58.6 million by 2020 [3]. The most common type of glaucoma is open-angle glaucoma, which develops slowly over time without pain, making it difficult to detect [1]. However, when the damage reaches to a degree that people feel uncomfortable, it is often too late and some severe consequences are inevitable. So the glaucoma is called "silent theft of eyesight" [4]. The disease has some common traits including high eye pressure, damage to the optic nerve, large cup to disc ratio, and gradual vision loss [1]. Currently, there is no cure for glaucoma, but early diagnosis and treatment is very important to prevent becoming worse. For example, if people are

© Springer International Publishing AG 2017
H. Chen et al. (Eds.): ICSH 2017, LNCS 10347, pp. 191–201, 2017.
https://doi.org/10.1007/978-3-319-67964-8_19

diagnosed with glaucoma at the early stage, they can control the eye pressure to prevent further vision loss [5].

Since doctor diagnosis process is costly and prone to error, some researches have been conducted to diagnose glaucoma automatically [5]. The prior research can be divided into two types. The first type segments glaucoma-related tissues such as the cup, disc, vessels and calculates features for classification [6, 7]. The second type applies computer vision algorithm to extract features such as textural features, higher order spectra features, wavelet features and trains classifiers such as SVM to get the result [8, 9].

With the development of deep learning, many impressive models have been proposed for image classification and object detection [10–13]. Recently, some studies have shown that analyzing medical image data automatically using deep learning algorithms can achieve good performance in medical diagnosis [14, 15]. However, these models are like a black-box and it is not easy to incorporate domain knowledge to them. They can work quite well when the data and the computing resource is so rich that we can build a rather complicated model to analyze enough useful features purely from data. However, the expensive computing resources and rich data are not available in some circumstances, which restrains wider use of deep learning. For example, when it comes to some medical images, the deep learning models sometimes perform relatively unsatisfying as inadequate data bounds the complexity of the model. Although Gulshan et al. [14] have applied deep learning to create an algorithm for automated detection of diabetic retinopathy and diabetic macular edema using more than 12,000 retinal images, such a large dataset cannot be obtained by everyone. What's more, some diseases are not very common, thus generating a limited amount of medical images. Long et al. [15] applied the deep learning model in a rare disease with hundreds of images. They applied transfer learning to build the model based on a model that has been trained using natural images. However, fine-tuning is not enough to mitigate this problem in some circumstances. In this paper, we study how to train an effective classifier based on a relatively small number of images, spending relatively less computation resource. Our solution takes advantage of domain knowledge. For example, not all part of medical images is useful for detection of a particular disease. To be specific, some tissues are more discriminative for a disease and their small change in appearance may lead to obviously different results. On the contrary, some tissues are not very important and different shapes do not mean a lot for specific diseases. Therefore, the information contained in different regions of medical image is uneven and some parts contain much more discriminative information than others. In such cases, we should pay more attention to the region containing discriminative information than other regions.

In this paper, we propose a deep-learning model incorporating medical domain knowledge. It can analyze the whole image and the discriminative region of the retinal images at the same time. Given the fact that the discriminative information for diagnosis of the glaucoma is mainly contained in the disc region, we propose to analyze the whole image and the local disc region simultaneously. To this end, a two-step approach is developed. First, an important local region of the medical image is extracted using a deep learning algorithm. And then a new two-branch convolutional neural network is proposed to analyze the extracted local region and the whole image simultaneously.

The main contribution of our paper is that we propose a two-branch convolutional neuron network model for glaucoma diagnosis by incorporating medical domain knowledge into the deep learning model. The model outperforms classical convolutional neuron networks using only a relatively small number of training data and spending less computational resource.

The remainder of the paper is organized as follows. In Sect. 2, we give a review of related works. Section 3 introduces our model in detail. We report on our experiments and results in Sect. 4. We conclude this paper in the last section.

2 Related Work

2.1 Glaucoma Diagnosis

The localization of Optic Disc is the initial step for many further tasks such as locating other anatomical structures and extracting the Optic Disc boundary. Chaudhuri et al. [16] noticed that the Optic Disc region is the brightest region on the retinal image, so they detected it by thresholding out the pixels with the intensity values below a certain level. Lalonde et al. [17] proposed an Optic Disc center detection method by combining a Hausdorff-based template matching technique and the pyramidal decomposition for large-scale object tracking.

Many efforts have been made to diagnose glaucoma based on the retinal images automatically. The methods proposed can be divided into two types. One is segmentation-based approach, usually including Optic Disc detection. These methods make use of medical knowledge and try to get some common glaucoma features such as cup, disc, RNFL defect and so on. Nayak et al. [6] applied morphological operations on the green channel of RGB images to segment Optic Disc and cup, which were used to calculate cup to disc ratio for glaucoma diagnosis. Babu and Shenbagadevi [7] used fuzzy c-means clustering on the wavelet transformed green plane image after removal of blood vessels. They calculated the cup to disc ratio values and compared them with those of golden standard obtained from the ophthalmologists for glaucoma classification. Lee et al. [18] also used the green plane of the retinal images for glaucoma diagnosis. They detected intensity decrease around the Optic Disc for RNFL detection, which is also a common trait of glaucoma. The other type is non-segmentation based methods. Dua et al. [8] trained a range of classifiers, including support vector machine, sequential minimal optimization, random forest, and naive Bayes classification models, based on the wavelet-based energy features which were calculated from various wavelet filters. Mookiah et al. [9] calculated higher order spectra (HOS) and discrete wavelet transform (DWT) features from retinal images and trained SVM classifier for automated classification of normal and glaucoma images. Yadav et al. [19] calculated texture features from the area localized around the optic cup in the retinal images. After that, they trained neural network classifier on the extracted features for image classification.

However, there are three drawbacks in the previous works. First, for the segmentation-based methods, the segmentation of some tissues such as cup is challenging and the mistake in segmentation can accumulate to lead to poor results in classifications. Second, the non-segmentation based methods fail to make use of medical knowledge and the process is like a black box. Finally, both of them cannot make full use of the image data compared with deep learning models that have shown great advantages in image processing.

2.2 Deep Learning Models

Deep learning has achieved superior results in a wide range of fields, especially in computer vision. Since the impressive results were achieved from Alexnet in ImageNet Large Scale Visual Recognition Competition (ILSVRC) in 2012 [10], many successful models such as VGG net [11], GoogLenet [12], Deep Residual Net [13] have appeared and demonstrated the advantages of deep learning over traditional methods. Besides images classification, various deep learning models have been proposed for a wide range of tasks such as object detection [20], semantic segmentation [21], instance segmentation [22], image annotation [23] and so on.

Inspired by the superior performance of deep learning models, many researchers have designed or transferred the deep learning models to medical research. Xu et al. [24] extracted feature representation through deep learning and proposed the multiple instances learning (MIL) framework in classification. They conducted experiments on dataset consisting of colon cancer histopathology images and concluded that automatic feature learning outperforms manually constructed featured. Bar et al. [25] used a CNN that was trained with ImageNet and then transferred it to the medical field to identify different types of pathologies in chest x-ray images. The results they got, an area under curve (AUC) of 0.79 for classification between healthy and abnormal chest x-ray, showed that deep learning with large-scale non-medical image databases can be transferred for general medical image recognition tasks. Gulshan et al. [14] built a deep learning model for automated detection of diabetic retinopathy and diabetic macular edema in retinal fundus images and achieved a high sensitivity and specificity. Long et al. [15] adopted transfer learning to design a model based on the championship model in ILSVRC 2014 for accurate diagnosis and provided treatment decisions for a rare disease, congenital cataracts. Chen et al. [26] designed and trained convolutional neuron networks on ORIGA and SCES datasets for glaucoma diagnosis and got better results than state-of-the-art algorithms. Although these researchers have achieved better results, their proposed models are usually very complicated to avoid overfitting. Transfer learning can help mitigate the limited medical images problem. However, it works unsatisfactorily sometimes. What's more, they treated each part of the images equally and failed to make use of medical knowledge.

3   Model

Glaucoma has some common traits including larger Cup-to-Disc ratio, Retinal Nerve Fibre Layer Detection (RNFLD), Peripapillary Atrophy (PPA) and vasculature hemorrhage [1]. All of these can be concluded from the Optic Disc region. So the Optic Disc region, though relatively small, contains much more discriminative information than other regions. This domain knowledge inspires us to design a model that analyzes the whole image, and at the same time, pay more attention to the Optic Disc region. We achieve this by designing a two-branch convolutional neuron network to analyze both the whole image and the Optic Disc region automatically extracted by another deep learning model.

Figure 1 shows the whole framework of our proposed method for glaucoma diagnosis.

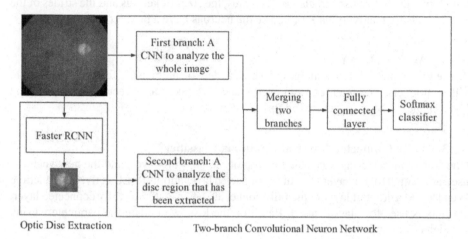

Optic Disc Extraction   Two-branch Convolutional Neuron Network

Fig. 1. The framework of our model

3.1 Optic Disc Region Extraction

To obtain discriminative information of retinal fundus images, we need to extract the region of interest, the Optic Disc region. A technical method to achieve this goal is to conduct object detection. We choose *Faster-RCNN* to complete this task [20]. *Faster-RCNN* can be divided into two stages. The first stage is region proposal stage, which is fed with an image as an input and outputs a set of rectangular object proposals. The second stage is object detection stage, which uses the object proposals to produce the rectangle boxes of the object. *Faster-RCNN* accelerates the test time of the first stage by taking the advantage of GPU, so real-time object detection goal can be achieved [20]. What's more, *Faster-RCNN* is one of the state-of-art methods in the field of object detection.

3.2 Two-Branch Neuron Networks

We design a two-branch convolutional neuron network. One branch is used to analyze the whole image and the other is to analyze the extracted region. Then we concatenate the two branches by combining the features extracted from each one. Following that, we add one fully connected layer for classification.

3.2.1   Branch of the Model

Each branch is a classical convolutional neuron network that contains five convolutional layers. We also add dropout layer and max pooling layer to avoid over-fitting problem [10]. Rectified Linear Units (ReLU) activation function is applied to the output of each neuron, which has been proved to perform better than sigmoid function [10]. As we hope the branch that deals with the whole images focuses on the global features and that deals with Optic Disc regions extracts local features, the sizes of kernels and the strides of the first branch are relatively larger to make the neurons have a broader receptive filed.

3.2.2   Merging Layer

At the top of each branch, a merging layer is added to combine the features extracted in different levels. The features from each branch are taken as a vector, so the merging layer connects the two vectors and forms a new vector.

3.2.3   Fully Connected Layer and Softmax Classifier

One fully connected layer is added on top of the merging layer, and the new vector is used as an input for the layer. The fully connected layer adopts ReLU activation function. We also add a dropout layer to the fully connected layer. After the fully connected layer, softmax is used for classification. Based on the loss, we update the parameters using Adadelta as optimizers.

Figure 2 shows the framework of the two-branch neuron network. Each branch contains 5 convolutional layers. "C1: Feature maps 32, 7 * 7 * 3" means there are 32 kernel layers of size 7 * 7 * 3 in the first convolutional layer. The network structures of the two branches are similar except that the sizes of kernels and strides in the first branch are relatively larger. The sizes of the kernels of that branch are 7 * 7 * 3, 5 * 5 * 32, 3 * 3 * 32 and 3 * 3 * 32 and the strides in that branch are 2, 2, 1, 1, and 1. The sizes of

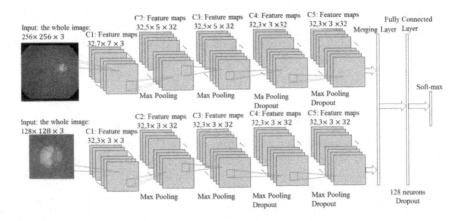

Fig. 2. The framework of the two-branch convolutional neuron network

strides in the second branch are all equal to 1. Max-pooling layers follow all the convolutional layers. Dropout is used in the third and fourth convolutional layer and the fully connected layer.

4   Experiment

4.1   Data

We collected data from Beijing Tongren Hospital, one of the best hospitals in China. Our data includes retinal fundus images and diagnosis results, including 3554 retinal fundus images from about 2000 patients who suffered from various kinds of eye diseases such as glaucoma, cataract, diabetic retinopathy and so on. Among the 3554 retinal images, 1391 images are diagnosed with glaucoma while 2163 images are not.

Figure 3 shows an image of our dataset, which is a standard image usually taken to help doctor to diagnose eye disease, from which we can see the tissues such as Optic Disc in the bright circle area.

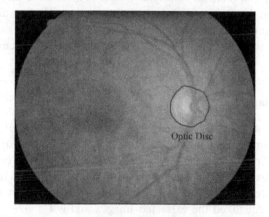

Fig. 3.   One example of retinal fundus images

4.2   Optic Disc Detection

For the optic disc detection task, we first manually labeled 1,500 retinal fundus images. These images were then divided into training set and testing set randomly, with 1,200 and 300 images respectively. Then, we built *Faster-RCNN* based on caffe, which is a popular framework in the field of deep learning. The parameters we used in training the model were all by default. We achieved good performance on the test set. Among all the retinal fundus images in the test dataset, no more than 10 images failed to be extracted the right region because of relatively poor image quality. Then we applied the model to the remaining images to extract Optic Disc automatically. In Fig. 4, rectangles show two example optic disc regions extracted using model *Faster-RCNN*.

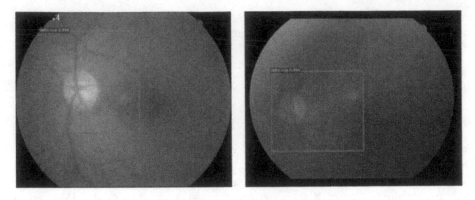

Fig. 4. Examples of extracted optic disc regions

By the way, object detection can bring another bonus for us. It can be used to distinguish the left eye from the right eye. As each image is not labeled as left and right, it is necessary to distinguish them as usually not both of them have disease. But they are usually been taken at the same time and we need to distinguish them automatically. The principle is rather simple: if the center of the rectangle detected is on the left, it is the left eye; otherwise, it is the right eye. This is a quite effective principle, and with only 2% error.

4.3   Glaucoma Diagnosis

We split our data into training set and testing set randomly with a ratio 0.8. As the original images are taken from different equipment, they have a various size such as 1924 * 1556 pixels, 1572 * 1308 pixels, 3048 * 2432 pixels, etc. So we need to equalize the size of these images. We first cropped the image into a square according to the shorter edge of the image. Then we reduced the square image to the same size and got a 256 * 256 image. Similarly, we also equalized the extracted images and got a size of 128 * 128. We implemented the two-branch convolutional neuron network based on the Keras with Tensorflow as backend. The early stopping technique was added to avoid overfitting problem.

We implemented different classification methods to compare the performance. We fine-tuned the well-known Alexnet for the glaucoma diagnosis. We also trained our model with just one branch for the whole image or optic disc regions. Besides the CNN model, we also extracted rotation-invariant local binary patterns (LBP) features and scale-invariant feature transform (SIFT) and then fed them to logistic regression classifier respectively [8, 27]. On top of that, we computed the visual words using the method proposed by Niebles and Li [28], which was fed to the logistic regression classifier for glaucoma classification. Table 1 compares the accuracy.

Table 1. The accuracy of classification results obtained from different approaches

	Accuracy
Logistic regression with SIFT features	60.84%
Logistic regression with LBP features	62.67%
Visual words classification	63.49%
Fine-tuned Alexnet	71.83%
One-branch CNN for the whole image (5-conv layers)	71.36%
One-branch CNN for the extracted images (5-conv layers)	74.95%
Two-branch CNN for the extracted images (4-conv layers)	75.83%
Two-branch CNN for the extracted images (6-conv layers)	74.89%
Two-branch CNN for the extracted images (5-conv layers)	**81.69%**

As we can see from the table, the performance of the deep learning models is obviously better than the traditional methods. What's more, the two-branch convolutional neuron network gets the highest accuracy, which demonstrates the advantages of the proposed model. We also notice that the two-branch convolutional neuron networks with 5 convolutional layers performs better than that with 6 convolutional layers, which may suffer from the over-fitting problem due to the limited data.

4.4 Number of Parameters

We estimate the number of parameters of the model. The parameters of our model include kernel parameters and the fully connected layer parameters. The number of the kernel parameters is about 12 thousand and the figure for the fully connected layer is about 1.3 million. So the total is about 1.4 million. Although it is slightly higher than the traditional convolutional neuron networks with similar architecture, which contains about 1.1 million parameters, the performance of the two-branch neuron network is obviously better. What's more, our model contains much fewer parameters than the Alexnet, which contains about 60 million parameters [10]. This means our model can achieve a better result with relatively less computing resources.

5   Conclusion

In this paper, we make use of medical domain knowledge that the Optic Disc region contains much more important information than other regions for glaucoma diagnosis. Based on this knowledge, we propose to analyze the local optic disc region and the whole image simultaneously. To do that, the Optic Disc region is extracted using *Faster R-CNN* model first, and then a convolutional neuron network with two branches is proposed to perform the glaucoma diagnosis, analyzing the features from the whole image and the disc region respectively. The *Faster R-CNN* performs well in Optic Disc detection, which provides a reliable support for the two-branch convolutional neuron network. Experiments conducted on real dataset shows that our model outperforms the classification methods based on the traditional computer vision algorithm and the classical convolutional neuron networks.

In the future, we plan to enlarge our dataset to build a deeper model so that we will be able to extract more discriminative features for glaucoma diagnosis to improve the diagnosis accuracy further.

Acknowledgements. This work is supported in part by the National Natural Science Foundation of China (NSFC) with grant numbers 71432004 and 71490724.

References

1. Schacknow, P.N., Samples, J.R.: The Glaucoma Book: A Practical, Evidence-Based Approach to Patient Care. Springer, New York (2010). doi:10.1007/978-0-387-76700-0
2. Mantravadi, A.V., Vadhar, N.: Glaucoma. Prim. Care **42**(3), 437–449 (2015). Saunders (Elsevier)
3. Quigley, H.A., Broman, A.T.: The number of people with glaucoma worldwide in 2010 and 2020. Br. J. Ophthalmol. **90**(3), 262–267 (2006)
4. Javitt, J.C.: Preventing blindness in Americans: the need for eyehealth education. Surv. Ophthalmol. **40**(1), 41–44 (1995)
5. Haleem, M.S., Han, L., Van, H.J., Li, B.: Automatic extraction of retinal features from colour retinal images for glaucoma diagnosis: a review. Comput. Med. Imaging Graph. **37**(7–8), 581–596 (2013)
6. Nayak, J., Acharya, R., Bhat, P.S., Shetty, N., Lim, T.C.: Automated diagnosis of glaucoma using digital fundus images. J. Med. Syst. **33**(5), 337–346 (2009)
7. Babu, T.G., Shenbagadevi, S.: Automatic detection of glaucoma using fundus image. Eur. J. Sci. Res. **59**(1), 22–32 (2001)
8. Acharya, U.R., Dua, S., Du, X., Sree, S.V., Chua, C.K.: Automated diagnosis of glaucoma using texture and higher order spectra features. IEEE Trans. Inf. Technol. Biomed. **15**(3), 449–455 (2001)
9. Dua, S., Acharya, U.R., Chowriappa, P., Sree, S.V.: Wavelet-based energy features for glaucomatous image classification. IEEE Trans. Inf Technol. Biomed. **16**(1), 80–87 (2012)
10. Krizhevsky, A., Sutskever, I., Hinton, G.E.: Imagenet classification with deep convolutional neural networks. In: Advances in Neural Information Processing Systems, pp. 1097–1105 (2012)
11. Simonyan, K., Zisserman, A.: Very deep convolutional networks for large-scale image recognition (2014). arXiv:1409.1556
12. Szegedy, C., Liu, W., Jia, Y., et al.: Going deeper with convolutions. In: Proceedings of the IEEE Conference on Computer Vision and Pattern Recognition, pp. 1–9 (2015)
13. He, K., Zhang, X., Ren, S., et al.: Deep residual learning for image recognition. In: Proceedings of the IEEE Conference on Computer Vision and Pattern Recognition, pp. 770–778 (2016)
14. Gulshan, V., Peng, L., Coram, M., et al.: Development and validation of a deep learning algorithm for detection of diabetic retinopathy in retinal fundus photographs. JAMA **316**(22), 2402–2410 (2016)
15. Long, E., Lin, H., Liu, Z., Wu, X., Wang, L., Jiang, J., An, Y., Lin, Z., Li, X., Chen, J., Li, J., Cao, Q., Wang, D., Liu, X., Chen, W., Li, J.: An artificial intelligence platform for the multihospital collaborative management of congenital cataracts. Nat. Biomed. Eng. **1**(0024), 1–8 (2017)

16. Chaudhuri, S., Chatterjee, S., Katz, N., Nelson, M., Goldbaum, M.: Automatic detection of the optic nerve head in retinal images. In: Proceedings of the IEEE International Conference on Image Processing, vol. 1 (1989)
17. Lalonde, M., Beaulieu, M., Gagnon, L.: Fast and robust Optic Disc detection using pyramidal decomposition and Hausdorff-based template matching. IEEE Trans. Med. Imaging **20**, 1193–2000 (2001)
18. Lee, S.Y., Kim, K.K., Seo, J.M., Kim, D.M., Chung, H., Park, K.S., Kim, H.C.: Automated quantification of retinal nerve fiber layer atrophy in fundus photograph. In: 26th Annual International Conference of the IEEE Engineering in Medicine and Biology Society, pp. 1241–1243 (2004)
19. Yadav, D., Sarathi, M.P., Dutta, M.K.: Classification of glaucoma based on texture features using neural networks. In: Seventh International Conference on Contemporary Computing (IC3), pp. 109–112 (2014)
20. Ren, S., He, K., Girshick, R., et al.: Faster R-CNN: towards real-time object detection with region proposal networks. In: Advances in Neural Information Processing Systems, pp. 91–99 (2015)
21. Farabet, C., Couprie, C., Najman, L., et al.: Learning hierarchical features for scene labeling. IEEE Trans. Pattern Anal. Mach. Intell. **35**(8), 1915–1929 (2013)
22. Dai, J., He, K., Sun, J.: Instance-aware semantic segmentation via multi-task network cascades. In: Proceedings of the IEEE Conference on Computer Vision and Pattern Recognition, pp. 3150–3158 (2016)
23. Wu, J., Yu, Y., Huang, C., et al.: Deep multiple instance learning for image classification and auto-annotation. In: Proceedings of the IEEE Conference on Computer Vision and Pattern Recognition, pp. 3460–3469 (2015)
24. Xu, Y., Mo, T., Feng, Q., et al.: Deep learning of feature representation with multiple instance learning for medical image analysis. In: 2014 IEEE International Conference on Acoustics, Speech and Signal Processing (ICASSP), pp. 626–1630. IEEE (2014)
25. Bar, Y., Diamant, I., Wolf, L., et al.: Deep learning with non-medical training used for chest pathology identification. In: SPIE Medical Imaging. International Society for Optics and Photonics, pp. 94140V–94140V-7 (2015)
26. Chen, X., Xu, Y., Yan, S., Wong, D.W.K., Wong, T.Y., Liu, J.: Automatic feature learning for glaucoma detection based on deep learning. In: Navab, N., Hornegger, J., Wells, W.M., Frangi, A.F. (eds.) MICCAI 2015. LNCS, vol. 9351, pp. 669–677. Springer, Cham (2015). doi:10.1007/978-3-319-24574-4_80
27. Lowe, D.G.: Distinctive image features from scale-invariant keypoints. Int. J. Comput. Vis. **60**(2), 91–110 (2004)
28. Niebles, J.C., Li, F.-F.: A hierarchical model of shape and appearance for human action classification. In: IEEE Conference on Computer Vision and Pattern Recognition, pp. 1–8 (2007)

Regression Analysis and Prediction of Mini-Mental State Examination Score in Alzheimer's Disease Using Multi-granularity Whole-Brain Segmentations

Jinzhi Zhang[1,2], Yuan Luo[1,2], Zihan Jiang[3], and Xiaoying Tang[1,2,4,5](✉)

[1] Sun Yat-sen University-Carnegie Mellon University (SYSU-CMU)
Joint Institute of Engineering, Sun Yat-sen University,
Guangzhou, Guangdong, China
[2] Department of Electrical and Computer Engineering,
Carnegie Mellon University, Pittsburgh, PA, USA
[3] School of Data and Computer Science, Sun Yat-sen University,
Guangzhou, Guangdong, China
[4] Sun Yat-sen University-Carnegie Mellon University (SYSU-CMU) Shunde
International Joint Research Institute, Shunde, Guangdong, China
[5] School of Electronics and Information Technology, Sun Yat-sen University,
Guangzhou, Guangdong, China
tangxiaoy@mail.sysu.edu.cn

Abstract. We presented and evaluated three sparsity learning based regression models with application to the automated prediction of the Mini-Mental State Examination (MMSE) scores in Alzheimer's disease(AD) using T1-weight magnetic resonance images (MRIs) from 678 subjects, including 190 healthy control (HC) subjects, 331 mild cognitive impairment (MCI) subjects, and 157 AD subjects. The raw features were obtained from a validated multi-granularity whole-brain analysis pipeline, providing multi-level whole-brain segmentation volumes. We employed the ridge, lasso, and elastic-net as our regression algorithms, with the whole-brain volumes at each level being the independent variables and the MMSE score being the dependent variable. We used 10-fold cross-validation to evaluate the prediction performance and another 10-fold inner loop to estimate the optimal parameters in each model. According to our results, the combination of elastic-net and the second level of whole-brain segmentation volumes (a total of 137 volumes) worked the best compared to all other possible combinations. The work presented in this paper provides a potentially powerful and novel non-invasive biomarker for AD.

Keywords: MMSE · AD · Sparsity learning · Multi-granularity · Whole-brain segmentation

© Springer International Publishing AG 2017
H. Chen et al. (Eds.): ICSH 2017, LNCS 10347, pp. 202–213, 2017.
https://doi.org/10.1007/978-3-319-67964-8_20

1   Introduction

Alzheimer's disease (AD), the most common form of dementia, is an irreversible
and progressive neurodegenerative brain disorder that is characterized by impairment in memory, thinking, and behavior, which usually occurs in middle or late
life [1, 2]. In clinical practice, a main approach for AD diagnosis is based on psychometric tests, which is considered as the defacto gold standard. The mental
and behavioral abnormalities associated with AD can be quantified by severity rating scales [3, 4]. One of the most commonly used measures for evaluating
cognitive impairment is the Mini-Mental State Examination (MMSE) [5].

MMSE provides a continuous scale, with scores ranging from 0 to 30, to
examine the progression in AD. It provides us a quantitative criterion to assess
the degree of impairment in certain primary cognitive functions such as orientation to time and place, registration, attention, the immediate and delayed recall,
calculation, language, and constructional praxis [6, 7]. MMSE has been suggested
to be one of the most successful criteria in AD monitoring [8].

The advent of advanced neuroimaging techniques provides new tools for
examining and monitoring the neurodegeneration in AD. Structural neuroimaging measures have been shown to be sensitive to the AD-induced brain degener-
ation. During the past decade, a variety of structural AD biomarkers have been
proposed and validated, including three main categories. The first type of structural AD biomarkers is designed based on cortical thickness [9, 10]. The second
type is the volumes of specific structures of interest [11]. And the third one is
usually obtained from whole-brain analyses such as voxel-based morphometry
(VBM) [12]. Some research showed that the gray matter and white matter den-
sities derived in VBM may be potential neuroimaging markers when evaluating
cognitive functioning in AD [13]. Another approach is region of interest (ROI)
based whole brain analysis. The whole brain is first segmented into multiple
ROIs. And then, biomarkers are obtained from those whole-brain ROIs, typically the volumetric measurements of all ROIs. The whole-brain segmentation
volumes have also been shown to be useful in the prediction of clinical scores in
AD [14].

Structural imaging biomarkers would not be useful in clinical applications if
they could not correctly predict the cognitive impairment in AD. In other words,
a robust and reliable AD biomarker is desired to be able to predict the MMSE
score accurately. In the work of Duchesne and colleagues [15], the MMSE scores
were predicted by using a multiple linear regression model with the independent variables being the average T1-weighted (T1w) MR image intensity within
each of multiple ROIs. The T1w images of all subjects have been transformed
to a common space via affine registration. In another work [16], a sparse random forest (RF) based regression framework was presented to predict clinical
scores, including the MMSE score, in AD using features (such as cortical thickness, cortical volumes, and the total cortical surface area) from high-resolution
structural T1w MRI scans from the Alzheimer's Disease Neuroimaging Initiative
(ADNI) study. In both of those two works, the authors estimated multiple clinical variables separately, without considering the common information shared

across those variables, and have only used a single modality MRI image (T1w) for regression. Recently, a Multi-Modal Multi-Task (M3T) learning method has been proposed to jointly predict multiple variables using multi-modality MRI data with key techniques including a multi-task based feature selection, a kernel-based fusion of multi-modality data, and a support vector regression [17]. However, the research on sparse learning based regression methods, such as ridge regression, lasso regression, and elastic-net regression has been very limited, especially with multi-granularity whole-brain segmentation volumes being the input features.

In this paper, we propose to automatically predict the MMSE scores in AD based on multi-granularity whole-brain segmentation volumes [18] obtained from T1w images by using ridge, lasso, and elastic-net as the regression algorithms. The data came from the ADNI database, including a total of 190 healthy control (HC) subjects, 331 mild cognitive impairment (MCI, a middle stage between normal aging and AD) subjects and 157 AD subjects. We first segmented each T1w image into 5-level whole-brain segmentations using the multi-atlas likelihood fusion (MALF) algorithm [20] and then used the whole-brain segmentation volumes at each level to serve as inputs to the three sparsity learning based regression models (ridge, lasso, and elastic-net). We employed 10-fold cross-validation to assess the prediction accuracy in each case. The underlying motivation is to automatically predict MMSE scores in AD via a simple structural MR scanning rather than a set of complicated cognitive tests.

2   Method

2.1   Subjects

The structural MRI data used in this article was obtained from the ADNI study (adni.loni.usc.edu), a large five-year study launched in 2004 by the National Institute on Aging, the National Institute of Biomedical Imaging and Bioengineering, the Food and Drug Administration, private pharmaceutical companies and non-profit organizations, as a $60 million, 5-year public-private partnership.

We included a total of 678 subjects, including 157 AD subjects, 331 MCI subjects, and 190 HC subjects. The demographic characteristics of each of the three groups are presented in Table 1. Specifically, subjects were 55 to 92 years old and had MMSE scores ranging from 20 to 30. There were significant group differences in terms of MMSE between HC and MCI ($p - value = 1.1E - 43$) as well as that between HC and AD ($p - value = 1.2E - 118$). In terms of age, HC and MCI differed significantly ($p - value = 0.0303$), but not between HC and AD ($p - value = 0.1166$).

2.2   Multi-granularity Whole-Brain Segmentations

In order to obtain features used in the regression analysis, we performed multi-atlas whole-brain segmentation [20] and multi-granularity analysis [18] for each

Table 1. Demographic characteristics of the sample involved in this study

	HC (n = 190)	MCI (n = 331)	AD (n = 157)
Subject age (year)	76.23 ± 4.96	74.93 ± 7.28	75.16 ± 7.63
No. male subjects	95	210	83
No. female subjects	95	121	74
MMSE score	29.17 ± 0.96	27.06 ± 1.76	23.38 ± 1.96

subject. From the T1w image of each subject, 289 ROIs were obtained using (MALF) [20] with only 274 remained after removing the ROIs of skull, bone marrow, optic tract and cerebrospinal fluid. According to their ontological relationship [18], the 274 ROIs defined in the segmentation map were recombined to form 5 levels during the multi-granularity analysis. As the level goes from 1 to 5, the number of ROIs decreases in the following order: 274-137-54-19-8. Each level was created by merging certain individual ROIs of the previous level. Hierarchical relationship was defined at those 5 levels with each level linked through ontology-based hierarchical structural relationships [18,19]. At the sparsest ontology level (level 5), it defines 7 classical definitions of the brain ontology (telencephalon (right and left), diencephalon (right and left), mesencephalon, metencephalon, and myelencephalon). The telencephalon is sub-divided into 3 single structures, namely cerebral cortex, cerebral nuclei, and white matter at level 4. Cerebral cortex is then sub-divided into frontal cortex, parietal cortex, occipital cortex, temporal cortex, limbic, and insula at level 3. After that, Limbic is sub-divided into cingulate cortex and hippocampus at level 2, and the cingulate cortex is sub-divided into another 3 structures at level 1, including anterior cingulate, dorsal cingulate, and posterior cingulate. In Fig. 1, we demonstrate the five level whole-brain segmentations of one subject at three different axial slices. The volume of each ROI at each level was calculated after segmentation. The volumes of all ROIs at each level were used as the raw features for automated predictions of MMSE scores, being the multiple independent variables in each regression model.

2.3 Cross Validation and Feature Normalization

10-fold cross validation was applied throughout the entire procedure for each of the five levels and each regression algorithm. Feature normalization and parameter estimation were conducted on the training data within each cross validation iteration.

For each feature f_i of the training samples in one cross validation iteration, the following feature normalization scheme was applied:

$$f_i = \frac{f_i - \bar{f}_i}{\sigma_{f_i}}$$ (1)

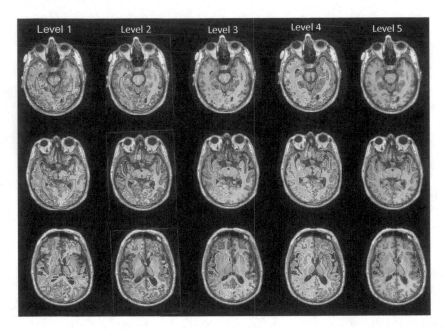

Fig. 1. Demonstration of the five-level whole-brain segmentations of one representative subject for three axial views

where $\bar{f}_i$ and σ_{f_i} are respectively the mean and corrected sample standard deviation of the feature across the entire training set. This step is to center the sample points and to avoid the features with large variance dominating the regression procedure. To ensure the samples in both training and testing sets are applied of the same transformation, the $\bar{f}_i$ and σ_{f_i} were used to normalize the corresponding feature in the testing samples as well.

2.4   Regression Analysis

Linear regression is a frequently-used approach for modeling the relationship between a scalar dependent variable y and one or more explanatory variables (or independent variables) X in a way such that

$$y = X\beta + \varepsilon \qquad (2)$$

where $y = \{y_1, y_2, ..., y_n\}^T$, $X = \{x_1^T, x_2^T, ..., x_n^T\}$, $x_i^T = \{x_{i1}, x_{i2}, ..., x_{im}\}$, $\beta = \{\beta_1, \beta_2, ..., \beta_m\}^T$, and $\varepsilon = \{\varepsilon_1, \varepsilon_2, ..., \varepsilon_n\}^T$, with n denoting the total number of samples in the training data and m denoting the total number of the independent variables. In our case, n is equivalent to 610 or 612 and m is equivalent respectively to 274, 136, 54, 19, and 8 at level 1, level 2, level 3, level 4, and level 5. β is an m-dimensional parameter vector, and ε_i is the error term. The parameters β are usually obtained via maximum likelihood estimation by minimizing the cost function

$$j\left(\beta\right) = \left(X\beta - y\right)^2. \tag{3}$$

To avoid overfitting, we employed three sparsity learning based regression methods, including the ridge regression, the lasso regression, and the elastic-net regression.

Ridge Regression. Ridge regression is known as weight decay. It adds an L2-norm regularization term to the cost function, resulting in

$$j\left(\beta\right) = \left(X\beta - Y\right)^2 + \lambda \|\beta\|_2^2, \tag{4}$$

where the L2-norm was computed by $\|\beta\|_2^2 = \sum_{i=1}^{m} |\beta_i|^2$. In ridge regression, the coefficients of some variables will tend towards 0 infinitely.

Lasso Regression. Lasso (least absolute shrinkage and selection operator) is a regression analysis method that performs variable selection and regularization simultaneously in order to enhance the prediction accuracy and interpretability of the statistical model. It adds an L1-norm regularization term to the cost function such that

$$j\left(\beta\right) = \left(X\beta - Y\right)^2 + \lambda \|\beta\|_1, \tag{5}$$

where $\|\beta\|_1 = \sum_{i=1}^{m} |\beta_i|$. Different from the ridge regression, lasso will set the coefficients to 0 for certain independent variables (features).

Elastic-Net Regression. Elastic-net addresses several shortcomings of lasso [21]. When $m > n$ (the number of independent variables is greater than the sample size) lasso can select only n variables (even when more features are associated with the outcome) and it tends to select only one variable from a set of highly correlated variables. Additionally, even when $n > m$, if the independent variables are strongly correlated, lasso does not perform as well as ridge does. The elastic-net combines the advantages of ridge and lasso by adding both an L2-norm term and an L1-norm term to the cost function such that

$$j\left(\beta\right) = \left(X\beta - Y\right)^2 + \lambda \|\beta\|_1 + \lambda \|\beta\|_2^2. \tag{6}$$

Elastic-net makes use of both the L1 and L2 regularization.

2.5   Implementation

We implement the three regression algorithms in Matlab using the built-in lasso function. The function was given by

$$cost(\beta) = \min_{\beta 0, \beta}(\frac{1}{2N} \sum_{i=1}^{N} (y_i - \beta_0 - x_i^T \beta)^2 + \lambda P_\alpha), \tag{7}$$

where

$$p_\alpha^\beta = \frac{1-\alpha}{2} \|\beta\|_2^2 + \alpha \|\beta\|_1 = \sum_{j=1}^{p} (\frac{(1-\alpha)}{2} \beta_j^2 + \alpha |\beta_j|). \qquad (8)$$

for an α strictly between 0 and 1, and a nonnegative λ. It reduces to the lasso model when $\alpha = 1$. And as α shrinks toward 0, elastic-net approaches ridge regression. When we set $0 < \alpha < 1$, it becomes an elastic-net regression model.

In lasso and ridge regression, we implemented a 10-fold cross validation. We partitioned the 678 subjects into 10 parts, with each of 9 parts containing 68 subjects and the 10th part containing 66 subjects, and thus there are either 610 or 612 subjects in our training samples. We used one part to be the testing data and the other 9 parts to be the training data in each of 10-fold cross validation. We estimated the optimal λ with another 10-fold inner-loop cross validation using the training subjects. The range of candidate λ is from 10^{-2} to 10^5, with a step size of $10^{0.01}$. Then, we used this optimal λ to obtain the parameter vector β in each fold. Finally, we used the model to predict the MMSE scores for the testing subjects left at the very beginning. In elastic-net regression, there are three 10-fold loops, with the most outer 10-fold being the same as that in lasso and ridge. The most inner 10-fold loop was used to estimate the optimal α with its candidate values ranging from 0.01 to 1.00 and a step size of 0.01. After obtaining the optimal α, we used the middle-loop 10-fold to estimated the optimal λ. Then we computed the parameter vector β using the optimal α and the optimal λ in the most outer 10-fold loop. Finally, we applied the resulting model to predict the MMSE scores for the testing subjects left out at the very beginning.

2.6   Evaluation Metrics

We employed two types of quantitative metrics to evaluate the prediction accurary: (1) The average relative error, as given by

$$Error = \frac{\sum_{i=1}^{n} (|y_{i_{true}} - y_{i_{predict}}| / y_{i_{true}})}{n} \qquad (9)$$

where $y_{i_{true}}$ is the real MMSE score of the $i-th$ testing subject and $y_{i_{predict}}$ is the corresponding predicted MMSE score; (2) The Pearson's correlation coefficient (PCC), in terms of both strength and significance, between $y_{predict}$ and y_{true}.

3   Results

The errors obtained from the four regression methods, with each of the five-level whole-brain segmentation volumes being the features for predicting MMSE, are tabulated in Table 2. We observe that the discrepancy between the estimated MMSE scores and the true values when using the second level of whole-brain segmentation volumes was the minimum, regardless of the regression model

Table 2. The mean error obtained from each of the four regression methods when using each of the five-level whole-brain segmentation volumes as the input features.

Regression/level	Level 1	Level 2	Level 3	Level 4	Level 5
Linear	9.35%	7.67%	7.67%	8.01%	8.15%
Ridge	7.04%	6.99%	7.52%	7.99%	8.16%
Lasso	7.09%	6.93%	7.60%	7.98%	8.19%
Elastic-net	7.07%	6.92%	7.56%	7.99%	8.17%

employed. As expected, linear regression was inferior to any of the three sparsity learning based regression methods, with the lowest error obtained at level 2 and level 3. For any of the three sparsity learning based regression methods, the prediction performance in terms of the discrepancy follows level 2 > level 1 > level 3 > level 4 > level 5, with all errors below or around 8%. Comparing the performance across levels, they are very similar to each other, with the lowest error obtained when applying elastic-net to the second level of whole-brain segmentation volumes. The performance in terms of the correlation between the predicted MMSE scores and the true values had similar patterns. As shown in Table 3, in all cases, the estimated MMSE scores and the true values are significantly positively correlated. However, for each of the four methods, level 2 outperformed all the other ones in terms of both correlation strength and correlation significance. Similar to the error patterns, level 2 and level 3 worked the best for linear regression and level 2 > level 1 > level 3 > level 4 > level 5 for any of the three sparsity methods. Again, a combination of the elastic-net regression and the second level of whole-brain segmentation volumes worked the best in the correlation respect, similar to that when evaluated by the error criterion.

Table 3. The PCC values (r) and the $p-values$ obtained in correlating the estimated MMSE scores and the true values.

		Linear	Ridge	Lasso	Elastic-net
Level 1	r	0.318	0.530	0.520	0.527
	$p-value$	$2.2E-17$	$2.5E-50$	$3.2E-48$	$1.3E-49$
Level 2	r	0.453	0.542	0.550	0.554
	$p-value$	$1.3E-35$	$4.1E-53$	$6.4E-55$	$9.1E-56$
Level 3	r	0.388	0.427	0.419	0.424
	$p-value$	$9.2E-26$	$2.0E-31$	$3.6E-30$	$6.7E-31$
Level 4	r	0.309	0.318	0.324	0.322
	$p-value$	$1.8E-16$	$2.2E-17$	$4.9E-18$	$9.0E-18$
Level 5	r	0.266	0.273	0.262	0.268
	$p-value$	$2.0E-12$	$4.8E-13$	$3.9E-12$	$1.3E-12$

Table 4. The mean and standard deviations of λ for all three methods with each of the five-level whole-brain segmentation volumes.

Regression/level	Level 1	Level 2	Level 3	Level 4	Level 5
Ridge (λ)	1.166±0.15	0.496±0.08	0.193±0.05	0.074±0.02	0.110±0.02
Lasso (λ)	0.080±0.01	0.071±0.01	0.046±0.01	0.028±0.01	0.025±0.02
Elastic-net (λ)	0.168±0.08	0.139±0.05	0.093±0.03	0.046±0.03	0.043±0.03

The results of λ, measuring the weight of the regularization term, in all cases are shown in Table 4. It is worth noting that in each case we had 10 λ values given that we have 10 folds of model training. According to results presented in Table 4, for each regression method, as the granularity of whole-brain segmentation decreased, the value of λ on average decreased accordingly. In elastic-net regression, the values of α, weighting between the L2-norm regularization and the L1-norm regularization, are respectively 0.57 ± 0.23, 0.45 ± 0.24, 0.38 ± 0.27, 0.59 ± 0.38, 0.52 ± 0.29 for level 1, level 2, level 3, level 4, and level 5. This suggests that a 1-to-1 balance between the two regularization terms in elastic-net generally worked the best in MMSE prediction.

The estimated coefficients, β, of all features (independent variables) in all cases, as shown in Fig. 2. We notice that the relative values of the coefficients for different ROIs within the same level of whole-brain segmentation are similar across different levels as well as different methods. In other words, the coefficient of a specific ROI is large at each of the other 4 levels if it is large at level 1, as compared to the coefficients of other ROIs within the same level. Similarly, if the coefficient of a specific ROI at a specific segmentation level is large in ridge regression, it is also large in both lasso regression and elastic-net regression.

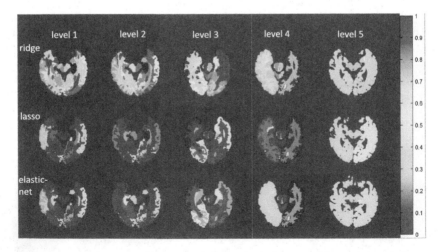

Fig. 2. The estimated coefficient, β, for each of the input volumes from each of the 5-level whole-brain segmentations for all three regression methods.

4 Discussion

In this paper, we have evaluated three sparsity learning based regression algorithms for predicting the MMSE scores in AD using multi-granularity whole-brain segmentation volumes for a total of 678 subjects. Several important findings emerged from our results: (1) Among the three regression algorithms, elastic-net outperformed the other two using any of the five levels of whole-brain segmentation volumes. This agrees with the general understanding that elastic-net provides a good balance between the L2-norm regularization and the L1-norm regularization, which benefits the prediction system. The weights of those two types of regularization terms in our optimal elastic-net model was about 1-to-1 as measured from our 10-fold cross validation. (2) Overall speaking, the combination of elastic-net and the second level of whole-brain segmentation volumes worked the best compared to all other ..possible combinations, in terms of either the discrepancy or the correlation between the estimated MMSE and the true MMSE. (3) For all three regression methods and all five-level whole-brain segmentation volumes, they worked actually very well with relative low errors (below 8%) and strong as well as significant correlations (PCC > 0.5, $p - value < 1E - 11$). (4) For each of the three regression algorithms (ridge, lasso, and elastic-net), as the granularity decreased (from level 1 to level (5), the coefficient (λ) for the regularization term decreased accordingly. This is because the feature space became sparser as the granularity decreased and thus less features will be assigned of a small coefficient (in ridge and elastic-net) or a zero coefficient (in lasso and elastic-net).

Sparsity learning based regression methods have been used in other works as well. In the work of Huang and his colleagues [16], they presented a non-linear supervised sparse RF based regression framework to predict a variety of longitudinal AD clinical scores. A soft-split technique was employed to assign probabilities to the test sample in the RF framework so as to enhance the prediction accuracy. Different from our regression algorithms, they used support vector regression [17] to predict MMSE scores. Not only the MRI data but also the PET and CSF data, from ADNI subjects, were used. They also used multi-model multi-task strategy for more accurate predictions. Another work [14] applied the relevance vector regression (RVR) algorithm [22] to predict MMSE scores based on four different datasets. However, other than the work presented in this paper, combining sparsity learning based regression methods with multi-granularity whole-brain volumetrics has not been explored yet. The procedure proposed in this work, taking advantage of the hierarchical whole-brain structural information and sparsity learning based regression, may have the potential of providing a robust and reliable AD biomarker that is able to predict the MMSE scores accurately. The MMSE score is related to the 3 categories of clinical states in the neuropathology of AD (HC, MCI and AD). Diagnosing the clinical status of a patient based on the predicted MMSE score is one of our future developments and we will explore more substantially in this research direction.

There are another two future directions based on the work presented here. Firstly, kernel based sparsity learning methods, such as kernel ridge regression

[23], have been successfully applied to the automated prediction of MMSE in AD. One of our future endeavors will be investigating various kernel based sparsity learning methods and apply them to our multi-granularity whole-brain segmentation volumes in terms of MMSE prediction. Secondly, in this work, we analyzed the five-level whole-brain segmentation volumes separately. A potential combination of those multi-level volumetrics may further boost the performance of our MMSE prediction.

Acknowledgments. This work is supported by the National Natural Science Foundation of China (81501546) and the SYSU-CMU Shunde International Joint Research Institute Start-up Grant (20150306). We would like to thank Yuanyuan Wei, Jingyuan Li, and Huilin Yang for valuable discussions.

References

1. Michael, S., Mega, M.D., Jeffrey, L., Cummings, M.D., Tara, F., Jeffrey, G.D.: The spectrum of behavioral changes in Alzheimer's disease. Neurology **46**, 130–135 (1996)
2. Howard, C., Daniel, B.S.: Priming and semantic memory loss in Alzheimer's disease. Brain Lang. **36**, 420–446 (1989)
3. Morris, J.C.: The clinical dementia rating (CDR): current version and scoring rules. Neurology **43**, 2412–2414 (1993)
4. Reisberg, B.F., Erris, S.H., De Leon, M.J., Crook, T.: The global deterioration scale for assessment of primary degenerative dementia. Am. J. Psychiatr. **139**, 1136–1139 (1982)
5. Folstein, M.F., Folstein, S.E., McHugh, P.R.: Mini-mental state: a practical method for grading the cognitive state of patients for the clinician. J. Psychiatr. Res. **12**, 189 (1975)
6. Guy, M., Drachman, D., Folstein, M., Katzman, R., Price, D., Stadlan, E.M.: Clinical diagnosis of Alzheimer's disease report of the NINCDS-ADRDA work group under the auspices of Department of Health and Human Services Task Force on Alzheimer's disease. Neurology **34**, 939 (1984)
7. Tom, N., Tombaugh, C., Nancy, J., McIntyre, M.A.: The mini-mental state examination: a comprehensive review. J. Am. Geriatr. **40**, 922–935 (1992)
8. Mitchell, A.J.: A meta-analysis of the accuracy of the mini-mental state examination in the detection of dementia and mild cognitive impairment. J. Psychiatr. Res. **43**, 411–431 (2009)
9. Querbes, O., Aubry, F., Parient, J., Lotterie, J.A., Demonet, J.F., Duret, V., Puel, M., Berry, I., Fort, J.C., Celsis, P.: Individual early diagnosis of alzheimer's disease using cortical thickness measurement: impact of cognitive reserve. Neuroimage **47**(Suppl1), S79 (2009)
10. Hartikainen, P., Rsnen, J., Julkunen, V., Niskanen, E., Hallikainen, M., Kivipelto, M., Vanninen, R., Remes, A.M., Soininen, H.: Cortical thickness in frontotemporal dementia, mild cognitive impairment, and Alzheimer's disease. J. Alzheimers Dis. (JAD) **30**(4), 857–874 (2012)
11. Convit, A., Leon, M.J.D., Tarshish, C., Santi, S.D., Tsui, W., Rusinek, H., George, A.: Specific hippocampal volume reductions in individuals at risk for Alzheimer's disease. Neurobiol. Aging **18**(2), 131–138 (1997)

12. Ashburner, J., Friston, K.J.: Voxel-based morphometry: the methods. Neuroimage **11**(1), 805–821 (2000)
13. Baxter, L.C., Sparks, D.L., Johnson, S.C., Lenoski, B., Lopez, J.E., Connor, D.J., Sabbagh, M.N.: Relationship of cognitive measures and gray and white matter in Alzheimer's disease. J. Alzheimers Dis. **9**, 253–260 (2006)
14. Cynthia, M., Stonnington, M., Carlton, C., Stefan, K., Cliord, R., Jack, J., John, A., Richard, S.J., Frackowiak, M.: Predicting clinical scores from magnetic resonance scans in Alzheimer's disease. Neuroimage **51**(4), 1405–1413 (2010)
15. Duchesne, S., Caroli, A., Geroldi, C., Frisoni, G.B., Collins, D.L.: Predicting clinical variable from MRI features: application to MMSE in MCI. In: Duncan, J.S., Gerig, G. (eds.) MICCAI 2005. LNCS, vol. 3749, pp. 392–399. Springer, Heidelberg (2005). doi:10.1007/11566465_49
16. Huang, L., Jin, Y., Gao, Y., Thung, K., Shen, D.: Longitudinal clinical score prediction in Alzheimer's disease with soft-split sparse regression based random forest. Neurobiol. Aging **46**, 180–191 (2016)
17. Zhang, D., Shen, D.: Multi-modal multi-task learning for joint prediction of clinical scores in Alzheimer's disease. In: Liu, T., Shen, D., Ibanez, L., Tao, X. (eds.) MBIA 2011. LNCS, vol. 7012, pp. 60–67. Springer, Heidelberg (2011). doi:10.1007/978-3-642-24446-9_8
18. Djamanakova, A., Tang, X., Li, X., Faria, A.V., Ceritoglu, C., Oishi, K., Hillis, A.E., Albert, M., Lyketsos, C., Miller, M.I., Mori, S.: Tools for multiple granularity analysis of brain MRI data for individualized image analysis. Neuroimage **101**, 168–176 (2014)
19. Wu, D., Ceritoglu, C., Miller, M.I., Mori, S.: Direct estimation of patient attributes from anatomical MRI based on multi-atlas voting. Neuroimage Clin. **12**, 570–581 (2016)
20. Tang, X., Oishi, K., Faria, A.V., Hillis, A.E., Albert, M.S., Mori, S., Miller, M.I.: Bayesian parameter estimation and segmentation in the multi-atlas random orbit model. PLoS One **8**(6), e65591 (2013)
21. Zou, H., Trevor, H.: Regularization and variable selection via the elastic net. J. R. Statist. Soc. Ser. B (Statist. Methodol.) **67**(2), 301–320 (2005). Wiley
22. Michael, E.T.: Sparse bayesian learning and the relevance vector machine. J. Mach. Learn. Res. **1**, 211–244 (2001)
23. Chu, C., Ni, Y., Tan, G., Saunders, C.J., Ashburner, J.: Kernel regression for fMRI pattern prediction. Neuroimage **56**, 662–673 (2011)

Apply Convolutional Neural Network to Lung Nodule Detection: Recent Progress and Challenges

Jiaxing Tan[1(✉)], Yumei Huo[1], Zhengrong Liang[2], and Lihong Li[1]

[1] City University of New York, New York, NY, USA
jtan@gradcenter.cuny.edu, {Yumei.Huo,Lihong.Li}@csi.cuny.edu
[2] Stony Brook University, Stony Brook, NY, USA
Jerome.Liang@sunysb.edu

Abstract. Convolutional Neural Network has shown great success in many areas. Different from the hand-engineered feature based classification, Convolutional Neural Network uses self-learned features from data for classification. Recently, some progress has been made in the area of Convolutional Neural Network based lung nodule detection. This paper gives a brief introduction to the problems in such area reviews the recent related results, and concludes the challenges met. Besides some technical details, we also introduce some available public packages for a fast development and some public data sources.

1 Introduction

American Cancer Society [1] showed that lung cancer is the leading cause of cancer-related deaths with 158,080 deaths estimated for the United States in 2016. Early detection of lung cancer is the key to prevent lung cancer and thus help in a sharp increase in the survival rate. A popular detection tool, computer tomography (CT), has been analyzed subjectively by radiologists. The anticipated large amount interpretation effort demands a computer-aided detection (CAD) scheme to help radiologists to efficiently diagnose lung cancer. As a result, automated CAD of lung cancer has been developed, which is typically a classifier based on hand engineered features.

Convolutional Neural Network (CNN) has shown a great success in computer vision on the ImageNet challenge. Since AlexNet [2] was proposed, the performance improvement has been achieved for almost every year with deeper and deeper structures supported by high performance computing facilities. Compared with manually selected feature based classifier, CNN could learn features from data itself, which turns out to be more efficient and automatic [3]. Also, some progress has been made in medical imaging using CNN to solve real-life problems, especially lung nodule detection. In this paper, we aim at giving a brief introduction on what is happening in the area of CNN based lung nodule detection with typical methods. Also, we provide lists of available public packages for fast development and public datasets.

© Springer International Publishing AG 2017
H. Chen et al. (Eds.): ICSH 2017, LNCS 10347, pp. 214–222, 2017.
https://doi.org/10.1007/978-3-319-67964-8_21

The rest of this paper is organized as follows: In Sect. 2, we give a general picture of CNN with a list of commonly used public packages. Then typical recent methods are shown in Sect. 3. In Sect. 4, we demonstrate some challenges and their possible solutions. At last, the conclusion is given in Sect. 5.

2   Convolution Neural Network

In this section, we first give a general picture about CNN, then we provide a list of commonly used packages for fast implementing a CNN model.

2.1   What Is Convolutional Neural Network

Generally speaking, CNN is a deep neural network, inspired by the biology study of human cortex, constructed by four types of layers: input layer, multiple convolution layers and several fully-connected layers in the end. Each convolution layer is followed by a subsampling layer. A CNN example is shown in Fig. 1. We will introduce CNN with this example.

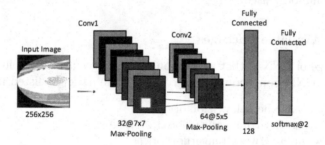

Fig. 1. A CNN example

Input Layer. The Input layer is in charge of reading data with a predefined size without performing any changes to it. In Fig. 1, the input layer reads in a CT scan image with size 256 × 256.

Convolution Layer. A convolution layer has k different kernels, and each has the shape $m \times n$ and performs convolution operation (denoted as $\star$) on each of j sub-images of the input image i. A non-linear function g will be applied to the convolution result with a bias b added. The whole procedure is shown in Eq. 1.

$$f = g((W_i * i_{1:j}) + b) \qquad (1)$$

The output of the convolution layer is k feature maps, each generated by a convolution operation with one kernel applied on the whole image. In Fig. 1, there are 2 convolution layers. Conv1 has 32 kernels, each of size 7 × 7, conv2 has 64 kernels, each of size 5 × 5.

Subsampling Layer. Subsampling layer, following a convolution layer, performs a down-sampling operation on the feature maps generated by the convolution layer. There are several ways to perform sub-sampling, such as average-pooling, median-pooling and max-pooling. In Fig. 1, the network uses max-pooling strategy.

Fully Connected Layer. A fully connected layer is the same as the layers in a traditional Multi Layer Perceptron (MLP). The input is an image i with operations shown in Eq. 2, where b denotes the bias. The last layer of a CNN model is usually a fully connected layer which serves as an output layer. In the output layer, the number of neurons denotes the number of classes in the classification task.

$$f = g((W_i \times i_{1:j}) + b) \tag{2}$$

Non-linear Function. Non-linear function g is used in both convolution and fully connected layer. Functions like Tanh, Sigmoid and Relu are often used as a Non-linear Function. For the output layer, i.e. the last layer of a CNN, a softmax function is commonly used.

2.2 Some Available Packages

One advantage of CNN is that several public packages are available. Instead of building your CNN from scratch, you could try the packages listed below:

- Caffe: http://caffe.berkeleyvision.org/
- Lasagne: https://lasagne.readthedocs.io/en/latest/
- TensorFlow: https://www.tensorflow.org/
- Theano: http://deeplearning.net/software/theano/
- Torch: http://torch.ch/

All these packages are publicly available online with multi-platform and GPU support, which reduce the workload of implementing a CNN based task. Also, the packages have been optimized to be efficient.

3   Some Recent CNN Based Methods

In this section, we demonstrate some typical recent methods on CNN based lung nodule detection. In the literature, various CNN designs have been proposed. We classify them into three groups: 2D CNN based, 3D CNN based and Holistic CNN based. We will introduce these three groups in this section.

3.1 2D CNN Based Lung Nodule Detection

Given a set of CT scans of a patient, which usually contains more than 300 slices depending on the body size of the patient, radiologists will check the scan slice by slice to detect the nodule. For each scan, radiologists will observe every sub-region in it. This procedure is performed in 2D slices.

In this procedure, each slice could be viewed as a 2D image and the inspection could be viewed as image classification on sub-regions. So we could use a 2D CNN based classifier to simulate it. After applying some pre-processing such as lung segmentation and noise elimination, the slice would be cut into small sub-regions. Each region is an input into CNN and the output is a decision whether such region contains a nodule or not. The combined result shows if a nodule exists in this slice.

Most recently, Tajbakhs et al. [4] compares the performance of several CNN structures on lung nodule detection with MTANN. Several models, including a shallow CNN, rd-CNN, famous LeNet [6] and AlexNet [2], are compared in this paper, which gives some guidance on how to design CNN. Although MTANN outperforms CNN, MTANN is a group of neural networks, and each is in charge of a certain situation, while CNN only has one network for all situations. It could be very interesting to know if we design a group of CNN, each to deal with a certain situation, will them give us a better result than MTANN?

Also, we would like to mention the work of Shin et al. [5], where they use transfer learning to take advantage of the pre-trained CNN model from computer vision to perform CT scan analysis. Although they lung disease detection instead of lung nodule detection, we think this paper is complimentary to [4]. In [5] three very deep CNN structures achieve good result while in [4] only shallow CNN structures have good performance. They developed a strategy of transform the single channel CT scan into a 3 channel image. In this way, people can use some pretrained model from computer vision instead of training their model from scratch. We will further explain pretrain in the challenge section. They experiment on three famous CNN structures and compare variants in the number of parameters and different training strategies: train the model from scratch, transfer learning and "off-the-shelf". The results show that too deep CNN could have its performance limited by the size of dataset. When use a deep CNN from computer vision, reduce the number of parameters could possibly increase the performance. The idea of Transfer learning provides a way to use pretrained model to perform CT scan analysis.

3.2 3D CNN Based Lung Nodule Detection

When radiologists check each scan, for a better inspection, besides going through each region of the scan, they will also check the same region on the slices before or after the current slice to decide whether there is a nodule inside. Such detection procedure takes advantage of the 3D nature of the CT scan, which could also be an inspiration on the design of CNN based detection.

Traditionally, a CNN takes a 2D matrix as an input. However, there are some recent publications in computer vision introduce 3D CNN. Tran et al. [7] has applied a 3D CNN for video scene recognition to take advantage of the third dimension of the video, time property, for a better performance. To recognize 3D object, Maturana et al. [8] has applied a 3D CNN which achieved promising performance.

In the area of lung nodule detection, due to the 3D nature of CT scan, it will be reasonable to apply 3D CNN. Some efforts have also been made. Anirudh [9] has applied 3D CNN on a weakly labelled lung nodule dataset. He uses a voxel $\hat{v}$ as a input into the CNN to decide whether the center point v located at (x, y, z) to be a nodule or not. $\hat{v}$ is defined as $(x - w : x + w, y - w : y + w, z - h : z + h)$, which means not only neighbors of v in the same slice but also the neighbors on the previous and latter slice are considered to make the decision. This design is closer to how radiologist performs lung nodule detection. A sensitivity of 80% for 10 false positives per scan has been given on their weakly labelled dataset as a result.

In [10], Golan et al. developed a 3D CNN based lung nodule detector using votes for nodule locating. Normally in a detection procedure, the type of each pixel in the scan only decides once. In their work, the detection result for each pixel is acquired by a combination of multiple votes. The votes are generated by sliding windows in the 3D space. Each sliding window would provide one vote for all the pixels inside by its classification result, where all the pixels inside are considered to have the same type as the classification result. In this way, there are multiple votes for a single pixel coming from different sliding windows. The final decision is made by a comparison of the total votes from different sliding windows with a predefined threshold. Such strategy could reduce the prediction error by an ensemble of multiple detection results.

3.3   Holistic CNN Lung Nodule Detection

All the methods we have mentioned in the previous two sections mainly obey the pipeline so that the detection result of a given slice is based on the results from a group of sub-tasks which perform nodule detection in each region of the slice with a sliding window. Such pipeline is not very efficient. The concern is whether we could perform nodule detection on the whole image to achieve the detection result without dividing it into sub-tasks.

Gao et al. [11] has applied a holistic classification on lung CT scans to detect 6 different kinds of diseases. Although the task is lung disease detection instead of lung cancer, this paper casts some light on using a different pipeline to perform nodule detection. Their methods takes the whole lung CT image as an input and the output is whether this patient is healthy or has some kinds of lung disease. Their method reaches a descent result in the experiment. Besides efficiency, another advantage of taking the whole CT scan as an input is that the noise affect less as more information is available.

Apart from the area of biomedical image analysis, some methods published in computer vision could also cast some light on this part. For example, recently, Yolo [12] proposed that object detection is performed with only one scan. With an input image, the output given by the CNN shows the type and the location, in the form of the boundary, of the object. Such method is very similar to the lung nodule detection in theory. It is very interesting to know whether it is more efficient to perform a holistic CNN detection than a sliding window based pipeline.

4   Some Challenges

Despite of the success of applying CNN for lung nodule detection, challenges also remain. In this section, we discuss some challenges presented in some papers and experienced in our practice. As CNN is a highly data-oriented method, a majority of the challenges lie in the data part. So we discuss data related challenges in the first two parts and other challenges in the third part.

4.1   Data Source

CNN, as some other big data technologies, requires a large enough dataset to learn the classification rules. Different from computer vision area, where large and clean benchmark dataset is available, limited lung nodule dataset is available to the public. Most people have their own datasets containing different numbers of patients from various sources. Where to get data is a big challenge to perform a deep learning based detection. Here we list some public lung nodule dataset used by recent publications as a reference.

- SPIE-AAPM-LUNGx dataset: a dataset used for a lung challenge originally to decide whether a nodule is benign or malignant.
- LIDC-IDRI: contains 1018 cases, the largest public database founded by the Lung Image Database Consortium and Image Database Resource Initiative. On the website lung nodule CT scan is available for download.
- ELCAP Public Lung Image Database: contains 50 low-dose thin-slice chest CT images with annotations for small nodules.
- NSCLC-Radiomics: contains 422 non-small cell lung cancer (NSCLC) patients.

4.2   Data Preparation

The major purposes of the data preparation are to make the training data less confusing, more fit to CNN and enrich data size.

To make the data less confusing, some literature perform lung segmentation to reduce noise. Then possible smooth methods could be applied to the segmented lung parts. Also, some other unnecessary parts, like some light dots or air, could be filtered out with threshold or other techniques.

For the purpose of modifying the data to be more fit for CNN, one challenge to be mention is the difference between CT scan and a RGB image. For a RGB image, it contains three channels, each channel has data ranging from 0 to 255. For a CT scan, it has only one channel with data ranging from $[-1000, 3000]$, which is much larger. Based on our experiments, if one directly puts CT scan with such large range into CNN, the performance will be limited. To make CT scan more similar to the image originally processed by CNN in computer vision, one solution is to rescale the data range of CT scan to $[0, 255]$. This could definitely cause information loss. In [5,11], an idea has been raised that turn the one channel CT scan into three channels by separating attenuation into three levels: low, normal and high. Then the three channeled image would be rescaled into $[0, 255]$. One benefit of this method is that the CT image now is in the same format with a RGB image. People can use pretrained CNN model to enhance detection performance. The pretrained model could be viewed as: first, we train a CNN to learn from normal RGB image so that it could extract some strong features from RGB image, in other words, these features are very good at recognizing RGB images of different classes; then we finetune the CNN on the transformed CT image. This is like training an expert with a new task, the difficulty of which is much less than training a newbie from scratch.

To enlarge the size of dataset to meet the need of big data by CNN, some methods such as image translation could be applied to enlarge dataset. The generated ones are considered different from the original image. Also, adding random noise, such as white noise, to the original image, could also be a solution to enlarge dataset.

One more thing is the issue of imbalanced dataset. As nodule detection is a binary classification problem (Nodule or Non-nodule), to train a classifier, the dataset should be a balanced one, which means both classes have equal number of samples. However, obviously, in a set of CT scans, the number of slices containing nodule is much smaller than that of slices do not contain nodules. So when preparing the training dataset, we need to balance the dataset to make the number of two types of samples, containing nodule or not, to be equal.

4.3 Some Other Challenges

Besides the data-related challenges mentioned above, there remains some other challenges. Below we list some of them:

- HPC support: The training of CNN based model requires huge amount of calculations on huge amount of data. Even with the help of HPC can the CNN model be trained in a durable length of time. Nowadays, besides training CNN purely on CPU, CUDA accelerated GPU has also been used for training as well.
- High Cost: As with the need of HPC, another challenge is cost. The support of HPC consumes large amount of energy and requires facilities. The concept of energy aware computing could be considered when designing a HPC system for CNN.

– Multi-disciplinary Cooperation Required: The design of a CNN based lung
  nodule detection system requires the cooperation from multiple disciplinary
  such as medical, radiology and computer science. Each expert from a certain
  area provides their own domain knowledge. The knowledge from different
  domains could guide how to perform data preparation, how to design the
  CNN model and how to make the system user friendly to radiologists. So it
  is very important for people from different areas to understand each other.
  Also, how to protect the data privacy is also a big concern in the cooperation.

5   Conclusion

In this paper, we give a brief introduction on the recent progress of using CNN
for lung nodule detection. A list of public packages as well as a list of public data
are given. We can see that CNN has shown great potential in the area of lung
nodule detection with either 2D or 3D convolution and the trend to simplify
the detection pipeline. Meanwhile, challenges still remain and researchers are
working on solving them. We can see a very promising future for the CNN based
lung nodule detection.

References

1. American Cancer Society. http://www.cancer.org/cancer/lungcancer-non-small
   cell/detailedguide/non-small-cell-lung-cancer-key-statistics
2. Krizhevsky, A., Sutskever, I., Hinton, G.E.: Imagenet classification with deep convolutional neural networks. In: Advances in Neural Information Processing Systems
   (2012)
3. LeCun, Y., et al.: Deep learning. Nature **521**(7553), 436–444 (2015)
4. Tajbakhs, N., et al.: Comparing two classes of end-to-end machine-learning models
   in lung nodule detection and classification: MTANNs vs. CNNs. Pattern Recognit.
   63, 476–486 (2017)
5. Shin, H.-C., et al.: Deep convolutional neural networks for computer-aided detection: CNN architectures, dataset characteristics and transfer learning. IEEE Trans.
   Med. Imaging **35**(5), 285–1298 (2016)
6. LeCun, Y., et al.: Gradient-based learning applied to document recognition. Proc.
   IEEE **86**(11), 2278–2324 (1998)
7. Tran, D., et al.: Learning spatiotemporal features with 3D convolutional networks.
   arXiv preprint arXiv:1412.0767 (2014)
8. Maturana, D., Scherer, S.: Voxnet: a 3D convolutional neural network for real-
   time object recognition. In: 2015 IEEE/RSJ International Conference on Intelligent
   Robots and Systems (IROS). IEEE (2015)
9. Anirudh, R., et al.: Lung nodule detection using 3D convolutional neural networks
   trained on weakly labeled data. In: SPIE Medical Imaging. International Society
   for Optics and Photonics (2016)
10. Golan, R., et al.: Lung nodule detection in CT images using deep convolutional
    neural networks. In: 2016 International Joint Conference on Neural Networks
    (IJCNN). IEEE (2016)

11. Gao, M., et al.: Holistic classification of CT attenuation patterns for interstitial lung diseases via deep convolutional neural networks. In: Computer Methods in Biomechanics and Biomedical Engineering: Imaging & Visualization, pp. 1–6 (2016)
12. Redmon, J., et al.: You only look once: unified, real-time object detection. arXiv preprint arXiv:1506.02640 (2015)

Using Machine Learning to Diagnose Bacterial Sepsis in the Critically Ill Patients

Yang Liu[1] and Kup-Sze Choi[2(✉)]

[1] Faculty of Health and Social Sciences,
The Hong Kong Polytechnic University, Hong Kong, China
14117476g@connect.polyu.hk
[2] Centre for Smart Health, School of Nursing,
The Hong Kong Polytechnic University, Hong Kong, China
hskschoi@polyu.edu.hk

Abstract. Sepsis is a life-threatening organ dysfunction caused by a dysregulated host response to infection. Early antibiotic therapy to patients with sepsis is necessary. Every hour of therapy delay could reduce the survival chance of patients with severe sepsis by 7.6%. Certain biomarkers like blood routine and C-reactive protein (CRP) are not sufficient to diagnose bacterial sepsis, and their sensitivity and specificity are relatively low. Procalcitonin (PCT) is the best diagnostic biomarker for sepsis so far, but is still not effective when sepsis occurs with some complications. Machine learning techniques were thus proposed to support diagnosis in this paper. A backpropagation artificial neural network (ANN) classifier, a support vector machine (SVM) classifier and a random forest (RF) classifier were trained and tested using the electronic health record (EHR) data of 185 critically ill patients. The area under curve (AUC), accuracy, sensitivity, and specificity of the ANN, SVM, and RF classifiers were (0.931, 90.8%, 90.2%, 91.6%), (0.940, 88.6%, 92.2%, 84.3%) and (0.953, 89.2%, 88.2%, 90.4%) respectively, which outperformed PCT where the corresponding values were (0.896, 0.716, 0.952, 0.822). In conclusion, the ANN and SVM classifiers explored have better diagnostic value on bacterial sepsis than any single biomarkers involve in this study.

Keywords: Sepsis · Bacterial sepsis · Machine learning · Artificial neural network · Support vector machine · Diagnostic value

1 Introduction

Sepsis is a complex, fatal disease and mainly occurs after serious infections. The latest International Consensus defined sepsis as a life-threatening organ dysfunction caused by a dysregulated host response to infection [1]. It is one of the most common reasons for intensive care unit (ICU) attendance, and can be easily found in non-ICU departments as well (10.9% of hospitalizations in U.S.; 95% CI) [2, 3]. Meanwhile, it is associated with high mortality, 34.7% to 52.0% of inpatient deaths in U.S. (95% CI) occurred among patients with sepsis [3].

In clinical practice, it is difficult to diagnose sepsis accurately. In 1991, the American College of Chest Physicians and the Society of Critical Care Medicine defined sepsis as

© Springer International Publishing AG 2017
H. Chen et al. (Eds.): ICSH 2017, LNCS 10347, pp. 223–233, 2017.
https://doi.org/10.1007/978-3-319-67964-8_22

infection, or suspected infection, meeting two or more systemic inflammatory response syndrome (SIRS) criteria (Sepsis 1.0) [4]. However, latter studies criticized that the Sepsis 1.0 criteria lacked both sensitivity and specificity [5, 6]. After the release of the Sepsis 2.0 criteria, which was too complicated and impractical for clinic usage, the new Sepsis 3.0 criteria was released in February 2016. The Sequential Organ Failure Assessment (SOFA) score in ICU or the qSOFA score outside ICU were recommended to replace SIRS criteria. Although Seymour's research showed that SOFA and qSOFA score has a higher predictive validity for in-hospital mortality [7], the reliability is uncertain and should be tested and verified by future research. Therefore, patients meeting any of those criteria could be considered as suspected sepsis.

Guidelines recommend that the early antibiotic therapy should be administered to patients with suspected sepsis [8]. Every hour of antibiotic usage delay would decrease the survival chance of patients with severe sepsis by 7.6% [9]. However, since it takes at least 48 h to obtain the results of a blood culture test, which is the gold standard of bacteria detection, even for an experienced physician, it is difficult to choose the effective antibiotics in early treatment. Usually, physicians have to speculate the possible source of infection under limited resources, and then be forced to use several types of empiric, broad-spectrum antibacterial agents in order to cover all the possible bacteria. Yet, the excessive usage of antibiotics may lead to unwanted liver and kidney damage, and extra medical spending as well [10].

There are certain biomarkers that can be referenced in the early hours of sepsis infection, such as blood routine (include total and differential white blood cell (WBC) count, platelet count, erythrocyte & reticulocyte count, and hemoglobin), and C-reactive protein (CRP), but their sensitivity and specificity are not sufficient for physicians to distinguish bacterial infection. Specifically, the sensitivity and specificity of CRP and WBC are (75%, 67%) and (46.4%, 46.7%) respectively [11]. Platelet Count (PLT) and Hemoglobin (Hgb) were also proven to be associated with the occurrence and development of disease [12, 13] but cannot diagnose bacterial infection alone [14].

On the other hand, procalcitonin (PCT) showed the best diagnostic value so far, with a sensitivity of 88% and a specificity of 81% [15] and had the ability to identify Gram-positive and Gram-negative bacterial infection [16]. Therefore, the newest guideline recommends using PCT level to diagnose sepsis. However, some studies also pointed out that PCT level may increase after surgery [17], trauma [18], heatstroke [19], burn [20], severe pancreatitis [21], anaphylactic shock [22] or cardiogenic shock [23] without obvious infection, which would affect its diagnostic value on sepsis.

Artificial neural networks (ANN), as one of the machine learning technologies, can be used for classification in this context. The structure of ANN is similar to the human brain, with nodes and links that simulate the functions of neuron bodies, axons, and dendrites. Some research showed that ANN exhibit better performance than other statistical classifier methods [24, 25]. Lammers et al. [26] showed that ANN was capable of discriminating wound infection with sensitivity of 70% and a specificity of 76% (as compared to 54% and 78% of physicians), and Heckerling et al. [27] developed an ANN model with sensitivity of 82.1% and specificity 74.4% for identifying urinary tract infection. Thus, ANN classifier may have the capacity to indicate bacterial infection with the various infection-related biomarkers as input. Similar to ANN, support vector machine (SVM) is a supervised machine learning method where the training a SVM model is a process trying to identify the widest gap that can separate the data mapped in a high-dimensional coordinate system by different categories [28]. Previous researches showed the SVM classification models had powerful performances on tasks related to biomarker data [29–31]. Besides, random forest (RF), developed by Breiman [32], is an ensemble learning method that using bagging algorithm to build multiple decision trees ensemble with random subsets and variables. Studies showed that RF method could predict diseases with good accuracy [33–36]. In the paper, these three machine learning methods are exploited to diagnose bacterial sepsis in the critically ill patients.

2 Methods

2.1 Subjects

EHR data of 185 inpatients in the ICU and Medical ICU (MICU) departments with suspected sepsis in the General Hospital of Guangzhou, China, were collected through the convenience sampling method in this study. 13 patients among were diagnosed with heatstroke; 27 with trauma; 9 with severe pancreatitis and 15 with postoperation. Meanwhile, 102 cases of them were diagnosed with bacterial sepsis by a physician through the medical records.

The inclusion criteria are as follows: 16–80 years of age with a suspected diagnosis of infection (admitting or discharge diagnoses for infection or taking antibiotic treatment during hospitalization), or fulfilling SIRS criteria or the SOFA score > 2; with the results of blood routine, PCT, CRP, and blood culture tests. Subjects will be excluded if they are pregnant; have any diseases that affect their immune system seriously (e.g., autoimmune disease, AIDS, cachexia); taking immunosuppressive therapy; with a discharge diagnosis of virus or fungal infection.

2.2 Data Collection

General information (gender, age), medical history, progress note (temperature, heart rate, respiratory rate, blood pressure, Glasgow coma scale, SOFA score), prescription, and admitting and discharge diagnoses of subjects were recorded through a de-identified processing following the HIPAA Privacy Rule's De-Identification Standard [37]. The following biomarker measurements will be obtained from the clinical laboratory: Blood Routine Examination (Total leukocyte count, Neutrophils Count, Eosinophils Count, Lymphocytes Count, Monocytes Count, Basophils Count, Erythrocyte Count, Hemoglobin, Hematocrit Value, Platelet Count), PCT, CRP, PaO2, FIO2, Bilirubin, and Creatinine.

3 Dataset

Generally, values of blood routine, PCT and CRP will be applied as the input; attributes that can be calculated from other test results in the blood routine test have been ignored by the study, such as Neutrophils percent (NE/WBC), Eosinophils percent (EOS/WBC), Basophils percent (BAS/WBC), Lymphocytes percent (LYM/WBC), Monocytes percent (MON/WBC), Mean Corpuscular Volume (Hct/RBC), Mean Corpuscular Hemoglobin (Hgb/RBC), and Mean Corpuscular Hemoglobin Concentration (Hgb/Hct). Since gender or age could affect the normal range of some biomarkers, they were considered as inputs as well. Thus, there were fourteen inputs and two outputs contained in the final dataset (Table 1). Also, a normalization method was applied to scale the numerical values into the range [0, 1].

Table 1. Dataset

Input	Attributes	Input values of the algorithms
1	Gender	1 (Male), 0 (Female)
2	Age	Normalized to [0,1]
3	Total Leukocyte Count (WBC)	
4	Neutrophils Count (NE)	
5	Eosinophils Count (EOS)	
6	Basophils Count (BAS)	
7	Lymphocytes Count (LYM)	
8	Monocytes Count (MON)	
9	Erythrocyte Count (RBC)	
10	Hemoglobin (Hgb)	
11	Hematocrit Value (Hct)	
12	Platelet Count (PLT)	
13	Procalcitonin (PCT)	
14	C-reactive protein (CRP)	
Output	Attributes	Output values of the algorithms
1	Bacterial sepsis	1 (Yes), 0 (No)

3.1 Machine Learning Models

A backpropagation neural network model of fourteen neurons in the input layer, seventeen in the first hidden layer, two in the second hidden layer and one in the output layer was trained through the Fast Artificial Neural Network Library (FANN) [38] using linear activation function at the output and sigmoid activitaiton functrion at the hidden layer (Fig. 1).

The SVM classifier model was trained using the Matlab LIBSVM toolbox [39]. The parameters c = 1.414 and g = 4 were optimized by a grid search under a 10-fold cross-validation process. The RF model was built using the Matlab RF tool [40, 41], the tree number was set to 800 after a parameter performance evaluation under a 10-fold cross-validation process.

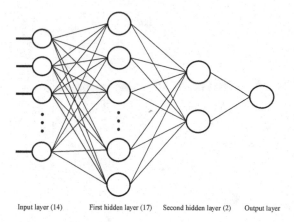

Input layer (14)   First hidden layer (17)   Second hidden layer (2)   Output layer

Fig. 1. The neural network structure.

3.2 Evaluation

The performance of the classifications was tested using leave-one-out cross-validation (LOOCV), where the classifier used single observation to test the performance of model trained by the remaining observations. The process was then repeated to ensure that all observation was tested. Then, sensitivity, specificity, and accuracy were calculated from the results. In addition, receiver operating characteristic (ROC) curves were plotted, and AUC was calculated to determine the overall performance of the machine learning models. Meanwhile, in order to compare the diagnostic values of the machine learning methods and the biomarkers, the ROC curve was studied for each biomarker, and the sensitivity, specificity, and accuracy of the three biomarkers with the largest AUC were determined based on the best cutoff point that maximizes the Youden's index (i.e. sensitivity + specificity − 1) [42].

4 Result

The ROC curves of the selected biomarkers have been plotted as Fig. 2. PCT got the highest diagnostic value, with an AUC of 0.896 (95% confidence interval [CI], 0.81 to 0.942) via biomarkers, followed by CRP (AUC, 0.832; 95% CI, 0.7743 to 0.890) and NE (AUC, 0.681; 95% CI, 0.603 to 0.759). At a cutoff value at 8.56 ng/ml of PCT, 87.5 mg/l of CRP, and 14.34 of Neutrophil count, they yielded sensitivity, specificity, and accuracy of (71.6%, 95.2%, 82.0%); (75.5%, 78.3%, 76.8%); and (56.9%, 75.0%, 64.9%), respectively. PCT was the most powerful biomarker for diagnosing sepsis syndrome in this analysis (Table 2).

To explore the diagnostic performance between single biomarker and machine learning models, ROC curves of PCT, ANN, SVM, and RF were plotted (Fig. 3). As shown in Table 3, all three machine learning models yielded a higher AUC value (ANN: 0.931, 95% CI 0.889–0.973; SVM: 0.940, 95% CI 0.903–0.977; RF: 0.953, 95% CI 0.924–0.981) than the most valuable biomarker, PCT (0.896, 95% CI 0.851–0.942).

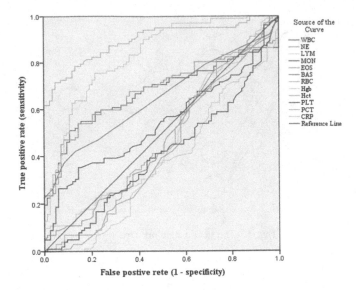

Fig. 2. ROC curves of biomarkers

Table 2. AUC and CI of biomarkers

Test result variable(s)	Area	Asymptotic 95% Confidence interval	
		Lower bound	Upper bound
WBC	0.672	0.593	0.751
NE	0.681	0.603	0.759
LYM	0.418	0.336	0.500
MON	0.540	0.457	0.623
EOS	0.476	0.392	0.561
BAS	0.648	0.570	0.727
RBC	0.462	0.376	0.547
Hgb	0.429	0.343	0.515
Hct	0.431	0.346	0.516
PLT	0.408	0.326	0.490
PCT	0.896	0.851	0.942
CRP	0.832	0.774	0.890

Both the accuracy and sensitivity of ANN (90.8%, 90.2%), SVM (88.6%, 92.2%), and RF(89.2%, 88.2%) were better than those of PCT (82.2%, 71.6%) at a cutoff value of 8.56 ng/ml determined by Youden's index (see Table 4), where the specificity of ANN (91.6%), SVM (84.3%), RF (90.4%) were lower than that of PCT (95.2%). However, when we set the cutoff PCT concentration with identical 88.2% sensitivity at 3.40 ng/mL, both its accuracy (78.4%) and specificity (66.3%) were clearly lower than those of ANN, SVM, and RF models (see Table 4).

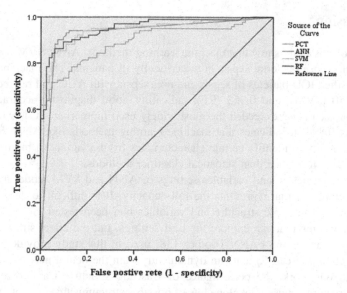

Fig. 3. ROC curves of PCT, ANN, and SVM

Table 3. AUC and CI of ANN, SVM, PCT and CRP

Test result variable(s)	Area	Asymptotic 95% Confidence interval	
		Lower bound	Upper bound
PCT	0.896	0.851	0.942
ANN	0.931	0.889	0.973
SVM	0.940	0.903	0.977
RF	0.953	0.924	0.981

Table 4. Performance of ANN, SVM, RF, and PCT

	ANN	SVM	RF	PCT (Cutoff = 8.56)	PCT (Cutoff = 3.40)
True positive	92	94	90	73	90
False positive	7	13	8	4	28
True negative	76	70	75	79	55
False negative	10	8	12	29	12
Accuracy	90.8%	88.6%	89.2%	82.2%	78.4%
Sensitivity	90.2%	92.2%	88.2%	71.6%	88.2%
Specificity	91.6%	84.3%	90.4%	95.2%	66.2%

5 Discussion

The results of this study show that machine learning methods, ANN, SVM, and RF can be used to diagnose bacterial sepsis in the critically ill patients. The machine learning models classified ICU patients of sepsis and non-sepsis with AUC that ranged at 0.931 (ANN), 0.940 (SVM), and 0.953 (RF), indicating good diagnostic accuracy. These classification accuracies exceeded the most widely used biomarker, PCT, which had a ROC area of 0.896. It indicates that machine learning methods like ANN, SVM, and RF have the ability to identify certain characteristics from a variety of biomarkers and exhibit better performance than statistical classifier methods.

The current structure and variables settings of ANN and SVM model may not be the best combination that represents the full capacity. It is difficult to detect the best settings unless all possible structure and variables had been tested. Some tools have provided algorithms that can explore the best settings, but the effect still needs to be verified. For example, the FANN Toolbox [38] used in this study provide a topology training function (Cascade2) that can dynamically train the neural network. However, according to our work, the performance of Cascade structure was worse than the 14-17-2-1 structure we used, let alone lots of possible structures that are not explored in general. Another simple example is that many methods are available to determine the best c and g value when building a SVM classifier, such as Grid Search, Genetic Algorithm (GA) and Particle Swarm Optimization (PSO) method. However, out tests show that even though the overall performances of the SVM models built based on these methods were similar, the best c and g value generated by different methods could vary a lot. Meanwhile, when new data were added into models, the variables could be changed again. Therefore, it is a challenging task to find out or even evaluate the best structure and variables.

Moreover, the sample size of this study may still be not enough for the machine learning methods to identify sufficiently specific characteristics. Sepsis is always associated with other medical conditions, which in turn affects the biomarkers that diagnose sepsis [17–21]. In this study, the number of subjects with burn, anaphylactic shock or cardiogenic shock were lower than 10. Along with individual variations, the feature of these samples might not be learned by the algorithms completely. To solve this problem, it is necessary to enlarge the sample size in the future work. A sufficient sample size will not only resolve the current problem but also meet the requirements of applying more advanced methods in the fields of deep learning, e.g. stacked autoencoder (SAE) [43] and multi-layer convolutional neural networks (CNNs) [44].

6 Conclusion

ANN, SVM, and RF methods were explored in this study for diagnosing bacterial sepsis in the critically ill patient. All the proposed classifiers, using 14 biomarkers as the input, evaluated by the leave-one-out cross-validation technique, showed better performance in AUC, accuracy, sensitivity and specificity, when compared to those obtained by using a single biomarker. This study has shown that ANN, SVM, and RF classifiers can improve the diagnostic quality of bacterial sepsis. However, studies with larger sample size are necessary in future study to improve the performance of classifiers. Further research on the structure and setting of the models in the machine learning methods concerned will also be conducted.

Acknowledgement. This work is supported in part by the Hong Kong Research Grants Council (PolyU 152040/16E), the Hong Kong Polytechnic University (G-UC93, G-YBKX) and the YC Yu Scholarship for Centre for Smart Health.

References

1. Singer, M., Deutschman, C.S., Seymour, C., et al.: The third international consensus definitions for sepsis and septic shock (sepsis-3). JAMA **315**, 801–810 (2016). doi:10.1001/jama.2016.0287
2. Angus, D.C., Linde-Zwirble, W.T., Lidicker, J., Clermont, G., Carcillo, J., Pinsky, M.R.: Epidemiology of severe sepsis in the United States: analysis of incidence, outcome, and associated costs of care. Crit. Care Med. Baltim. **29**, 1303–1310 (2001)
3. Liu, V., Escobar, G.J., Greene, J.D., Soule, J., Whippy, A., Angus, D.C., Iwashyna, T.J.: Hospital deaths in patients with sepsis from 2 independent cohorts. JAMA **312**, 90–92 (2014)
4. Bone, R.C., Balk, R.A., Cerra, F.B., Dellinger, R.P., Fein, A.M., Knaus, W.A., Schein, R., Sibbald, W.J.: Definitions for sepsis and organ failure and guidelines for the use of innovative therapies in sepsis. The ACCP/SCCM Consensus Conference Committee. American College of Chest Physicians/Society of Critical Care Medicine. Chest J. **101**, 1644–1655 (1992)
5. Sprung, C.L., Sakr, Y., Vincent, J.-L., Le Gall, J.-R., Reinhart, K., Ranieri, V.M., Gerlach, H., Fielden, J., Groba, C.B., Payen, D.: An evaluation of systemic inflammatory response syndrome signs in the sepsis occurrence in acutely ill patients (SOAP) study. Intensive Care Med. **32**, 421–427 (2006)
6. Vincent, J.-L., Opal, S.M., Marshall, J.C., Tracey, K.J.: Sepsis definitions: time for change. Lancet Lond. Engl. **381**, 774 (2013)
7. Seymour, C.W., Liu, V.X., Iwashyna, T.J., Brunkhorst, F.M., Rea, T.D., Scherag, A., Rubenfeld, G., Kahn, J.M., Shankar-Hari, M., Singer, M.: Assessment of clinical criteria for sepsis: for the third international consensus definitions for sepsis and septic shock (Sepsis-3). JAMA **315**, 762–774 (2016)
8. Dellinger, R.P., Levy, M.M., Rhodes, A., Annane, D., Gerlach, H., Opal, S.M., Sevransky, J. E., Sprung, C.L., Douglas, I.S., Jaeschke, R.: Surviving sepsis campaign: international guidelines for management of severe sepsis and septic shock, 2012. Intensive Care Med. **39**, 165–228 (2013)
9. van Zanten, A.R.: The golden hour of antibiotic administration in severe sepsis: avoid a false start striving for gold*. Crit. Care Med. **42**, 1931–1932 (2014)
10. Gross, P.A., Patel, B.: Reducing antibiotic overuse: a call for a national performance measure for not treating asymptomatic bacteriuria. Clin. Infect. Dis. **45**, 1335–1337 (2007)
11. Harbarth, S., Holeckova, K., Froidevaux, C., Pittet, D., Ricou, B., Grau, G.E., Vadas, L., Pugin, J.: Diagnostic value of procalcitonin, interleukin-6, and interleukin-8 in critically ill patients admitted with suspected sepsis. Am. J. Respir. Crit. Care Med. **164**, 396–402 (2001)

12. Miglietta, F., Faneschi, M., Lobreglio, G., Palumbo, C., Rizzo, A., Cucurachi, M., Portaccio, G., Guerra, F., Pizzolante, M.: Procalcitonin, C-reactive protein and serum lactate dehydrogenase in the diagnosis of bacterial sepsis, SIRS and systemic candidiasis. Infez. Med. Riv. Period. Eziologia Epidemiol. Diagn. Clin. E Ter. Delle Patol. Infett. 23, 230–237 (2015)

13. Wang, K., Bhandari, V., Chepustanova, S., Huber, G., Stephen, O., Corey, S., Shattuck, M.D., Kirby, M.: Which biomarkers reveal neonatal sepsis? PLoS ONE 8, e82700 (2013)

14. Becchi, C., Al Malyan, M., Fabbri, L., Marsili, M., Boddi, V., Boncinelli, S.: Mean platelet volume trend in sepsis: is it a useful parameter? Minerva Anestesiol. 72, 749–756 (2006)

15. Guven, H., Altintop, L., Baydin, A., Esen, S., Aygun, D., Hokelek, M., Doganay, Z., Bek, Y.: Diagnostic value of procalcitonin levels as an early indicator of sepsis. Am. J. Emerg. Med. 20, 202–206 (2002). doi:10.1053/ajem.2002.33005

16. Charles, P.E., Ladoire, S., Aho, S., Quenot, J.-P., Doise, J.-M., Prin, S., Olsson, N.-O., Blettery, B.: Serum procalcitonin elevation in critically ill patients at the onset of bacteremia caused by either Gram negative or Gram positive bacteria. BMC Infect. Dis. 8, 1 (2008)

17. Meisner, M., Tschaikowsky, K., Hutzler, A., Schüttler, J., Schick, C.: Postoperative plasma concentrations of procalcitonin after different types of surgery. Intensive Care Med. 24, 680–684 (1998). doi:10.1007/s001340050644

18. Mimoz, O., Edouard, A.R., Samii, K., Benoist, J.F., Assicot, M., Bohuon, C.: Procalcitonin and C-reactive protein during the early posttraumatic systemic inflammatory response syndrome. Intensive Care Med. 24, 185–188 (1998). doi:10.1007/s001340050543

19. Hausfater, P., Hurtado, M., Pease, S., Juillien, G., Lvovschi, V.-E., Salehabadi, S., Lidove, O., Wolff, M., Bernard, M., Chollet-Martin, S., Riou, B.: Is procalcitonin a marker of critical illness in heatstroke? Intensive Care Med. 34, 1377–1383 (2008). doi:10.1007/s00134-008-1083-y

20. Mann, E.A., Wood, G.L., Wade, C.E.: Use of procalcitonin for the detection of sepsis in the critically ill burn patient: a systematic review of the literature. Burns. 37, 549–558 (2011). doi:10.1016/j.burns.2010.04.013

21. Rau, B.M., Kemppainen, E.A., Gumbs, A.A., Büchler, M.W., Wegscheider, K., Bassi, C., Puolakkainen, P.A., Beger, H.G.: Early assessment of pancreatic infections and overall prognosis in severe acute pancreatitis by procalcitonin (PCT): a prospective international multicenter study. Ann. Surg. 245, 745 (2007). doi:10.1097/01.sla.0000252443.22360.46

22. Kim, Y.J., Kang, S.W., Lee, J.H., Cho, J.H.: Marked elevation of procalcitonin level can lead to a misdiagnosis of anaphylactic shock as septic shock. Int. J. Infect. Dis. 37, 93–94 (2015). doi:10.1016/j.ijid.2015.06.012

23. Geppert, A., Steiner, A., Delle-Karth, G., Heinz, G., Huber, K.: Usefulness of procalcitonin for diagnosing complicating sepsis in patients with cardiogenic shock. Intensive Care Med. 29, 1384–1389 (2003). doi:10.1007/s00134-003-1827-7

24. Patil, S., Henry, J.W., Rubenfire, M., Stein, P.D.: Neural network in the clinical diagnosis of acute pulmonary embolism. CHEST J. 104, 1685–1689 (1993)

25. Tu, J.V.: Advantages and disadvantages of using artificial neural networks versus logistic regression for predicting medical outcomes. J. Clin. Epidemiol. 49, 1225–1231 (1996)

26. Lammers, R.L., Hudson, D.L., Seaman, M.E.: Prediction of traumatic wound infection with a neural network-derived decision model. Am. J. Emerg. Med. 21, 1–7 (2003). doi:10.1053/ajem.2003.50026

27. Heckerling, P.S., Canaris, G.J., Flach, S.D., Tape, T.G., Wigton, R.S., Gerber, B.S.: Predictors of urinary tract infection based on artificial neural networks and genetic algorithms. Int. J. Med. Inf. 76, 289–296 (2007). doi:10.1016/j.ijmedinf.2006.01.005

28. Cortes, C., Vapnik, V.: Support-vector networks. Mach. Learn. 20, 273–297 (1995). doi:10.1023/A:1022627411411

29. Abeel, T., Helleputte, T., Van de Peer, Y., Dupont, P., Saeys, Y.: Robust biomarker identification for cancer diagnosis with ensemble feature selection methods. Bioinformatics **26**, 392–398 (2010). doi:10.1093/bioinformatics/btp630
30. Liu, J.J., Cutler, G., Li, W., Pan, Z., Peng, S., Hoey, T., Chen, L., Ling, X.B.: Multiclass cancer classification and biomarker discovery using GA-based algorithms. Bioinformatics **21**, 2691–2697 (2005). doi:10.1093/bioinformatics/bti419
31. Wang, G., Lam, K.-M., Deng, Z., Choi, K.-S.: Prediction of mortality after radical cystectomy for bladder cancer by machine learning techniques. Comput. Biol. Med. **63**, 124–132 (2015). doi:10.1016/j.compbiomed.2015.05.015
32. Breiman, L.: Random forests. Mach. Learn. **45**, 5–32 (2001). doi:10.1023/A: 1010933404324
33. Hsieh, C.-H., Lu, R.-H., Lee, N.-H., Chiu, W.-T., Hsu, M.-H., Li (Jack), Y.-C.: Novel solutions for an old disease: diagnosis of acute appendicitis with random forest, support vector machines, and artificial neural networks. Surgery **149**, 87–93 (2011). doi:10.1016/j. surg.2010.03.023
34. Özçift, A.: Random forests ensemble classifier trained with data resampling strategy to improve cardiac arrhythmia diagnosis. Comput. Biol. Med. **41**, 265–271 (2011). doi:10. 1016/j.compbiomed.2011.03.001
35. Nguyen, C., Wang, Y., Nguyen, H.N.: Random forest classifier combined with feature selection for breast cancer diagnosis and prognostic (2013). doi:10.4236/jbise.2013.65070
36. Azar, A.T., Elshazly, H.I., Hassanien, A.E., Elkorany, A.M.: A random forest classifier for lymph diseases. Comput. Methods Programs Biomed. **113**, 465–473 (2014). doi:10.1016/j. cmpb.2013.11.004
37. Lawrence, D.: Health insurance portability and accountability act (HIPAA) privacy rule and the national instant criminal background check system (NICS). Final rule. Fed. Regist. **81**, 382–396 (2016)
38. Nissen, S.: Implementation of a fast artificial neural network library (FANN). Rep. Dep. Comput. Sci. Univ. Cph. DIKU. 31, 29 (2003)
39. Chang, C.-C., Lin, C.-J.: LIBSVM: a library for support vector machines. ACM Trans. Intell. Syst. Technol. **2**, 27:1–27:27 (2011). doi:10.1145/1961189.1961199
40. Google Code Archive - Long-term storage for Google Code Project Hosting. https://code. google.com/archive/p/randomforest-matlab/
41. Liaw, A., Wiener, M.: Classification and regression by random forest. R. News **2**, 18–22 (2002)
42. Youden, W.J.: Index for rating diagnostic tests. Cancer **3**, 32–35 (1950)
43. Miotto, R., Li, L., Kidd, B.A., Dudley, J.T.: Deep patient: an unsupervised representation to predict the future of patients from the electronic health records. Sci. Rep. **6**, 26094 (2016). doi:10.1038/srep26094
44. Nguyen, P., Tran, T., Wickramasinghe, N., Venkatesh, S.: Deepr: a convolutional net for medical records (2016). ArXiv160707519 Cs Stat

Data/Text Mining in Healthcare

A Deep Learning Based Named Entity Recognition Approach for Adverse Drug Events Identification and Extraction in Health Social Media

Long Xia[1], G. Alan Wang[1], and Weiguo Fan[2(✉)]

[1] Department of Business Information Technology, Pamplin College of Business, Virginia Tech, 1007 Pamplin Hall, Blacksburg, VA 24061, USA
[2] Department of Accounting and Information Systems, Pamplin College of Business, Virginia Tech, 3007 Pamplin Hall, Blacksburg, VA 24061, USA
wfan@vt.edu

Abstract. Drug safety surveillance plays a significant role in supporting medication decision-making by both healthcare providers and patients. Extracting adverse drug events (ADEs) from social media provides a promising direction to addressing this challenging task. Prior studies typically perform lexicon-based extraction using existing dictionaries or medical lexicons. While those approaches can capture ADEs and identify risky drugs from patient social media postings, they often fail to detect those ADEs whose descriptive words do not exist in medical lexicons and dictionaries. In addition, their performance is inferior when ADE related social media content is expressed in an ambiguous manner. In this research, we propose a research framework using advanced natural language processing and deep learning for high-performance ADE extraction. The framework consists of training the word embeddings using a large medical domain corpus to capture precise semantic and syntactic word relationships, and a deep learning based named entity recognition method for drug and ADE entity identification and prediction. Experimental results show that our framework significantly outperforms existing models when extracting ADEs from social media in different test beds.

Keywords: Adverse drug events · Pharmacovigilance · Social media · Deep learning · Word embeddings · Named entity extraction

1 Introduction

Adverse drug events (ADEs) are injuries/side effects caused by taking medical treatments related to a drug. In the United States, ADEs account for over 3.5 million physician visits, 1 million emergency department visits, and more than 2 million injuries, hospitalizations, and deaths [1]. The surging cases and costs make patients and clinical experts believe the importance of effective ADEs surveillance systems which not only provide more reliable evidence for risky drug identification to healthcare providers, but also warn other patients about the potential issues and side effects for better risk control. Thus, a great attention has been drawn to this research field from pharmacovigilance community

© Springer International Publishing AG 2017
H. Chen et al. (Eds.): ICSH 2017, LNCS 10347, pp. 237–248, 2017.
https://doi.org/10.1007/978-3-319-67964-8_23

to detect, assess, understand and prevent ADEs [2]. Pharmacovigilance, according to World Health Organization (WHO), is defined as "the science and activities relating to the detection, assessment, understanding and prevention of adverse effects or any other drug-related problem" [3].

Currently, reporting ADEs mainly relies on online and open data sources, including the U.S. Food and Drug Administration (FDA) Adverse Event Reporting System (FAERS) and VigiBase maintained by the WHO [4]. However, these systems rely on spontaneous reporting and ignore the large amount of discussions related to ADEs in the open Internet space such as social media. With the prevalence of social media, the way in which people learn about health and disease topics and share their medical conditions, diagnosis, treatment, and medications is changing dramatically. This increased availability of health social media data also provides an intriguing research opportunity to health analytics researchers [5].

Given the large amount of user generated content scattered around hundreds of health social networking sites and forums available on the Internet, it is infeasible for patients or medical practitioners to manually identify ADEs and aggregate online patient reports [6]. Thus, automated processing of online patient reports from social media can alleviate the information overload problem and provide useful information for health decision-making. A great effort has been devoted to developing effective and efficient methods to automatically extract ADEs from online patient reports in social media. A widely used method is to utilize lexicon-based extraction using existing dictionaries of medical lexicons including Unified Medical Language System (UMLS), the medical terms in FDA's FAERS, Consumer Health Vocabulary (CHV), Side Effect Resource (SIDER), etc. This approach achieves a satisfactory performance in automatically extracting ADEs from online patient reports [7].

However, there are several limitations with the lexicon-based approach. First, social media contains a large amount of online patient colloquial vocabulary, including abbreviation, buzzwords, special expressions, typos and misspellings. Also, drug issues and ADEs mentioned by patients are sometimes highly specific, and they might be quite different from the lexicons in medical dictionaries, which are normally more generic. Second, since the medical lexicon dictionaries are built on passive reporting systems, it cannot be used to dynamically capture new ADEs and cannot be used to monitor ADEs in real time. Last but not the least, informal language used in social media postings can cause confusion for lexicon-based text mining algorithms. A deeper understanding of the context is needed. Table 1 illustrates these issues with online drug reviews extracted from WebMD.

From Table 1, we observe some data characteristics of social media postings. In post 1, the user uses an abbreviation: 'wght loss' to represent 'weight loss'. This is different from professional medical lexicons. In post 2, the ADE is presented in a highly specific manner. However, the standard medical lexicon dictionaries use 'weight gain'. In post 3, there is a misspelling ('weight', which should be 'weight'). In post 4, 'powdery taste' is a new ADE which does not exist in medical lexicon dictionary. In post 5, although there is a negation word 'never', it does not negate the sentence. In post 6, the word 'never' actually negates the ADEs and drug indications. When facing the first five situations in Table 1, the current lexicon based extraction would fail.

Table 1. Examples of patient self-reports in social media

No.	Review content	Contain ADE
1	I get so **weak [ADE]** and **lethargic [ADE]** and it does cause **wght loss [ADE]**	Yes
2	**Gained 40 lbs [ADE]** in 2yrs on oral meds	Yes
3	I have a **heart condition [ADE]** and was not made aware of the **wieght gain [ADE]** side effect	Yes
4	**Stomach pain [ADE], bad smell [ADE], powdery taste [ADE]**, and **loose bowels [ADE]**	Yes
5	I have never had a problem with **cramping legs, feet, extremely achey muscles [ADE],** until taking this pill	Yes
6	I never had any nausea with it	No

From the discussion above, despite current research progresses, mining high quality ADEs information from social media is still challenging and requires more advanced techniques. We are motivated to design and implement a new ADE identification and extraction method that can be applied to health social media postings to improve medication decision-making and facilitate preventive care. We adapt a deep learning based named entity recognition (NER) approach, which utilizes word embeddings trained on medical corpus to capture syntactic and semantic relationships between words and inside sentences, for automatic and effective ADE extraction.

Our contributions to literature are 3-fold: (1) To the best of our knowledge, this is the first study that develops an advanced deep learning based NER approach for drug entity and ADE entity extraction; (2) We are also the first to construct word embeddings trained on the largest medical domain corpus that we created for the purpose of ADE extraction. Because of the words relations learned from medical domain corpus, this approach features a high level of generalizability and is robust to capture new ADEs to achieve real-time monitoring of ADEs in social media; (3) Moreover, our system can learn both syntactic and semantic relations in the sentences of social media postings and extract drug and ADE entities in the same step, which provides a simplified (one step) yet highly efficient and effective way for ADE extraction.

The rest of the paper is organized as follows. Section 2 reviews related work in ADE extraction and highlight the research gap. Section 3 describes our proposed research framework. Section 4 presents the experiments and evaluation results. Section 5 discusses the contributions of this study and directions for future work.

2   Related Work

2.1   Pharmacovigilance in Social Media

Recognizing the value of patient intelligence on pharmacovigilance in social media and the demand of advanced techniques for analyzing health social media contents, researchers had conducted extensive studies in this field. Some of the recent studies are listed in Table 2. As shown in Table 2, those studies differ in three aspects: social media data source, medical lexicon dictionary, and ADE extraction method.

Table 2. Previous studies on pharmacovigilance in social media

Apply biomedical relation extraction	Studies	Lexicon dictionaries	Social media data source	Results
Not applied	Leaman et al. [8]	Lexicons: UMLS, MedEffect, SIDER	Daily strength	Precision: 78:3%; Recall: 69:9%; F-measure: 73:9%
Not applied	Nikfarjam and Gonzalez [9]	Association rule mining	Daily strength	Precision: 70%; Recall: 66.3%; F-measure: 68.0%
Co-occurrence analysis	Benton et al. [10]	Lexicons: CHV, FAERS	Breast cancer forums	Not applied
Rule-based analysis	Wu et al. [11]	Lexicon constructed by authors	Online discussions	Precision: 70%; Recall: 69%
Not applied	Bian et al. [12]	Lexicon: FAERS	Twitter	Accuracy: 74%; AUC value: 0.82
Learning-based analysis	Liu and Chen [7]	Lexicons: UMLS, FEARS, CHV	Diabetes and heart disease forums	Precision: 82%; Recall: 56.5%; F-measure: 66.9%

Prior studies mainly focused on three types of social media data sources, including general discussion forums [8, 9, 11], general social media (e.g., Twitter) [12], and disease-specific discussion forums [7, 10]. Medical lexicon dictionaries were used to identify medical entities in the posts for further analysis. This lexicon-based entity recognition approaches were widely used mainly because of the existence of well-developed medical lexicon dictionaries, including UMLS [7, 8], FEARS [7, 10, 12], CHV [7, 10], and MedEffect [8], SIDER [8].

To determine if there is a causal relationship between the drug and medical issues, medical relation extraction techniques were utilized during ADE extraction. Benton et al. used a co-occurrence analysis approach to identify relations [10]. Wu et al. developed a rule-based approach to determine the probability that a user would mention the ADE when he/she is discussing the drug [11]. Liu and Chen utilized shortest dependency path kernel based statistical learning and semantic filtering to extract the medical relations to improve their ADE extraction results [7].

2.2 Word Embeddings

Many current healthcare information systems treat words in text data as indices in a vocabulary. Although this word representation features several advantages such as simplicity and robustness, it does not capture the similarity as well as semantic and syntactic relations between words [13]. For example, if "diabetes" and "hypertension" appear in the text, the system only considers the existences but ignores their internal similarities and relations. A solution to this problem is to use distributed representation of words. Distributed representation of words as continuous vectors can capture the similarities between words by calculating their distances in the vector space. Thus, the vectors for "diabetes" and "hypertension" should be close in vector space. This distributed representation of words as vectors, defined as word embeddings, helps learning algorithms achieve better performance in many natural language processing (NLP) tasks by grouping similar words [14]. Recently, Mikolov et al. developed the Skip-gram model, an efficient method for learning high quality word embeddings [13]. The word embeddings have succeeded in capturing fine-grained semantic and syntactic regularities.

The word relations represented in word embeddings could be a useful property in ADE recognition because we could learn the medical specific word-vectors that capture a large number of precise semantic and syntactic word relationships in the medical domain from a large unlabeled medical corpus. For example, we can group the ADE key words together to help extract ADE. Also, using this unsupervised deep learning, we can dynamically feed in any available data to the learning process to refine the learned word embeddings, which provides the capability for dynamic updates from new data. We expect the word embeddings trained on text documents in the medical domain will perform better than traditional word representations in tackling various healthcare text mining tasks.

2.3 Named Entity Recognition

Named entity recognition (NER) is a very important NLP task to find and cluster named entities in text data into different categories. It has been used to identify various entities such as locations, organizations, and person names from text data. Various methods have been used in the past for NER tasks. But they mainly relied on manual features and focused on improving feature selection and engineering [16–18].

Collobert et al. proposed an effective neural network model that requires little feature engineering and instead learns important features from word embeddings trained on large quantities of unlabeled text [15]. Though an improvement has been achieved by this model, there are a few limitations. The most important one is that it uses a window-based context to classify the word in the center, thus it only considers the surrounding words close to the target word, but completely discards the relations between center word and words far away from it. However, these long-distance relations could be helpful for various NLP tasks [17]. This problem can be solved by applying the recurrent neural network (RNN), which can process variable length inputs and consider long distance word dependencies [16]. A variant of RNNs, the long-short term memory (LSTM), achieved a great success to tackle many NLP tasks as it is able to leverage both short-distance and long-distance dependencies [17]. For tasks such as NER, which is deal with sequential classification, a bi-directional LSTM model that can consider all the words on both sides of the target word is expected to give better performance compared with the fixed-size window classification [18].

2.4 Research Questions

We have identified several research gaps based on the discussions above. First, previous research heavily relies on medical lexicon dictionaries, which greatly limited their capabilities in dynamically and robustly monitoring ADE. Second, learning-based approach was proved to outperform rule-based and co-occurrence based methods in extracting ADE [7]. However, only simple and shallow learning techniques were applied in prior research. Few advanced learning based methods have been adopted in health social media analytics. Third, despite the availability of massive health social media data on the Internet, few prior studies identify its significance and usefulness to help improve the performance of current health information systems.

Based on the research gap identified, our study addresses three questions.

1. How to develop a research framework that can outperform existing ADE extraction methods, and achieve dynamically real-time monitoring of ADE in social media?
2. Can the word embeddings trained on a medical corpus capture semantic and syntactic word relationships and help improve the performance of ADE extraction?
3. How can a model trained on one test bed achieve comparable performance on another test bed? In other words, how to develop an ADE extraction framework that can be generally applied to different corpuses?

To address our research questions, we develop a novel ADE extraction framework, which is distinctly different from the existing extraction models. We are using RNN based NER approach for ADEs recognition and extraction, incorporating pre-trained word embeddings using a large medical corpus. Our approach achieves significantly improved extraction performance compared with baseline methods. Our findings can benefit all stakeholders related to pharmacovigilance, including regulators, drug companies, patients, and doctors, in identifying potential drug side effects and risks.

3   Research Framework

Figure 1 shows our overall research framework for pharmacovigilance in health social media. There are two major components: word embeddings training and RNN based NER. The detailed steps are explained below.

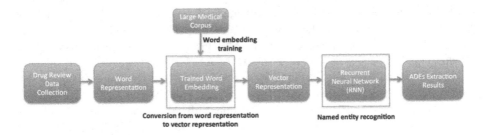

Fig. 1. Research framework for pharmacovigilance in health social media

3.1 Data Collection

For the word embeddings training purpose, we downloaded the Open Access Subset of PubMed Central (PMC), which contains 1.25 million articles and 3.5 billion tokens. PMC is an online digital database of freely available full-text biomedical literature. We also developed automated crawlers to download text contents of posts from various online healthcare websites, to have a better coverage of different types of health social media, including general health discussion forum (Daily Strength), drug review website (WebMD), doctor review website (HealthGrades), and disease-specific discussion forum (American Diabetes Association).

3.2 Word Embeddings Training

We trained our word embeddings using the 4 billion tokens found in our medical corpus. This is an unsupervised learning process, which does not require human labeling. Different dimensions of word vector can be tested to identify the best setting. After training, a set of word vectors will be generated, which will serve as a lookup table to replace words to vector representations in the next step (Sect. 3.4).

3.3 Converting from Word Representation to Vector Representation

As discussed in previous section, word embeddings trained from the large corpus should be able to capture semantic and syntactic relations between words. The learned relationships and similar words groupings could be useful to improve various NLP tasks. This step is to convert every word in the raw text data to vector representation. From Sect. 3.2, we obtain a dictionary of trained word vectors, whose keys are the word and values are the vectors. All words from drug reviews are lowercased and passed through the dictionary to convert a sequence of words to a sequence of vectors.

3.4 Named Entity Recognition

As RNN is able to capture both short-distance and non-trivial long-distance word dependencies, and learn the sentences as a whole, we believe it would give improved performance over previous lexicon and rule-based approach. We use word-vectors learned from a large unlabeled medical corpus to incorporate the precise semantic and syntactic word relationships, and combined with NER to accomplish ADE extraction.

4 Experiment and Results

4.1 Research Test Bed

Recognizing the prevalence and significant impact of chronic diseases, we choose diabetes and hypertension in our study. These two diseases cover a large population. Patients with either one or both diseases normally rely on medications treatments to control and improve their medical conditions. We chose online reviews for our study, rather than tweets, Facebook or forum postings, in order to be more focused on drug related contents. For building ADE extraction model purpose, we developed a crawler to download drugs reviews from WebMD, which is the leading publisher in the United States and has the largest amount of online drug reviews. We include following fields from the website, review ID, drug name, URL, ratings, and review text content.

4.2   Tagging Scheme

We randomly selected 5,600 diabetes drug reviews and 800 hypertension drug reviews. We used a simple protocol (provided in Appendix), each word in the sentence was labeled to one of three entity groups: D, S, or O (which stand for Drug Entity, ADE entity, and Others, respectively). Four graduate students were separated into two groups with each group annotating every word in the dataset separately. A third rater will make a final decision whenever the two groups disagree. A summary of the annotated relation instances is provided in Table 3.

Table 3. Labeled entity distributions of three datasets

	Entity classes	Total count	Percentage
Training set (Diabetes drug)	Others	212,638	91.44%
	Drug	7,472	3.21%
	ADEs	12,432	5.35%
Testing set (Diabetes drug)	Others	43,522	92.31%
	Drug	1,396	2.96%
	ADEs	2,231	4.73%
Testing set (Hypertension drug)	Others	37,934	90.69%
	Drug	1,221	2.92%
	ADEs	2,674	6.39%

4.3   Evaluation Metrics

We use standard evaluation metrics, precision, recall and f-measure, which are widely used in information system research [8], to evaluate the performance of ADE extraction using our proposed framework.

4.4   Experiments and Results

In this study, we conduct our experiments on extracting patient reports of ADEs by performing three tasks: RNN and NER based ADE extraction, helpfulness of medical word embeddings and generalizability testing.

ADE Recognition and Extraction.   To build and train the model for drug entity and ADEs entity recognition, we selected 5,600 reviews of drugs for diabetes and 800 reviews of drugs for hypertension, and the entity class of each word was tagged based on the tagging scheme introduced in Sect. 4.2. We trained a bi-directional LSTM model consisted of two recurrent layers that can consider all the words on both sides of the target word for NER task. We compared the results from our RNN based ADEs recognition and extraction method with lexicon-based approach to demonstrate the efficacy of our framework. We show some examples of our predictions in Table 4.

Table 4. Examples of predicted results and error analysis

No.	Predicted results	Correct prediction?	Implication
1	I have been taking **metaformin [Drug]** for 2 wks now	Yes	'Metaformin' is misspelled, but is correctly identified
2	I have also **gained 40 lbs [ADEs]** since I started taking it	Yes	'Gained 40 lbs' is very specific ADEs but is correctly identified
3	Some **heart pulsation [ADEs]** and **upset of stomach [ADEs]**	Yes	'Heart pulsation' does not exist in training set, but is correctly identified
4	After 3 month on **this med** I suffered a **stress fracture [ADEs]** in my left foot	No	'This med' is classified as drug entity

Based on our observation, our model is effective in identifying ADEs and drug entities, even with the presence of misspelling (post 1), abbreviation (post 2), highly specific (post 2) or new ADEs terms (post 3). Errors in drug entity identification mainly occurred mainly due to the fact that patients used pronouns to stand for a specific drug name in a review (post 4). In this case, "this med" was determined as drug entity. However, this actually makes sense because under the context in this sentence, "this med" should be the drug entity from a semantic perspective. This demonstrates the RNN based approach is able to capture the relations within sentence.

In Table 5 we compared the baseline lexicon-based statistical learning and semantic filtering approach developed by Liu and Chen [7] against our extraction method.

Table 5. Results of drug entity and ADE extraction

Approach	Testing dataset	Entity type	Precision (%)	Recall (%)	F1 (%)
RNN based NER	Diabetes	Drug	87.3	90.1	88.7
		ADEs	**78.1**	**75.8**	**76.9**
	Hypertension	Drug	84.7	86.2	85.4
		ADEs	76.2	72.4	73.8
Lexicon-based (baseline method)	Diabetes forum	**Drug**	**90.6**	**89.6**	**90.1**
		ADEs	54.3	64.8	59.1

Our approach achieved 88.7% in f-measure for drug entity identification and 76.9% in f-measure for ADE extraction. We compared our results with those obtained by lexicon-based method, which achieved 90.1% for drug entity identification and 59.1% for ADE extraction. The baseline result is lower than that reported by Liu and Chen [7], the major reason is because they performed a strict data selection step, while we used the complete data without any data selection. The results demonstrated that our method improves the performance for ADE extraction by a large margin, demonstrating the robustness of our approach. However, our approach got slightly lower performance in extracting drug entity compared with baseline method, indicating the lexicon-based method is quite effective to extract drug entity.

Helpfulness of Medical Word Embeddings. We hypothesize that word embeddings trained on in-domain text are able to capture domain-specific word relations, and they may perform better than the ones trained on general corpus. To test the helpfulness of medical word embeddings for ADE extraction task, we also download the publicly available word vectors trained on general Wikipedia corpus [14]. We compared our medical word vectors with the general word embeddings. All the three dimensions, 50, 100, and 300, were included for comparisons. Table 6 shows the results.

Table 6. Results of drug entity and ADE extraction with different word embeddings and vector dimensions

Training corpus	Vector dimensionality	Entity type	Precision (%)	Recall (%)	F1 (%)
Medical corpus	**50**	**Drug**	**87.3**	**90.1**	**88.7**
		ADEs	**78.1**	**75.8**	**76.9**
	100	Drug	86.8	87.8	87.2
		ADEs	78.9	70.2	74.3
	300	Drug	87.2	90.0	88.6
		ADEs	73.2	75.6	74.0
Wikipedia corpus	50	Drug	87.4	88.0	87.7
		ADEs	81.9	66.5	73.4
	100	Drug	87.9	86.0	86.9
		ADEs	77.3	69.5	73.2
	300	Drug	82.8	91.0	86.7
		ADEs	80.1	67.8	73.4

The best results were obtained by using medical corpus trained word embeddings with vector dimensionality of 50. Based on our evaluations, a consistent increase in f-measure can be observed by using word embeddings trained on medical domain corpus. This demonstrates that the medical in-domain semantic and syntactic relations between words can help improve ADE extraction task.

Generalizability Testing. One problem of many machine learning based approaches is that they do not generalize well across different datasets. Our model has the potential to generalize well since the word embeddings were trained on general medical corpus, they should be able to capture the word similarities across drugs with different indications. We trained our model on the diabetes dataset and tested it using diabetes dataset as wells as the hypertension drugs reviews to evaluate the generalizability and robustness of our model.

The results were shown in Table 5. From the results, we can observe that the model trained on diabetes drug reviews give a comparable performance on identifying drug entity and ADEs entity for hypertension drug reviews, compared to the results tested on diabetes drug reviews. This indicates our model is robust and can generalize well to drugs with different indications.

5   Conclusions and Future Research

In this study, we developed a novel research framework in the context of ADE extraction without using any medical lexicon dictionaries to do medical entities extraction, which is distinctly different with the prior lexicon-based models. We combined deep RNN based NER approach with large medical corpus trained word embeddings for ADEs recognition and extraction, by considering both semantic and syntactic relations between words captured by word embeddings, and both short and long-distance dependencies within sentences captured by deep RNN model.

The major contributions of our research is that we first applied the state-of-the-art deep RNN based NER technique for ADE extraction. The initial results from our relatively un-optimized approach are quite promising, our approach significantly improved the ADEs entity extraction performance compared with baseline methods by a large margin. Additional optimization will likely result in even better performance. Our proposed framework is highly efficient and effective to identify new or highly specific ADEs. Thus, our method can achieve dynamically real-time surveillance of ADEs in social media. We obtained a medical in-domain word embeddings trained on a large medical corpus we harvested, and confirmed their usefulness in one healthcare task. We also expect that high quality word vectors will become an important building block for future healthcare related applications, and the learning based approaches could generalize to other healthcare tasks.

Our ongoing works include collecting more ADEs data to fine-tune our model; establishing a comprehensive evaluation metrics for measuring the medical in-domain word embeddings; collecting more and diverse sources of healthcare corpus to extend the training corpus to improve the quality of word embeddings.

Appendix. Tagging Protocol

Entity Types: describe whether the entity class each word belongs to
For each word in the sentence:
Drug entity – If the word describes the name of a drug
ADE entity – If the word describes the ADE of a drug
Others – If the word neither describes the name nor the ADE of a drug.

References

1. Harpaz, R., DuMouchel, W., Shah, N.H., Madigan, D., Ryan, P., Friedman, C.: Novel data-mining methodologies for adverse drug event discovery and analysis. Clin. Pharmacol. Ther. **91**, 1010–1021 (2012). doi:10.1038/clpt.2012.50
2. Hauben, M., Bate, A.: Decision support methods for the detection of adverse events in post-marketing data. Drug Discov. Today **14**, 343–357 (2009). doi:10.1016/j.drudis.2008.12.012
3. World Health Organization. The importance of pharmacovigilance (2012)
4. Bate, A., Evan, S.: Quantitative signal detection using spontaneous ADR reporting. Pharmacoepidemiol. Drug Saf. **18**, 427–436 (2009). doi:10.1002/pds.1742
5. Miller, A.R., Tucker, C.: Active social media management: the case of health care. Inform. Syst. Res. **24**, 52–70 (2013). doi:10.2139/ssrn.1984973
6. Basch, E.: The missing voice of patients in drug-safety reporting. N. Engl. J. Med. **362**, 865–869 (2010). doi:10.1056/NEJMp0911494
7. Liu, X., Chen, H.: A research framework for pharmacovigilance in health social media: identification and evaluation of patient adverse drug event reports. J. Biomed. Inform. **58**, 268–279 (2015). doi:10.1016/j.jbi.2015.10.011
8. Leaman, R., Wojtulewicz, L., Sullivan, R., Skariah, A., Yang, J., Gonzalez, G.: Towards internet-age pharmacovigilance: extracting adverse drug reactions from user posts to health-related social networks. In: Proceedings of the 2010 Workshop on Biomedical Natural Language Processing. Association for Computational Linguistics (2010)
9. Nikfarjam, A., Gonzalez, G.H.: Pattern mining for extraction of mentions of adverse drug reactions from user comments. In: AMIA Annual Symposium Proceedings (2011)
10. Benton, A., Ungar, L., Hill, S., Hennessy, S., Mao, J., Chung, A., Leonard, C.E., Holmes, J.H.: Identifying potential adverse effects using the web: a new approach to medical hypothesis generation. J. Biomed. Inform. **44**, 989–996 (2011). doi:10.1016/j.jbi.2011.07.005
11. Wu, H., Fang, H., Stanhope, S.J.: Exploiting online discussions to discover unrecognized drug side effects. Methods Inf. Med. **52**, 152–159 (2013). doi:10.3414/ME12-02-0004
12. Bian, J., Topaloglu, U., Yu, F.: Towards large-scale twitter mining for drug-related adverse events. In: Proceedings of the 2012 International Workshop on Smart Health and Wellbeing. ACM (2012)
13. Mikolov, T., Chen, K., Corrado, G.S., Dean, J.: Efficient estimation of word representations in vector space (2013). arXiv preprint arXiv:1301.3781
14. Mikolov, T., Sutskever, I., Chen, K., Corrado, G.S., Dean, J.: Distributed representations of words and phrases and their compositionality. In: Advances in Neural Information Processing Systems (2013). arXiv:1310.4546
15. Collobert, R., Weston, J., Bottou, L., Karlen, M., Kavukcuoglu, K., Kuksa, P.: Natural language processing (almost) from scratch. J. Mach. Learn. Res. **12**, 2493–2537 (2011). arXiv:1103.0398
16. Goller, C., Kuchler, A.: Learning task-dependent distributed representations by backpropagation through structure. In: Neural Networks IEEE International Conference. IEEE (1996). doi:10.1109/ICNN.1996.548916
17. Gers, F.A., Schmidhuber, J., Cummins, F.: Learning to forget: continual prediction with LSTM. Neural Comput. **12**, 2451–2471 (2000). doi:10.1162/089976600300015015
18. Graves, A., Mohamed, A., Hinton, G.: Speech recognition with deep recurrent neural networks. In: 2013 IEEE International Conference on Acoustics, Speech and Signal Processing (ICASSP). IEEE (2013). arXiv:1303.5778

A Hybrid Markov Random Field Model for Drug Interaction Prediction

Haobo Gu[1,2] and Xin Li[1,2(✉)]

[1] Department of Information Systems, City University of Hong Kong,
Kowloon, Hong Kong
bohgu22222-x@my.cityu.edu.hk, Xin.Li@cityu.edu.hk
[2] City University of Hong Kong Shenzhen Research Institute,
Shenzhen, Hong Kong

Abstract. Drug interactions represent adverse effects when employing two or multiple drugs together in treatments. Adverse effects are critical and may be deadly in medical practice. However, our understanding of drug interactions is far from complete. In the medical study on drug interaction, the prediction of potential drug interactions will help reducing the experimental efforts. In this paper, we extend a hinge-loss Markov Random Field Model and propose hybrid model of it and logistic regression. In the model, we combine multiple types of chemical and biological evidence to infer the interactions between drugs. Logistic regression is used to learn weights of those evidences. Experiments shows that our approach achieves better performance than the state-of-the-art approaches on both prediction accuracy and time efficiency.

Keywords: Drug interaction · Markov random fields · Hybrid model

1 Introduction

Identification of potential Drug-Drug Interactions (DDIs) has a great value in clinical practice. Drug interactions are responsible for adverse drug reactions which may cause severe outcomes in treatment. Due to the large number of drugs and the high cost of experiments, it is difficult to test all possible drug pairs to identify interactions. The prediction of potential DDIs can help researchers to better use their efforts on a small number of candidate drugs for study, which is both economic and medical valuable and is an important direction in medical informatics research.

Drug interactions can be inferred based on different biological and chemical evidences and known interactions of drugs. For example, if two drugs have similar molecule structures, they may interact with a same set of drugs [1]. In this paper, we extend a hinge-loss Markov random field model for drug interaction prediction proposed by Sridhar et al. [2], in which we improve the model's capacity of leveraging multiple evidences to predict drug interactions. In our model, logistic regression is applied to learn weights of different drug similarities, which are then used as inputs of the Markov random field model. The experiment results show that our proposed algorithm has a better accuracy of identifying potential interactions and a better time efficiency as compared with the state-of-the-art drug interaction prediction algorithms.

© Springer International Publishing AG 2017
H. Chen et al. (Eds.): ICSH 2017, LNCS 10347, pp. 249–255, 2017.
https://doi.org/10.1007/978-3-319-67964-8_24

This paper is organized as follows: in Sect. 2, we review the literature about interaction prediction algorithms. Then we introduce our proposed interaction prediction algorithm in Sect. 3. Experiment result and analysis are in Sect. 4 and the conclusion is in Sect. 5.

2 Literature Review

The drug interaction prediction studies can be categorized into three streams. The first one is the classic biological approach, which is to directly test whether two drugs have interactions [3]. Obach summarized recent advances and challenges of this approach [4]. In general, the biological approach is costly due to the complexity of biological experiment. Only a few potential drugs can be examined under this approach.

The second steam of drug interaction prediction methods is text mining on clinical records and literature. This approach essentially is not a prediction method. It is a summarization of empirical evidence in practice. For example, Duke et al. constructed a template to retrieve FDA probe inhibitors and substrates from electrical medical records [5].

The last stream is statistical methods combining known drug interactions and drug similarities for prediction, which is the focus of this paper. For example, Fokoue et al. [6] built several similarity features from different sources and applied a modified logistic regression model to predict potential drug interactions. Zhang et al. [7] constructed a drug network based on drug similarity and interactions and applied a label spreading method to label possible interactions from known ones on the network. Sridhar et al. [2] proposed a probabilistic approach based on hinge-loss Markov random fields. The model defines similarity based rules as dependencies between drugs. The rules were represented as potential functions in Markov random fields. Those potential functions were combined linearly with weights in the framework.

3 Drug Interaction Prediction

In the drug interaction prediction problem, we assume a known drug interaction network $G = (V,E)$ in which V is a vector of nodes (i.e., drugs) and E is a vector of edges (i.e., drug interactions). Besides, there are a set of similarities between nodes $K = \{I_1,I_2,\ldots,I_k\}$ which are defined on chemical/biomedical evidences. The interaction prediction problem is thus a link prediction problem on G based on G and K.

In this problem, drug similarity plays a fundamental role. Because our focus is on the improvement of prediction algorithm, we use a same set of similarity functions established in literature to conduct the research. Upon the similarities, we model the drug interaction network using hinge-loss Markov random fields. In the model, the dependencies between drugs are modeled using similarity rules. We use logistic regression to learn the weights of those similarity rules. After all weights are optimized, potential drug interactions can be inferred using hinge-loss Markov random fields.

3.1 Hinge-Loss Markov Random Fields

Hinge-loss Markov random fields was proposed by Bach et al. [8] in 2013. In hinge-loss Markov random fields, a network structure upon random variables is leveraged to make predictions. Assume that $\mathbf{Y}$ is the target variables and $\mathbf{X}$ is the observed variables which are on the network. The joint probability density function can be represented as:

$$P(\mathbf{Y}|\mathbf{X}) = \frac{1}{Z}\exp\left(-\sum_{r=1}^{M}\lambda_r\phi_r(\mathbf{Y},\mathbf{X})\right),$$

where Z is a normalization coefficient, λ_r is the weight and $\phi_r(\mathbf{Y},\mathbf{X})$ is the hinge-loss potential function, which is defined upon dependencies of variables (i.e., drugs in our problem). For drug interaction prediction, dependencies between drugs needs to be defined as a series of rules. Assume that S_{ab} is the similarity between drug a and b, I_{ab} represents that there is an interaction between drug a and b. A straightforward rule is:

$$S_{ab} \cap I_{bc} \rightarrow I_{ac}$$

which means that if a and b are similar and b and c have an interaction, then a and c may have an interaction. The corresponding potential function can be formulated as:

$$\phi = \max\{S_{ab} + I_{bc} - I_{ac} - 1, 0\}$$

Because there are several types of similarity functions, there are multiple rules can be established in the Markov random field model. Assuming we have k similarity functions S^1 to S^k, we can establish a set of rules as follows:

$$\beta_1 : S_{ab}^1 \cap I_{bc} \rightarrow I_{ac}$$
$$\beta_2 : S_{ab}^2 \cap I_{bc} \rightarrow I_{ac}$$
$$\cdots$$
$$\beta_k : S_{ab}^k \cap I_{bc} \rightarrow I_{ac}$$

where $\boldsymbol{\beta} = [\beta_1, \beta_2, \ldots \beta_k]$ is the vector of weights. After the model structure and weights of potential functions are specified, a maximum a posteriori (MAP) inference can be used to make inference on potential drug interactions [9].

3.2 Weight Learning

In [2], Sridhar et al. took a weighted average method to combine the weights and use a maximum a posterior (MAP) method to optimize the weights.

In this paper, we propose to apply a logistic regression method to learn the weights. With k similarity functions S^1 to S^k, the model takes a form o

$$logit(p_{a,c}) = \beta_0 + \beta_1 S_{a\bar{b}}^1 + \ldots + \beta_k S_{a\bar{b}}^k$$

where $p_{a,c}$ is the probability for a and c to have an interaction. $S_{a\bar{b}}^k$ is the average of the kth similarity between a and the drugs interact with c. In other words, for $\mathbf{b} = \{b_1, b_2, \ldots b_m\}$ which is the vector of drugs interacting with drug c, the similarities between drug a and $b_1, b_2, \ldots b_m$ can be used as the evidences. $S_{a\bar{b}}^k$ is defined as:

$$S_{a\bar{b}}^k = mean(S_{ab1}^k, S_{ab2}^k, \ldots, S_{abm}^k)$$

Moreover, if the similarity between drug a and b is low, this similarity may contributes little on inference of interactions. To improve the time efficiency, we consider only some similarities which are larger than a threshold to compute the average similarity. In our experiment, a threshold of 0.4 performs best on predicting drug interactions.

To train the coefficients of the logistic regression, we randomly select some drug pairs with interactions and some drug pairs without interactions. After the logistic regression model is trained, the coefficients of features $\beta_1, \beta_2, \ldots \beta_k$ can be used as weights of similarity rules in Markov random fields.

4 Evaluation

4.1 Dataset

Following [2], we conduct our experiment on Drugbank's interaction data. We consider five similarity functions from [2] in our experiment, which are ATC similarity, protein target similarity, chemical similarity, Gene Ontology similarity and sequence similarity. ATC similarity is the semantic similarity calculated using ATC annotations of the World Health Organization ATC classification systems. Gene Ontology similarity is the semantic similarity based on the Gene Ontology annotations. Protein target similarity is the distance of drug's target in protein interaction network. Chemical similarity is the Jaccard similarity between the fingerprints of drugs. Sequence similarity is based on a Smith–Waterman sequence alignment score between drugs' targets. For more information about those similarities, please refer to [10].

Since not all drug pairs have interactions, after cross matching interaction data with similarity data, we get a dataset with 246 drugs and 3,978 interactions as our gold standard. The drugs have an average of 16 interactions. A half of drugs have less than 10 drugs. The drug with the most interactions has 98 interactions. The degree distribution of the drugs is shown in Fig. 1.

4.2 Experimental Framework

In the experiment, Sridhar et al.'s approach [2] is used as the baseline. It is a state-of-the-art algorithm which has better performance than other existing methods. In their work, maximum likelihood estimation is applied to estimate the parameters.

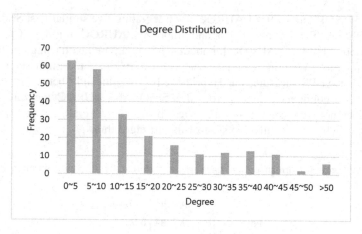

Fig. 1. Degree distribution

As the second baseline, we consider the MRF model use only one similarity function. In this research, we report the ATC similarity function since it provides the highest performance.

When using Markov random field for drug interaction prediction, to reduce the computational complexity, it is beneficial to apply a blocking method [2]. Instead of including all drugs into the consideration of the potential function of the model for parameter tuning, only the more similar drugs with the target drug are considered. In this research, we keep only the top 15 most similar drugs in the model.

10-fold cross validation is used to evaluate our prediction approach. We divide the known interactions of the dataset into 10 groups. In each group, the ratio of interaction pairs to non-interaction pairs is strictly controlled to reflect the prior distribution of the dataset. In each folder, 9 groups are used as the training sets and one group is used as the validation set. Interactions in the training data is considered known to predict interactions in the testing data. The overall performance of the method is averaged on the 10 folds.

We use the area under the receiver operating characteristic curve (AUROC) measure and the area under the precision and recall curve (AUPR) measure as evaluation metrics to assess the performance of our method by thresholding on prediction confidences of the model, we can make predictions with different true positive, false positive, true negative, and false negative value. Further, we can draw a ROC curve showing the change of true positive rate with false positive rate and a precision-recall curve showing the change of precision with recall. AUROC and AUPR calculates the percentage of region behind the ROC and PR curve on the entire diagram. In this work, AUROC and AUPR are calculated using the trapezoidal rule.

4.3   Results

Table 1 shows the prediction performance of 10-fold cross validation. As we can see, if we only use ATC similarity functions in the framework, the best performance we can get is 0.6757 AUPR and 0.9181 AUROC. By integrating five similarities, Sridhar et al. improves the AUPR for about 1% and improves AUROC for 4%. Our method improves both AUPR and AUROC for about 4% as compared with using one (the best) similarity function. We conduct a pair-wise t-test to evaluate the improvement of our algorithm. On AUPR measure, our Hybrid MRF is significantly better than the MRF model at 95% confidence interval (p = 0.025). On the AUROC measure, the two methods does not show significant difference (p = 0.76). Overall, the performance of our Hybrid MRF outperforms this state-of-the-art algorithm.

Table 1. Prediction performance (bold ones are not significantly different from the largest value at 95% confidence internal)

	AUPR	AUROC
Hybrid MRF	**0.7084**	**0.9561**
MRF	0.6856	**0.9552**
ATC similarity	0.6757	0.9181

Another significant advantage of our approach is the time efficiency. The computational complexity of the weight tuning method of the baseline method is polynomial when the number of nodes increases [2]. In our framework, the parameter tuning for Logistic regression for weight learning is about linear time on the size of training set. In practice, Sridhar et al.'s method for weight tuning is 9 h while our method is 180 s a machine with 64 GB memory and 8 core server in our experiments.

5 Conclusion

In this paper, we proposed a drug interaction prediction approach by combining hinge-loss Markov random fields and logistic regression. Several similarity rules are constructed in MRF to describe the drug network and logistic regression is applied to learn weights of similarity rules in MRF model. Experiment shows that our approach can achieve a better prediction performance and is significantly better than the traditional framework on time efficiency.

There is room to improve our approach in the future. First, we will improve the time efficiency of the model. Second, we will conduct further study and proposed new mathematical rules on interaction prediction. Third, we will study on how to better integrate different rules and different similarities by simultaneously considering two drug triples in one potential function.

Acknowledgements. The research is partially supported by GuangDong Science and Technology Project 2014A020221090 and the City University of Hong Kong Shenzhen Research Institute.

References

1. Klopmand, G.: Concepts and applications of molecular similarity. J. Comput. Chem. **13**(4), 539–540 (1992)
2. Sridhar, D., Fakhraei, S., Getoor, L.: A probabilistic approach for collective similarity-based drug-drug interaction prediction. Bioinformatics **32**(20), 3175–3182 (2016)
3. Chan, E., Tan, M., Xin, J., Sudarsanam, S., Johnson, D.E.: Interactions between traditional chinese medicines and western therapeutics. Curr. Opin. Drug Discov. Devel. **13**(1), 50–65 (2010)
4. Obach, R.S.: Predicting drug-drug interactions from in vitro drug metabolism data: challenges and recent advances. Curr. Opin. Drug Discov. Devel. **12**(1), 81–89 (2009)
5. Duke, J.D., et al.: Literature based drug interaction prediction with clinical assessment using electronic medical records: novel myopathy associated drug interactions. PLos Comput. Biol. **8**(8) 2012
6. Fokoue, A., Hassanzadeh, O., Sadoghi, M., Zhang, P.: Predicting drug-drug interactions through similarity-based link prediction over web data. In: proceedings of 25th International conference on companion world wide web, pp. 3–6 (2016)
7. Zhang, P., Wang, F., Hu, J., Sorrentino, R.: Label propagation prediction of drug-drug interactions based on clinical side effects. Sci. Rep. **5**, 12339 (2015)
8. Bach, S., Huang, B., London, B., Getoor, L.: Hinge-loss markov random fields: convex inference for structured prediction. Uai (2013)
9. Bach, S.H., Broecheler, M., Huang, B., Getoor, L.: Hinge-loss markov random fields and probabilistic soft logic. CoRR, vol. abs/1505.0, pp. 1–46 (2015)
10. Gottlieb, A., Stein, G.Y., Oron, Y., Ruppin, E., Sharan, R.: INDI: a computational framework for inferring drug interactions and their associated recommendations. Mol. Syst. Biol. **8**(592), 592 (2012)

EpiStrat: A Tool for Comparing Strategies for Tackling Urban Epidemic Outbreaks

Radhiya Arsekar[1], Durga Keerthi Mandarapu[2], and M.V. Panduranga Rao[2]([⊠])

[1] Goa University, Taleigão, India
radhiya.arsekar@gmail.com
[2] Indian Institute of Technology Hyderabad, Kandi, India
{cs15btech11024,mvp}@iith.ac.in

Abstract. Management and mitigation of epidemic outbreaks is a major challenge for health-care authorities and governments in general. In this paper, we first give a formal definition of a strategy for dealing with epidemics, especially in heterogeneous urban environments. Different strategies target different demographic classes of a city, and hence have different effects on the progression and impact of an epidemic. One has to therefore choose among various competing strategies. We show how the relative merits of these strategies can be compared against various metrics.

We demonstrate our approach by developing a tool that has an agent based discrete event simulator engine at its core. We believe that such a tool can provide a valuable what-if analysis and decision support infrastructure to urban health-care authorities for tackling epidemics. We also present a running example on an influenza-like disease on synthetic populations and demographics and compare different strategies for outbreaks.

1 Introduction

Significant progress has been made over the last century in mathematical modeling and analyses of epidemics, starting with the early work of Kermack and McKendrick [12,14] where they introduced compartmental models of epidemic and modeled epidemic progression through differential equations. Subsequent work introduced stochastic differential equations and stochastic processes [3]. The recognition that populations are not homogeneous resulted in the use of ideas from graph theory in the form of contact networks [13,15,18]. The advent of social media and the study of large graphs and complex networks resulted in a cross-breeding of ideas from both communities [1,20,21]. Ideas from physics have been applied to epidemiology as well, with good success [17,22]. Human mobility models have been incorporated to account for effects of traffic pattern on the spread of epidemics across geographies [6].

In this paper, we address a common problem faced by decision making health-care authorities during the outbreak of an epidemic in an urban setting. Large cosmopolitan cities exhibit great socio-economic and cultural diversity. While

H. Chen et al. (Eds.): ICSH 2017, LNCS 10347, pp. 256–267, 2017.
https://doi.org/10.1007/978-3-319-67964-8_25

there are slum areas that have higher population density, lower literacy rates and incomes, there are also upmarket areas that fare better in the above parameters. In addition, there are parameters associated with individuals, like age, nutrition levels etc. that influence the progression of an epidemic.

An epidemic outbreak poses the following dilemma to urban health-care authorities and policy makers: In what proportion should different demographics be paid attention to, to minimize various effects of an epidemic outbreak?

This paper is a step towards formalization of the problem statement and development of a decision support tool based on (agent based) modeling and simulation for solving the problem. Our contribution is twofold: (i) A formal definition of a *strategy* (ii) An agent based modeling and simulation approach for comparison of various strategies in terms of economic and demographic impact. To the best of our knowledge, this is the first attempt in this direction.

We now give a brief sketch of our approach. Details can be found in later sections. We first partition the entire population into different classes. This classification can be based on criteria like geographic location or socio-economic parameters. In our running example, we use a classification based on vulnerability of individuals to the epidemic. Next, we identify a set of measures that health-care authorities intend to take, to tackle the epidemic. We work with two different types of measures: abstract measures defined in terms of susceptibility lowering and concrete measures defined in terms of tangible steps like quarantine. Finally, we formally define a strategy in terms of the proportion and schedule of applying the measures on various demographic classes obtained previously.

Through agent based simulation, we can compare different strategies against epidemic metrics like peak incidence, cumulative incidence, duration of the epidemic, economic impact and the cost associated with implementing a strategy. We develop a tool for the simulation, as well as a comparison of these metrics. The tools allows fixing of various demographic and disease related parameters. In particular, if the costs of implementing a measure on different classes are available, the tool outputs the total cost of a strategy as a byproduct. We show *cumulative* infection plots and tabulate some other metrics for illustration.

We believe that such a tool would be useful to health-care policy makers in analyzing what-if scenarios before operationalizing a strategy for tackling an epidemic.

The rest of the paper is arranged as follows. In the next section, we briefly establish the preliminaries and terminology required for the rest of the paper and discuss relevant existing literature. In Sect. 3, we discuss our approach and the tool–a description of our agent based model, strategies and costing models. In Sect. 4, we demonstrate our approach through a synthetic scenario, and compare different strategies. We conclude in Sect. 5 with a discussion of future directions.

2   Preliminaries and Previous Work

Compartmental models have been the mainstay of epidemic analysis for almost a century [5]. These models partition the population into several compartments; the number of compartments depends on the disease. A common model is the SEIR, that classifies every individual into either the "Susceptible", the "Exposed" (but not symptomatic or infectious), the "Infectious" or the "Recovered" compartment. This models holds for several common diseases like influenza, measles, Ebola virus disease etc. Indeed, we use this model for our running example.

The transition dynamics of people from one compartment to another has been modeled in different ways, including deterministic and stochastic differential equations. Deterministic models, while being simple, have the limitation that they hold for large populations, with typically homogeneous mixing assumptions among the population.

The paradigm of modeling individual agents and their behavior has been used in recent times for analysis of epidemics. While being computationally expensive, these models gained traction in epidemiology community recently because of the higher degree of accuracy that they offer [4, 8, 9].

A lot of work has been done in studying sociological phenomena in the context of epidemics. For example, Mao [16] and Durham and Casman [7] investigate progressive decision making process and individual response to epidemics. Funk et al. [11] model the spread of awareness during an outbreak of an epidemic and discuss how this could result in a lowering of individual susceptibility, and therefore, a smaller outbreak size. There is also work on surveillance systems and mechanisms for targeting and monitoring various interventions during outbreaks [19]. The outcome of surveillance can then be used to formulate strategies to tackle the epidemics.

As mentioned earlier, there exist several tools based on various simulation and analysis paradigms for studying epidemic progression [2, 4, 6]. However, what is required is a tool that allows rapid evaluation and comparison of different strategies by health-care authorities. This paper is a first step in that direction.

3   Our Approach

3.1   Agent Based Model

The Usual Scenario, When There Is No Epidemic: We give a qualitative description of the agents and the environment. The parameters and actual values set for the simulation are detailed in the next section. We simulate a town on a square grid that has two areas: a "slum" area (Area 1) which is characterized by high population density, lower education, and an upmarket area (Area 2) with sparse population and higher education. Places consists of one or more grid points and an individual is located on one grid point. There are residential areas, workplaces, schools and market places in both areas. Individuals living in the town are characterized by features that are relevant to our experiments–home address, age, occupation, work place address etc., in addition to education level. In addition to the designated work places in the upmarket area, some of the slum dwellers also work in the residential areas in the upmarket area. The unit of time that we use is one hour. Movement of individuals in the city is modeled as movement from one grid point to another.

Each individual goes about his/her routine as defined by his/her age and occupation. Working hours are between 9AM and 5PM. Workplaces and schools consist of several grid points. The movement of the employees/students within the workplace/school is modeled as a random hops between the grid points within the workplace. Office-goers visit the market place in the evening with higher probability, while home-makers visit the market place with equal probability throughout the active day. In any case, everybody returns to his/her respective home at the end of the day (8:00 PM).

Outbreak of an Epidemic: The outbreak of the (influenza-like) epidemic proceeds as follows. We begin with an initial number of infected individuals. The epidemic comes to the notice of health-care authorities only after a certain threshold number of people are infected. After a delay δ that is defined by the strategy adopted by authorities, various measures (defined later) come into effect.

Regardless of their susceptibility, a healthy individual goes about his/her routine as usual. A healthy individual is exposed to infection if there is an infected individual sharing the same grid point at the same time. The probability that a healthy individual acquires the infection is given by [4]:

$$p_i = 1 - exp(\tau \sum_{r \in R} N_r ln(1 - rs_i\rho)) \tag{1}$$

where τ is the duration of exposure, R is the set of infectivities of the infected individual at that location, N_r is the number of infectious individual with infectivity r, s_i susceptibility of individual i and ρ is the transmissibility.

After acquiring the infection, he stays asymptomatic and non-infectious for a certain duration after which he becomes infectious. When infected, every individual stays at home with some probability.

The probability that an individual recovers after i_t units of time after entering the infectious stage is given by

$$p_r = 1 - (1 - (1/r_t))^{i_t}$$

where r_t is the average recovery time.

Health-Care Response: An alert is triggered to the health-care authorities only after a certain fraction of the population gets infected. In our simulations, we assume that it is triggered when $(1/25)$th of the population is infected. After a delay, the authorities respond with a strategy (defined later). This delay could be due to several reasons like lack of resources or systemic inertia.

3.2   The Strategy

Classification of the population can be done in several ways. A simple classification could be simply based on the locality of the individual–all individuals of Area 1 belong to one class, while those of Area 2 belong to another class.

A more sophisticated classification is given below. In this paper, we report simulation results for this classification. As mentioned earlier, we divide the entire population of n people into three demographic classes and assign different initial susceptibilities to each of these classes.

```
if a person A satisfies at least two of the following
conditions:
    1. A.age <=10 years
    2. A.age >=70 years
    3. A.MaxEducation <= High School
    4. A.residence = Area 1
then A.Class = 0

if A satisfies all of the following conditions:
    1. 11 <= A.age <= 69
    2. A.MaxEducation >= Graduation
    3. A.residence = Area 2
then A.Class = 2

otherwise
A.Class = 1
```

Let $|C_i| = n_i$, for $i \in \{0, 1, 2\}$. It is easy to see that the above routine partitions the population into the three classes $\{C_i\}$. Thus, $n_0 + n_1 + n_2 = n$.

We report experiments based on this classification method.

A *measure* is a step taken by the health care authorities that benefits an individual (of a certain class) with some probability. In this work, we consider two qualitatively different types of measures. The first is an abstract one, defined by a lowering of susceptibility. How this lowering is brought about, is not described. For example, for our simulations, we use the following abstract measures: for an individual with natural susceptibility s, lowering to (i) $2s/3$ (ii) $s/3$ and (iii) 0 (e.g., through vaccination).

The second type involves more concrete measures like closing schools, quarantine, minimizing transmission in health centers etc. While the latter type is easy to visualize, the former serves as a comparison point, and also leaves scope for including and combining other concrete measures. For example, for our simulations, we use the following concrete measures: (i) closing of schools and a reduction of transmission in hospitals to two-third of the individual's natural susceptibility (ii) quarantine of an infected individual with some probability and (iii) vaccination of an uninfected individual with some probability.

Definition 1. Given r demographic classes, and m "measures", a *strategy* is a $r \times m$ matrix S where $S_{i,j} = (p_{i,j}, t_{i,j})$ where $p_{i,j}$ is the probability that an individual of the demographic class C_i will benefit from measure j, and this measure will be taken after a delay of $t_{i,j}$ units after epidemic alert is raised.

Essentially, a strategy defines in what proportion are different demographics targeted by the health-care authorities. The delay $t_{i,j}$ accounts for the time needed to put various measures in place. While a strategy is intuitive in the context of abstract measures, we point out that even for concrete measures, the intuition holds. For example, it is more difficult (expensive) to bring down susceptibility among individuals of class C_0 even in hospitals. Similarly, it is also more difficult to impose quarantine on such an individual. Thus, it makes sense to associate the cost of such a measure with the probability of it being used on an individual of a certain class.

In our model, a person who is subjected to a measure is eligible to be subjected to subsequent measures. For example, in the case of abstract measures, if the person's susceptibility is lowered to $2s/3$, it can further be lowered to $s/3$ and 0 later.

Definition 2. Associated with a strategy is a $r \times m$ *expense* matrix E where each entry denotes the average expense of implementing the measure in an individual of class C_i.

Thus, the total expense of a strategy is $\sum_{i=0}^{r-1} \sum_{j=0}^{m-1} n_{i,j} E_{i,j}$, where $n_{i,j}$ is the number of individuals of class C_i who were subjected to measure j. Our partitioning of the population also allows to provide a rough estimate of the economic impact of the epidemic. For that, we associate an average economic value v_i with each individual of a demographic class C_i. Thus if l_i individuals of C_i get infected in a epidemic, we say that the economic impact of the epidemic is $\sum_i l_i v_i$.

Thus, different strategies yield different progressions of the epidemic. It results in different shapes of the epidemic curve, different economic impacts, and finally, different expenses.

3.3   The Tool

The tool is implemented in python 2.7. The simulator reads a configuration file that contains all necessary parameters to set up the environment, agents and disease specific parameters. The source code, instruction manual and examples are available at https://github.com/radh3110/EpiDemoSim-Project.

4   Simulation Results

To run the agent based simulation, we need to fix the properties of the disease, demographic and geographic settings of the model, and behavioral properties of the agents.

As mentioned earlier, we assume an influenza-like epidemic, and hence use values reported in literature for [10]. These are shown in Table 1. We emphasize that since populations are synthetic and so are some infection characteristics, the simulations results presented do not relate to any specific real life epidemic example. The examples are purely to demonstrate our approach and tool. Table 2 shows various parameters set in the agent model.

Recall that the classification scheme that we use in this paper results in three classes C_0, C_1 and C_2 of n_0, n_1 and n_2 individuals respectively, with decreasing

Table 1. Epidemic parameters

Transmissibility (ρ in Eq. 1)	0.029
Infectivity range (R in Eq. 1)	0.1–0.9
Expected duration of latent period	26 h
Incubation period duration	30–72 h
Recovery time	60 h

Table 2. Model parameters

People in Area 1	4000
People in Area 2	2000
Initially Infected	50
Probability of going to the market between 9AM to 5PM	0.05
Probability of going to the market between 6PM to 8PM	0.2
Probability of going to a hospital when symptomatic	0.4
Education Levels	0 to 4

natural susceptibilities. For the current simulation, we have $n_0 = 4029$, $n_1 = 1348$ and $n_2 = 623$. We assign a natural susceptibility of 0.8 to individuals of C_0, 0.5 to those of C_1 and 0.3 to those of C_2.

4.1 Measures

We begin by defining strategies that are agnostic to demographic classification. Any measure among the three (see Table 3) is implemented across all communities after the same delay. The delay depends on the measure–100, 80 and 50 time units for measures m_0, m_1 and m_2 respectively. We will first describe abstract strategies and then concrete strategies over which we report our simulations.

S_Φ is the "strategy" when there is no intervention on the part of health-care authorities. Therefore, susceptibility remain the same as their natural susceptibility for all individuals of all demographic classes. On the other hand, S_{m_0} is the strategy where we vaccinate every individual in the population. Finally, S_{red} is the strategy when the authorities do not intervene, but the susceptibilities of all individuals is one-third of the natural susceptibility associated to their respective class. This is to depict the situation when the general health-care, civic and educational infrastructure is so good that the susceptibilities are lower to begin with. Note that these strategies have the same interpretation in both abstract and concrete settings.

The abstract strategies S_{m_2} and S_{m_1} are strategies where the attempt is to lower individual susceptibilities to two-third and one-third respectively for all individuals of all classes.

The concrete strategy S_{m_2} is one where the susceptibilities of all people when in hospitals falls to $2s/3$ with probability 1 and schools close. The concrete strategy S_{m_1} is one where every symptomatic person is quarantined with probability 1.

Table 3. Common strategies

	m_0	m_1	m_2	m_Φ
S_Φ (for all classes)	0	0	0	1
S_{m_2} (for all classes)	0	0	1, 50	0
S_{m_1} (for all classes)	0	1, 80	0	0
S_{m_0} (for all classes)	1, 100	0	0	0

S_{red}: No intervention, susceptibility $1/3$ of respective natural susceptibilities of all classes.

Table 4 shows more complex strategies that target communities preferentially (and also, an example cost matrix). For example, the strategy in Table 4(a) targets community C_0. We explain the first row of this table, and leave the rest to the reader.

Table 4. Targeting specific demographics

(a) S_1: Focus on C_0.

	m_0	m_1	m_2
C_0	2/5, 100	1/5, 80	1/5, 50
C_1	1/5, 100	1/5, 80	2/5, 50
C_2	1/5, 100	1/5, 80	2/5, 50

(b) S_2: Focus on C_1.

	m_0	m_1	m_2
C_0	1/5, 100	1/5, 80	2/5, 50
C_1	2/5, 100	1/5, 80	1/5, 50
C_2	1/5, 100	1/5, 80	2/5, 50

(d) The cost matrix. These numbers are synthetic and chosen arbitrarily for purpose of illustration.

(c) S_3: Focus on C_2

	m_0	m_1	m_2
C_0	1/5, 100	1/5, 80	2/5, 50
C_1	1/5, 100	1/5, 80	2/5, 50
C_2	2/5, 100	1/5, 80	1/5, 50

	m_0	m_1	m_2
C_0	49	36	25
C_1	125	48	27
C_2	81	16	1

The abstract strategy reduces the susceptibility of a person of community C_0 to two-thirds with probability $1/5$ after a delay of 50 time units, to one-thirds with probability $1/5$ after a delay of 80 time units and gets vaccinated with probability $2/5$ after a delay of 100 time units.

On the other hand, the corresponding concrete strategy reduces the susceptibility of a person of community C_0 to two-thirds with probability $1/5$ after a delay of 50 time units, when in a hospital[1]. This concrete strategy also quarantines a symptomatic person of C_0 with probability 1/5 after a delay of 80 time units and finally, vaccinates with a probability of 2/5 after a delay of 100 time units.

In our simulations, we keep the probability of a measure being administered on a person independent of the previous measures administered on him/her. For example, the same person can get susceptibility lowered to s/3 and the subsequently get vaccinated. This assumption need not be true in general and can be relaxed. For example, in concrete strategies, it does not make sense for

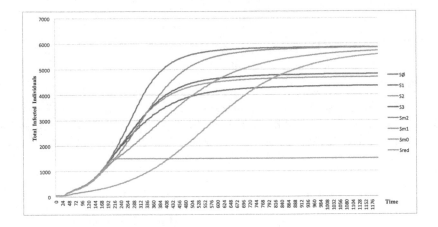

Fig. 1. Epidemic curves for abstract measures

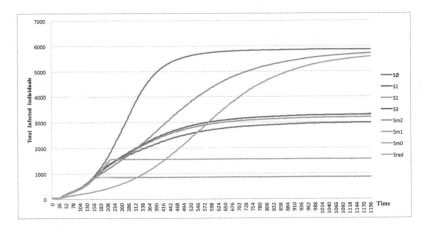

Fig. 2. Epidemic curves for concrete measures. Curves for S_Φ and S_{red} are reproduced here as well for easy comparison.

---

[1] Additionally, we close down all schools in our simulations.

Table 5. Auxiliary data generated for simulations with abstract measures

Strategy	Infected	Peak	Peak time	Alert triggered (hrs)	C_0 Infected	C_1 infected	C_2 Infected	C_0 Vaccinated	C_1 Vaccinated	C_2 Vaccinated	Total Vaccines	Economic impact	Total cost
S_ϕ	5862	46	297	–	3905	1288	617	0	0	0	0	8336	0
S_1	4349	33	206	76	2726	1063	508	1609	273	120	2002	6381	250295.5
S_2	4690	36	250	72	3289	873	507	827	527	123	1477	6528	292334.9
S_3	4812	37	264	75	3290	1072	399	805	265	249	1319	6633	260614
S_{m_2}	5853	36	293	69	3904	1285	612	0	0	0	0	8313	137744.0
S_{m_1}	5730	28	194	72	3861	1253	565	0	0	0	0	8065	241284.0
S_{m_0}	1502	32	190	77	1099	265	88	4029	1348	623	6000	1895	416384.
S_{red}	5586	25	556	–	3809	1194	532	0	0	0	0	7795	0

Table 6. Auxiliary data generated for simulations with concrete measures

Strategy	Infected	Peak	Peak time	Alert triggered (hrs)	C_0 Infected	C_1 infected	C_2 Infected	C_0 Vaccinated	C_1 Vaccinated	C_2 Vaccinated	Total vaccines	Economic impact	Total cost
S_1	2984	24	149	79	1890	718	326	1546	204	107	1857	4304	314077.5
S_2	3198	25	159	80	2243	586	318	764	479	111	1354	4371	354179.3
S_3	3295	24	183	84	2247	729	268	789	254	210	1253	4512	348965
S_{m_2}	5714	25	256	80	3876	1234	604	0	0	0	0	8160	278654.0
S_{m_1}	855	23	143	83	631	134	50	0	0	0	0	1019	425647.0
S_{m_0}	1559	34	199	84	1169	261	78	4029	1348	623	6000	1927	387781

the same person to be quarantined and later vaccinated, especially in SEIR epidemics.

We also associate an economic impact of $i + 1$ if an individual of class C_i gets sick. Figure 1 shows *cumulative* infection curves for abstract measures. It can be seen that but for universal vaccination, targeted strategies perform better than classification agnostic strategies. Table 5 shows various other auxiliary data generated, including how many people of each class get infected.

Figure 2 shows *cumulative* infection curves for concrete measures and Table 6 the corresponding auxiliary data. While targeted strategies outperform classification agnostic strategies here as well, the interesting observation here is that quarantine (with some probability, after 80 time units) is a better measure than vaccination (with some probability, after 100 time units).

It can also be seen that the infections are always less in the class targeted by a strategy.

5   Conclusion and Future Work

In this paper we introduced a formal definition of strategy for handling epidemics, and report a tool that allows evaluation of different strategies. This tool, we believe, will be very useful for performing what-if analyses during outbreaks. However, for the most part, the simulations that we report are over synthetic data. An immediate future goal is to incorporate real data into the model.

There are several features that can be added to the tool itself. One direction is to increase the set of strategies and measures. Another direction would be to allow a lot of configuration parameters to be specified by the user through a simple interface. This would include strategy and measure specification in addition specification of agent, environment and disease parameters.

References

1. Meyers, L.A., Newman, M.E.J., Pourbohloul, B.: Predicting epidemics on directed contact networks. J. Theoret. Biol. **240**(3), 400–418 (2006)
2. Apolloni, A., Kumar, V.S.A., Marathe, M.V., Swarup, S.: Computational epidemiology in a connected world. Computer **42**(12), 83–86 (2009)
3. Bailey, N.: The Mathematical Theory of Infectious Diseases and its Applications. Griffin, London (1975)
4. Barrett, C.L., Bisset, K.R., Eubank, S.G., Feng, X., Marathe, M.V.: Episimdemics: An efficient algorithm for simulating the spread of infectious disease over large realistic social networks. In: Proceedings of the 2008 ACM/IEEE Conference on Supercomputing (2008)
5. Brauer, F.: Compartmental models in epidemiology. In: Brauer, F., van den Driessche, P., Wu, J. (eds.) Mathematical Epidemiology. Lecture Notes in Mathematics, vol. 1945, pp. 19–79. Springer, Berlin (2008). doi:10.1007/978-3-540-78911-6_2
6. Broeck, W., Gioannini, C., Gonaçlves, B., Quaggiotto, M., Colizza, V., Vespignani, A.: The gleamviz computational tool, a publicly available software to explore realistic epidemic spreading scenarios at the global scale. BMC Infect. Dis. **11**(37) (2011)

7. Durham, D., Casman, E.A.: Incorporating individual health-protective decisions into disease transmission models: a mathematical framework. J. Roy. Soc. Interface **9**(68), 562–570 (2012)
8. Eubank, S.: Scalable, efficient epidemiological simulation. In: Proceedings of the 2002 ACM Symposium on Applied Computing. SAC 2002, pp. 139–145 (2002)
9. Eubank, S., Guclu, H., Anil Kumar, V.S., Marathe, M.V., Srinivasan, A., Toroczkai, Z., Wang, N.: Modelling disease outbreaks in realistic urban social networks. Nature **429**(6988), 180–184 (2004)
10. Frias-Martinez, E., Williamson, G., Frias-Martinez, V.: An agent-based model of epidemic spread using human mobility and social network information. In: Privacy, Security, Risk and Trust (PASSAT) and 2011 IEEE Third International Conference on Social Computing (SocialCom), pp. 57–64. IEEE (2011)
11. Funk, S., Gilad, E., Watkins, C., Jansen, V.A.A.: The spread of awareness and its impact on epidemic outbreaks. Proc. Nat. Acad. Sci. **106**(16), 6872–6877 (2009)
12. Hethcote, H.W.: The mathematics of infectious diseases. SIAM Rev. **42**(4), 599–653 (2000)
13. Keeling, M.J., Eames, K.T.D.: Networks and epidemic models. Interface **2**, 295–307 (2005)
14. Kermack, W., McKendrick, A.: A contribution to the mathematical theory of epidemics. Proc. R. Soc. A **115**, 700–721 (1927)
15. Lloyd, A.L., May, R.M.: How viruses spread among computers and people. Science **292**(5520), 1316–1317 (2001)
16. Mao, L.: Predicting self-initiated preventive behavior against epidemics with an agent-based relative agreement model. J. Artif. Soc. Soc. Simul. **18**(4), 6 (2015)
17. Meyers, L.A.: Contact network epidemiology: bond percolation applied to infectious disease prediction and control. Bull. Amer. Math. Soc. **44**, 63–86 (2007)
18. Newman, M.: The spread of epidemic diseases on networks. Phys. Rev. E **66**, 016128 (2002)
19. Nsubuga, P., White, M.E., Thacker, S.B., Anderson, M.A., Blount, S.B., Broome, C.V., Chiller, T.M., Espitia, V., Imtiaz, R., Sosin, D., Stroup, D.F., Tauxe, R.B., Vijayaraghavan, M., Trostle, M.: Public health surveillance: a tool for targeting and monitoring interventions. In: Disease Control Priorities in Developing Countries, 2nd edn. Washington (DC). The International Bank for Reconstruction and Development/The World Bank (2006). Chap. 53
20. Pastor-Satorras, R., Castellano, C., Van Mieghem, P., Vespignani, A.: Epidemic processes in complex networks. Rev. Mod. Phys. **87**, 925–979 (2015)
21. Pastor-Satorras, R., Vespignani, A.: Epidemic spreading in scale-free networks. Phys. Rev. Lett. **86**, 3200–3203 (2001)
22. Singh, S.: Branching processes in disease epidemics. Ph.D. Thesis, Cornell University (2014)

Mining Disease Transmission Networks from Health Insurance Claims

Hsin-Min Lu[✉] and Yu-Ching Chang

National Taiwan University, Taipei 106, Taiwan
{luim, r04725008}@ntu.edu.tw

Abstract. Disease transmission network can provide important information for individuals to protect themselves and to support governments to prevent and control infectious diseases. Current studies on disease transmission network mostly focus on scenarios in small, confined areas. We propose to construct disease transmission network using health status time series computed based on health insurance claims. We adopted Granger causality tests to identify potential links from the health status time series from all pairs of individuals. We evaluated our approach by predicting future health care seeking activates for similar diseases based on past health care seeking activates of neighbors in the disease network. The results suggest that the transmission network is able to improve prediction performance in a small random sample of 500 individuals.

Keywords: Disease transmission network · Health status time series · Health insurance claims

1 Introduction

Infectious diseases are a serious threat to the wellbeing of modern societies. While the advances of medications and technologies have helped us better manage and control some diseases such as small pox, we are still facing constant threats of emerging infectious disease every day.

An effective way to prevent infectious disease outbreak is to understand how diseases are transmitted from one patient to another. Understanding how a disease is transmitted can help us provide general guidelines to protect the public. For example, flu virus typically spreads through droplets when people with flu cough or talk, and we can protect ourselves by wearing masks.

The generic guidelines can be further enhanced if we know who are more likely to be the source of infection. We can then take extra cares when we need to be in contact with persons who have high chance of passing on the disease. Based on this idea, the goal of this study is to develop a data mining approach that identifies the potential sources of infection based on historical health insurance claim data. By doing so, we can provide "customized" disease prevention guidelines for each individual. Moreover, we can identify individuals who are at the key positions of the disease transmission network and take steps to reduce their contributions to the spread of a disease.

To achieve this goal, we propose to analyze large scale health insurance claim data and identify potential paths of infections based on diagnosis similarity and the timing of

© Springer International Publishing AG 2017
H. Chen et al. (Eds.): ICSH 2017, LNCS 10347, pp. 268–273, 2017.
https://doi.org/10.1007/978-3-319-67964-8_26

seeking healthcare services. We are facing several technical challenges in pursuing this line of research. First, developing and implementing algorithms for diagnosis similarity is a nontrivial task. Second, identifying meaningful paths of disease infection from all possible N^2 pairs of persons is critical to the ability of predicting future events of disease contraction at individual level. Finally, developing efficient infrastructure to search through all possible pairs of individual for disease transmission path is a challenging task if we plan to deploy our method at a metropolitan that involves millions of individuals.

We are at the early stages of the research, and have conducted small scale experiments to verify our initial design. Our initial results suggest that we can better predict future clinical visits for upper respiratory infection through inter-person links established from past health insurance claims. The improvement is small compared to using an individual past visit. We expect a better result if the experiments can be done at a larger scale.

This paper is organized as follows. Section 2 briefly introduces related works. Section 3 presents the data and methods adopted in this study. Section 4 summarizes the initial results. Section 5 concludes.

2 Related Work

The idea of identifying disease transmission network from various data sources such as locations, symptoms, and pathogen genome have been actively pursued in the past decades [1]. Most studies focused on a small population size less than two hundred. A common theme is to identify transmission trees from genetic similarity as well as other related data [2]. Given a set of individuals that are known to be infected with a given disease, we can assume that an individual acquired the disease from another individual in the sample. By looking at the data such as the symptom onset time and genetic similarity, we can model the problem of identifying the transmission tree as a statistical inference problem. By designing appropriate similarity measures for gene, onset time, and locations, relevant data from different sources can be combined to conquer the problem.

One limitation of these studies, however, is to focus on a small population in a confined area. Moreover, while various data types were adopted in the model, gene similarity played a critical role in identifying transmission tree. It is unclear whether the approach can work without pathogen genome.

Another line of research aims at identifying the dynamics of infectious disease at a sub-population level. For example, by performing Granger causality [3] on male and female HIV reported cases, Hsieh [4] was able to conclude that male HIV infection Granger-cause female HIV infection in a period of 36 months. Another similar study looked at the disease transmission network at a sub-population level by looking at the infection case time series at different locations [5].

While constructing inter-personal transmission network using genomic data can provide reliable results, obtaining pathogen genome at a large scale is expensive, and may not be a practical choice for a large population. Current studies that adopted surveillance data mostly focused on sub-population infection paths. There are few studies that construct inter-personal infectious network by using low cost personal health data that can be applied to construct large scale transmission networks.

3 Data and Method

The goal of this study is to design and evaluate a data analytic approach that constructs inter-personal disease infection network through personal health care records. This disease transmission network can then be used to predict future disease infections given the recent historical health records of persons who are connected in the network. To achieve this goal, we developed a design framework that takes health insurance claims as the data source, and construct a latent topic representations using diagnoses and medications of aggregated weekly visits. This latent topic representation captured the health status of an individual. Latent topics of our focal interests are combined to generate time series of weekly health status. These health status time series can then be analyzed to identify potential inter-personal pairs that are connected in the transmission network. The transmission network can then be further analyzed for it topology, and to predict future disease infection events based on connected nodes. Figure 1 summarizes our design framework.

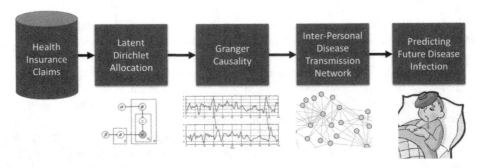

Fig. 1. A design framework to discover inter-personal infection network from health care insurance claims.

We adopted three years (2002 to 2004) of health insurance claims from the National Health Insurance Research Database and aggregated individual outpatient visits by week. The aggregation procedure simply combines all diagnoses and medications records in a week without removing duplications. We removed diagnoses and medications that appeared in less than five person-weeks. Moreover, diagnoses and medications that appeared in more than 20% of the records were deleted.

We trained a LDA model with 50 latent topics. The trained latent topic was applied to all weekly visits to compute the latent topic representation for each record. We manually identify 16 latent topics that are related to upper respiratory infection, and combined the probability of these topics to form a combined topic for upper respiratory infection.

To identify the potential inter-personal infection paths, we adopted Granger causality on the health status time series of all pairs of nodes, and keep all links with a p-value of less than 1%. Since we are at an early stage of the research, we filter the nodes by the following three criteria. We first count the weekly visits for each individual, and keep an individual if he or she has at least two records per year. Second, we only keep individuals who live in Taipei city. Finally, we draw a random sample of 500 individuals to perform Granger causality tests.

We ranked all directed links based on the p-value of Granger causality tests, and constructed the disease transmission networks based on the top N links with the smallest p-value. We set N to 50 and 100 in our preliminary study. This number can be treated as a tuning parameter in subsequent studies.

To evaluate the prediction performance of our approach, we further divide our dataset into a training period of first 104 weeks, and a testing period of subsequent four weeks. We constructed the infection network using time series data in the first 104 weeks, and predict whether an individual will visit a clinic for upper respiratory infection in the testing period. We adopted a simple baseline that predicts an individual's visit based on his or her past visit of the focal disease group.

4 Results

Figure 2 plots the disease transmission network estimated from the top 50 and 100 links identified using Granger causality tests. We can clearly see clusters of nodes that often contain male and female individuals of different ages. Verifying the correctness of the estimated disease transmission network is a challenging task, and we are still looking for an effective way to triangulate the result using other data sources. We are not expecting the network to be very dense since we are working on a small random sample of individuals. Another challenge is to efficiently finding most of the links since a comprehensive research required a time complexity of N^2.

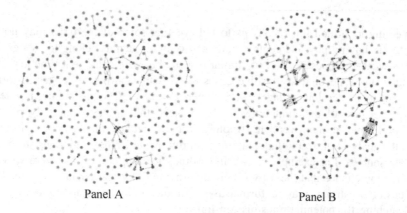

Panel A   Panel B

Fig. 2. Disease transmission network using top 50 links (Panel A) and top 100 links (Panel B). Blue and red dots represent male and female individuals; color tone represents age groups (darker for older individuals). (color figure online)

We evaluated the quality of the network by developing prediction models for future health care seeking activities. Figure 3 plots the ROC curve of the prediction model using the network showed in Panel B of Fig. 2. As can be seen from the figure. The red curve that represent the model using the transmission network is above the baseline model represented by the black line. The AUC of the network prediction model is 0.555 while the baseline has an AUC of 0.527. While the difference is small, we believe that the result indeed provide evidence that the estimated disease transmission network can provide useful information to prediction future health care seeking activities. One reason that the performance gain is small is because we are working on a small sample compared to the whole population in this metropolitan area (about three million). Moreover, we are using a lag period of one week to train models using time series of 104 weeks. As a result, links identified in current setting may be noisy, which may reduce the prediction performance.

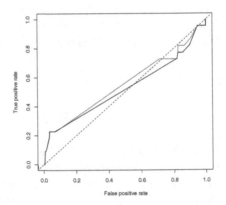

Fig. 3. ROC Curve of Prediction Performance. Blue line is the prediction performance using top 100 links. Block line is the baseline using last week's clinical visit to predict this week's visit. (color figure online)

Inspecting identified links leads us to believe that some of the links may not be interpreted as having physical contacts, and can only be seen as belong to two groups that often went to clinics because of similar disease but with consistent time lags. We can reduce this type of false positive cases if we can incorporate longer historical records and consider longer lag periods when conducting Granger causality tests. However, because of the limitations of the dataset, this strategy can only provide limited performance improvement. Another way to reduce false positive links is through the analysis of overall link patterns, and remove links that are inconsistent with other data sources. For example, if two individuals went to clinics that were very far away, then the chance that these two individual having physical contacts is very low. This types of constraints may be further used to reduce the computational complexity when searching for potential transmission links.

5 Conclusion

In this study, we investigated the problem of constructing disease transmission network using health insurance claims. We constructed health status time series by projecting the diagnoses and medications into a lower dimensional space. We can them identify potential relationships among individual through Granger causality tests.

Using three years of data from NHIRD, we conducted preliminary experiments that focused on 500 randomly sampled individuals. Our results suggest that the neighbors in disease transmission networks is able to better predict future health seeking activities compared to a baseline model using individual past activities. Our results suggest that the idea may have potential to be further expanded to be useful for real world scenarios.

References

1. Ray, B., Ghedin, E., Chunara, R.: Network inference from multimodal data: a review of approaches from infectious disease transmission. J. Biomed. Inform. **64**, 44–54 (2016)
2. Teunis, P., Heijne, J.C.M., Sukhrie, F., van Eijkeren, J., Koopmans, M., Kretzschmar, M.: Infectious disease transmission as a forensic problem: who infected whom? J. Roy. Soc. Interface **10**, 1–9 (2013)
3. Granger, C.W.J.: Investigating causal relations by econometric models and cross-spectral methods. Econometrica **37**, 424–438 (1969)
4. Hsieh, Y.-H.: Ascertaining the 2004–2006 HIV type 1 CRF07_BC outbreak among injecting drug users in taiwan. Int. J. Infect. Dis. **17**, e838–e844 (2013)
5. Yang, X., Liu, J., Zhou, X.-N., Cheung, W.K.: Inferring disease transmission networks at a metapopulation level. Health Inf. Sci. Syst. **2**, 8 (2014)

Semantic Expansion Network Based Relevance Analysis for Medical Information Retrieval

Haolin Wang[1,2,3] and Qingpeng Zhang[1,4(✉)]

[1] City University of Hong Kong, Hong Kong SAR, China
qingpeng.zhang@cityu.edu.hk
[2] University of Chinese Academy of Sciences, Beijing, China
[3] Chongqing Institute of Green and Intelligent Technology,
Chinese Academy of Sciences, Chongqing, China
[4] Shenzhen Research Institute of City University of Hong Kong, Guangdong, China

Abstract. Complex networks provide quantitative measures for complex systems, thus enabling effective semantic network analysis. This research aims to develop semantic relevance analysis methods for medical information retrieval to answer questions for clinical decision support system. We proposed a query based semantic expansion network for semantic relevance analysis in medical information retrieval tasks. Empirical studies of the network structure and attributes for discriminant relevance analysis revealed that expansion networks for relevant documents have a compact structure, which provides new features to identify relevant documents. We also found the existence of densely connected nodes as hubs in the associative networks for queries. Then, we proposed a novel rescaled centrality measure to evaluate the importance of query concepts in the semantic expansion network. Experiments with real-world data demonstrated that the proposed measure is able to improve the performance for relevance analysis.

Keywords: Complex networks · Semantic web · Knowledge-based systems

1 Introduction

Complex networks are widely used across different research areas because most of the real-world networks are complex systems. In this paper, we performed a preliminary study to utilize complex networks for semantic relevance analysis for medical information retrieval. Particularly, we focus on information retrieval for clinical decision support systems, which is important for better access to medical information. To find scientific evidence to support decision making, the first step is to obtain a set of possible relevant literatures.

For the medical domain, information at different levels can be extracted to build complex networks. At the disease network level, for instance, obesity is related to many other diseases such as diabetes, asthma and insulin resistance [1]. At the symptom level, symptom and disease relationships could be extracted from PubMed records [2]. The network-based approaches to human disease have multiple potential biological and clinical applications [3]. Medical knowledge bases such as Unified Medical Language

© Springer International Publishing AG 2017
H. Chen et al. (Eds.): ICSH 2017, LNCS 10347, pp. 274–279, 2017.
https://doi.org/10.1007/978-3-319-67964-8_27

System (UMLS) [4] developed by domain experts could be used to incorporate comprehensive domain knowledge. To improve the performance of semantic relevance analysis, we proposed the semantic expansion network to capture all explicit associations between queries and documents. The proposed networks and examples are presented in Sect. 2. The experiments and results are reported in Sect. 3. We conclude the paper in Sect. 4.

2 Semantic Expansion Network

To capture all possible associations between queries and documents, we extracted all concepts from the queries and documents respectively, and construct a *semantic expansion network* for each query-document pair. The workflow is illustrated in Fig. 1. First, concepts are extracted from document and query, respectively. Second, the system will retrieve all associated concepts from the external knowledge base (UMLS) to identify connected document concepts for current concepts. The loop stops when no associated concepts can be found for the expanded query concepts network. In summary, we expand the query using concepts from knowledge base incrementally and iteratively to extract the intersections between a document and the associative network of a query.

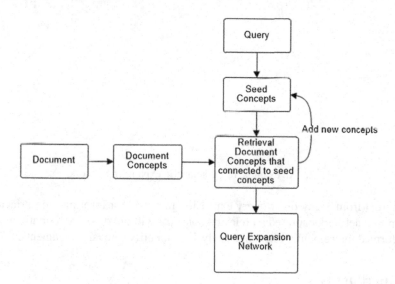

Fig. 1. Workflow to construct the semantic expansion network

For instance, a sample query provided by the 2014 TREC Clinical Decision Support (CDS) Track [5] with annotated concepts using MetaMap [6] is shown as below:

58-year-old *[Year, Temporal Concept; Old, Temporal Concept]* woman *[Women, Population Group]* with hypertension *[Hypertension, Disease or Syndrome]* and obesity *[Obesity Adverse Event, Finding]* presents *[Present, Quantitative Concept]* with exercise *[Exercise Pain Management, Therapeutic or Preventive Procedure]* – related

[Relationships, Qualitative Concept] episodic *[Episodic, Qualitative Concept]* chest pain radiating *[Chest Pain Radiating, Sign or Symptom]* to the back *[Dorsal, Spatial Concept]*.

Based on the proposed workflow, a semantic expansion network (Fig. 2) was constructed using a relevant document for the sample query.

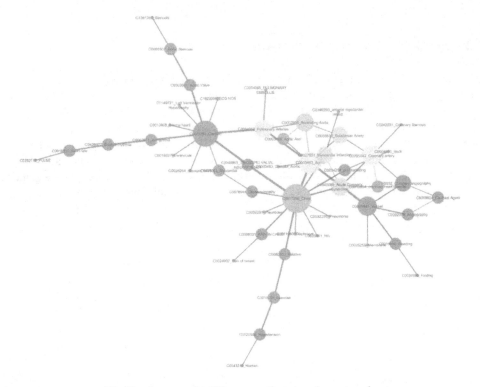

Fig. 2. An example of the semantic expansion network.

Different from many other query expansion methods for information retrieval [7], the proposed network captured all relevant concepts without distance limitations. Next, we performed the semantic relevance analysis to identify relevant documents.

3   Experiments

A subset of 2014 TREC CDS track data was used for the experiment. This track aims at answering clinical questions by retrieval of relevant biomedical literatures. 132 documents labelled as relevant or irrelevant to one sample query were used to evaluate the performance of proposed method in this preliminary study.

3.1 Empirical Analysis

In this section, we reported the comparison of the expansion networks constructed for the query with a set of relevant documents and irrelevant documents respectively. As shown in Table 1, the expansion network for relevant documents has a relatively compact structure. This is reasonable since these documents may have more related topics with the query.

Table 1. Network attributes of the semantic expansion networks for relevant documents and irrelevant documents

	Relevant documents	Irrelevant documents
# of nodes	540	836
# of edges	898	1233
Diameter	13	20
Network density	0.006	0.003

Real-world semantic networks are generally scale-free network [8, 9]. Similarly, in the expansion networks, a small proportion of concepts has much larger degree than other concepts (Fig. 3). It is worth noting that those concepts may not consistent with the query concepts, although the networks are expanded from query concepts (Fig. 3).

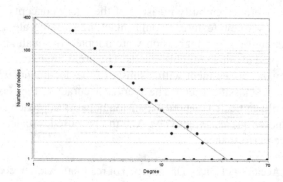

Fig. 3. Degree distribution of an expansion network.

3.2 Semantic Relevance Analysis

As mentioned in the last section, important nodes exist in the expansion network. We assume that the role query concepts play in the expansion network could contribute to relevance analysis. Centrality is widely used to measure the importance of a node. For instance, a topic labeling algorithm was proposed to identify the concepts that best represent the topics using graph centrality measures [10]. However, in the semantic networks, some widely used common concepts (usually domain-independent) may have many connections, while are not useful for relevance analysis. To address this, we proposed a rescaled centrality (w_i) to describe the importance of node in depicting the topic represented by the proposed expansion network.

$$w_i = \frac{c_i}{1 + \log d_i} \tag{1}$$

Where c_i is the closeness centrality for a concept in the proposed expansion network, and d_i is the degree (# of connections) of this concept in the semantic network extracted from the UMLS. The Eq. (1) adopts a similar form of the widely-used TF-IDF method, and is novel in terms of the incorporation of semantics hidden in the structure.

Finally, we evaluated the performance of relevance analysis based on the proposed semantic expansion networks. We used six attributes (listed in Table 2) to formulate a binary classification problem for the selected documents.

Table 2. Selected network features

	Network Attributes
1	# of nodes
2	# of edges
3	Average shortest path length
4	Diameter
5	Degree assortativity
6	Density

In addition, the average centrality measure of the query concepts in the expansion networks was used as a new feature. Popular machine learning algorithms including SVM, decision tree and logistic regression were adopted for evaluation. 5-fold cross validation was adopted to obtain reliable results. The preliminary experiment presented the results for relevance assessment with a subset of the documents with the accuracy metric (ratio of correct classifications). The average accuracy of the classifiers is shown in Table 3. The results indicated that the expansion network approach is able to identify relevant documents for queries effectively. And the proposed rescaled centrality could further improve the performance.

Table 3. Accuracy of binary classification of relevant/irrelevant documents

	Selected features	Selected features + closeness centrality	Selected features + rescaled centrality
SVM	0.703	0.724	**0.746**
Decision tree	0.652	0.797	**0.828**
Logistic regression	0.718	0.732	**0.748**

4 Conclusions

This paper presented the preliminary study of a complex network approach for semantic relevance analysis. A rescaled centrality measure was applied to describe the importance of query concepts in the semantic expansion network. The result demonstrated that the query based semantic expansion networks and the rescaled centrality measure are able to identify relevant documents effectively, and could be further explored to be integrated with existing information retrieval systems.

Acknowledgement. This work was supported by The National Natural Science Foundation of China (NSFC) Grant Nos. 71402157 and 71672163, the Guangdong Provincial Natural Science Foundation No. 2014A030313753, and The Theme-Based Research Scheme of the Research Grants Council of Hong Kong Grant No. T32-102/14 N.

The authors would like to thank Prof. Guanrong Chen for his constructive advice and guidance in this work.

References

1. Costa, L.D.F., Oliveira Jr., O.N., Travieso, G., Rodrigues, F.A., Villas Boas, P.R., Antiqueira, L., Viana, M.P., Correa Rocha, L.E.: Analyzing and modeling real-world phenomena with complex networks: a survey of applications. Adv. Phy. **60**, 329–412 (2011)
2. Zhou, X., Menche, J., Barabási, A.-L., Sharma, A.: Human symptoms–disease network. Nat. Commun. **5**, 4212 (2014)
3. Barabási, A.-L., Gulbahce, N., Loscalzo, J.: Network medicine: a network-based approach to human disease. Nat. Rev. Genet. **12**, 56–68 (2011)
4. Bodenreider, O.: The unified medical language system (UMLS): integrating biomedical terminology. Nucleic Acids Res. **32**, D267–D270 (2004)
5. Simpson, M.S., Voorhees, E.M., Hersh, W.: Overview of the trec 2014 clinical decision support track. DTIC Document (2014)
6. Aronson, A.R., Lang, F.-M.: An overview of metamap: historical perspective and recent advances. J. Am. Med. Inform. Assoc. **17**, 229–236 (2010)
7. Liu, Z., Chu, W.W.: Knowledge-based query expansion to support scenario-specific retrieval of medical free text. Inf. Retrieval **10**, 173–202 (2007)
8. Cong, J., Liu, H.: Approaching human language with complex networks Phy. life rev. **11**, 598–618 (2014)
9. Tachimori, Y., Iwanaga, H., Tahara, T.: The networks from medical knowledge and clinical practice have small-world, scale-free, and hierarchical features. Phys. A **392**, 6084–6089 (2013)
10. Hulpus, I., Hayes, C., Karnstedt, M., Greene, D.: Unsupervised graph-based topic labelling using dbpedia. In: Proceedings of the Sixth ACM International Conference on Web Search and Data Mining, pp. 465–474. ACM (2013)

Using Deep Learning to Mine the Key Factors of the Cost of AIDS Treatment

Dong Liu[1,2], Zhidong Cao[2(✉)], and Su Li[1]

[1] Beijing Key Laboratory of Big Data Technology on Food Safety,
Beijing Technology and Business University, Beijing 100048
People's Republic of China
[2] State Key Laboratory of Complex Systems Management and Control,
Institute of Automation, Chinese Academy of Sciences, Beijing 100190
People's Republic of China
zhidong.cao@ia.ac.cn

Abstract. The medical burden of AIDS is a significant public health problem. However, it is affected by the multiple factors, among which there is yet some vague cognition, and further exploration is necessary. Thus, the artificial neural network (ANN) and restricted Boltzmann machine (RBM) be treated as the infrastructure of deep neural networks (DNN), mainly based on the features of demography, pathology and clinical manifestation of AIDS patient's medical records to mine the impact factors of AIDS cost. And the proposed model could bring to light the previously uncharted latent knowledge and concepts. Based on reliable healthcare delivery, to inhibit the number of hospital days, intensive care and hospitalized frequency plus other sensitive factors, and avoid secondary infection and exposure to allergic reactions can obviously reduce the AIDS cost.

Keywords: ANN · RBM · AIDS cost · Impact factors

1 Introduction

AIDS (acquired immune deficiency syndrome, AIDS) is a significant public health problem. The joint assessment for AIDS indicated that as of September 2016 in China the cumulative number of deaths has exceeded 201,000 [1]. The patient life suffers a serious threat, but the biological technology resource of curbing AIDS is very scarce and precious. Thus, the scientific and efficient control in AIDS cost became a hot issue in decision-making of healthcare delivery.

The most widely used methods, such as linear regression, logistic regression(LR), clustering methods and SVM etc., have achieved some results [1–4]. However, the linear regression requires the normal distribution and variance homogeneity, plus a presumed linear relationship between the argument and dependent variables. Thus it performs feebly in nonlinear correlation. And the shallow machine learning models (e.g., SVM, LR, etc.) in complicated structure data is lack of expression ability, and could lead to dimension disaster [5]. Obviously, the traditional methods had been sinked into dilemma. Fortunately, the deep models which simulate the hierarchical structure in human brain can achieve the hierarchical expression of data [6]. This way

© Springer International Publishing AG 2017
H. Chen et al. (Eds.): ICSH 2017, LNCS 10347, pp. 280–285, 2017.
https://doi.org/10.1007/978-3-319-67964-8_28

can not only imitate the procedure of human thinking to improve efficiency overwhelmingly, but can identify and characterize implied knowledge and concepts [7, 8].

2 Materials and Methods

2.1 Data

The data sample in this study is derived from the AIDS-related HIS systems in China. A total of 2618 in hospitalized medical records were randomly selected from 2006 to 2010. The data items features include the age, gender, address, payment methods, hospitalized frequency, etc. More crucially, in this paper we put these features as the independent variable, and the actual AIDS cost was take as the dependent variable.

2.2 Methods

Primitively Hinton and Sejnowki were rooted in statistical mechanics research to propose the Boltzmann machine (BM) [5]. Although BM has excellent unsupervised learning ability, its pre-learning process is over complicated. Thus, the RBM come from the simplified BM, and has a prominent advantage, which has been rigorously proved by Bengio that RBM can fit any discrete distribution if the number of hidden layer units is enough [7]. Assuming that $(\mathbf{x}, \mathbf{h})$ represent the state of visible layer and hidden layer. Based energy function, we can deduce the joint probability distribution and marginal probability distribution (see formula (1)).

$$P(\mathbf{x}, \mathbf{h}|\theta) = \frac{e^{-E(\mathbf{x},\mathbf{h}|\theta)}}{Z(\theta)} \textbf{ under s.t. } Z(\theta) = \sum_{\mathbf{x},\mathbf{h}} e^{-E(\mathbf{x},\mathbf{h}|\theta)} \Rightarrow P(\mathbf{x}|\theta) = \frac{1}{Z(\theta)} \sum_{\mathbf{h}} e^{-E(\mathbf{x},\mathbf{h}|\theta)}$$

$$\textbf{Energy function} : E(\mathbf{x}, \mathbf{h}|\theta) = -\sum_{i=1}^{n} b_i x_i - \sum_{j=1}^{m} c_j h_j - \sum_{i=1}^{n} \sum_{j=1}^{m} x_i W_{ij} h_j$$

(1)

In order to obtain $P(x|\theta)$, it must require 2^{m+n} calculations to determine $Z(\theta)$, which is called as normalized factor. Therefore, the determination of probability distribution of RBM was still very hard. RBM had continued to be progression-free in technology till the invention of contrastive divergence algorithm (CD) and its improved algorithm [8, 9].

The initial design for DNN highlighted its hybrid strategy in model building, and Deng deeply analyzed this characteristic [10]. Combining with ANN, the unsupervised learning module can construct a deep model, such as Google's cat [5, 10]. Considering the existence theorem of mapping, that any continuous function can be approximated at a desired accuracy by a three layer perceptron network (ANN with one hidden layer) [11]. Moreover, the more layers in networks the more slow in convergence it will become. In light of this, as shown in Fig. 1, this study by cascading up two layer RBMs and a three layer ANN constructed a DNN. Those RBMs at the bottom of networks could deeply mine the information hidden in raw data, and then form the feature expressions which can act as the input of ANN. The top layer in ANN has regression forecast function, and can calculate the sensitivity of impact variables. In order to reveal how significant those variables, the variable sensitivity is defined as the important degree of input variables of networks. Namely the sensitivity analysis is to change a certain part of model, for observing the corresponding changes in network, so as to determine the important degree of this part for networks (formula (2)).

$$S_m = \frac{1}{n} \sum_{j=1}^{n} \frac{\max\limits_{i=1 \to n} \{f(x_i)\} - \min\limits_{i=1 \to n} \{f(x_i)\}}{\max\limits_{i=1 \to n} \{f(x_i)\}} \qquad (2)$$

In the training phase, we conduct layer-by-layer. Namely when it was RBM we adopted a modified CD algorithm [12] to train, while about ANN we take BP algorithm for pre-learning. In this way our networks can obtain better initial weights. In the fine-tuning stage, we used BP algorithm to fine tune the whole networks.

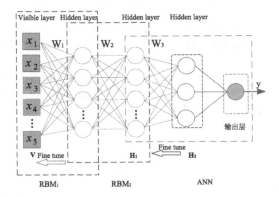

Fig. 1. Schematic diagram of model structure

3   Experimental Results

We primarily carried out a statistical description, which are shown in Tables 1 and 2. In this way, we can get the bottom feature operators. It indicated that the variables of AIDS cost affected each other. Among them there are a lot of complicated Non-linear relationships.

For eliminating the impact of different improved BP algorithms on the DNN performance and efficiency, this paper would use the LM algorithm, variable scale conjugate gradient algorithm. And the experiments noted that the LM algorithm is evidently best among them regardless of fitting and generalization ability. In Fig. 2, it indicated that: the sensitivity of hospital days, days of intensive care, days of sickness in danger, and hospitalized frequency are evidently exceed 0.6, plus rescue times, admission condition etc. are between 0.44 and 0.66, but ethnic, gender and whether follow-up are below 0.4.

Table 1. Discrete variables qualitative description

Var.	Categories	Qty.	Pct./%	Var.	Categories	Qty.	Pct./%
Gender	Man	1645	62.83	Admission Condition	Danger	116	4.43
	Woman	973	37.17		Urgent	867	33.11
Age	≤ 30	309	11.80		General	1640	62.64
	30 ~ 60	1497	57.18	Exchange department	Yes	627	23.95
	60 ~ 70	713	27.23		No	1991	76.05
	>70	99	3.78	Follow up	Yes	231	8.82
Marital status	Married	1725	65.89		No	2387	91.18
	Unmarried	307	11.80	Allergic drug categories	Chinese herb	1309	50
	Divorce	57	2.18		HIV antitoxin	491	18.75
	Widowed	529	20.21		Broad-spectrum antibiotics	572	21.85
Ethnic groups	Han	1797	68.64		Sulfonamides	157	6.01
	Minority	821	31.36		Penicillin	89	3.41
Work categories	Worker	312	11.92	Regions	North China	148	5.65
	Farmer	1184	45.23		South China	330	12.61
	Cadre	115	4.39		Central China	178	6.79
	Students	61	2.33		Northwest	669	25.55
	Children	10	0.38		Southwest	1075	41.06
	Other	936	35.75		Northeast	53	2.02
Payment methods	Basic medical insurance	1373	52.44		East China	165	6.30
				Admission methods	Outpatient clinic	1513	57.79
	Commercial insurance	20	0.76		Emergency	321	12.26
	Free	236	9.01				
	Self-funded	249	9.51		Referral	784	29.95
	Other	460	17.57				

Table 2. Continuous variables qualitative description

Var.	Min	Max	AVG.	SD.
Days of sickness in danger	0	43	15.17	48.37
Hospital days	1	88	23.16	26.54
Days of intensive care	1	56	6.39	27.61
Hospitalized frequency	1	10	4.27	4.13
Rescue times	0	12	0.83	0.821
Age	1	83	54.62	12.413

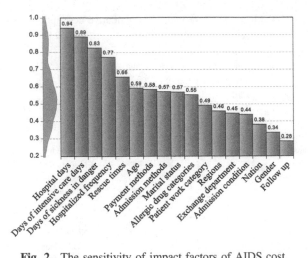

Fig. 2. The sensitivity of impact factors of AIDS cost

4 Conclusion and Discussion

However, the deep model is like a black box,which only focuses on input and output. Thus, we conducted the variables sensitivity analysis to explain the proposed deep model. The sensitivity is greater than 0.5 variables, can be considered very important; otherwise they can be considered more important, because they both are not strictly different. But AIDS is particular than general diseases after all, and here is some evidences: (1) the sensitivity of age was close to 0.6, because AIDS attacks the immune system in human body, and the older, the worse resistance. Once sick easily lead to complication, the medical cost will rapidly increase; (2) as AIDS is fatal, the patients' payment method and occupation categories for HIV aren't as sensitive as other diseases cost; (3) but the sensitivity of marital status is higher than other diseases cost to blame the AIDS's infectious mode; (4) also the allergic drugs categories are more sensitive, because the immune ability of patients is weak or disorder. In case of allergic reaction occurring, it can damage to the normal cell and tissue, and the medical expenses increased; (5) the sensitivity of intensive care is close to 0.9, mainly because of the expensive service. Initially AIDS cannot be spread, the patients with weak immunity who must prevent an infection from other diseases avoid endangering their lives, and thus they need the special care in quarantine. These indicated that the deep model can identify and characterize implied knowledge and concepts.

Based on reliable healthcare delivery, to reduce the hospital days, intensive care and hospitalized frequency is primary path for reducing AIDS's hospitalization cost effectively. Consciously we must commitment to preventing the infection (between patients and others around them, patients and patients with other virus), allergic reactions and related variables, such as age, allergic drug classification, etc. In this way, we can't reduce the unnecessary treatment program and economy burden, but also can improve the efficiency of hospital, even reducing unnecessary waste of medical resources.

Acknowledgement. This work is partially funded through NNSFC Grants #91546112. National Key R&D Program #2016YFC1200702 and #2016QY02D0200.

References

1. Zhang, Y.Q., Qin, X., Zhou, L., et al.: The AIDS epidemic and economic input impact factors in Chongqing, China, from 2006 to 2012: a spatial-temporal analysis. BMJ Open **5**(3) (2015)
2. Zhang, X.L., Zhang, Y.R., Aleong, T.H., et al.: Factors associated with the Household Income of Persons Living with HIV/AIDS in China. Global J. Health Sci. **4**(3), 108–116 (2012)
3. Harmon, T.M., Fisher, K.A., Mcglynn, M.G., et al.: Exploring the potential health impact and cost-effectiveness of AIDS vaccine within a comprehensive HIV/AIDS response in low and middle-income countries. PLoS ONE **11**(1), e0146387 (2015)
4. Stover, J., Bollinger, L., Izazola, J.A., et al.: What Is required to end the AIDS epidemic as a public health threat by 2030? The Cost and Impact of the Fast-Track Approach. PLoS ONE **11**(5), e0154893 (2016)
5. LeCun, Y., Bengio, Y., Hinton, G.: Deep Learing. Nature Mag. **521**(7553), 436–444 (2015)
6. Ryota, S., Shusuke, Y., Yasutaka, M., et al.: Deep learning application trial to lung cancer diagnosis for medical sensor systems. In: 2016 International SoC Design Conference (ISOCC), pp. 191–192 (2016)
7. Le, R.N., Bengio, Y.: Representational power of restricted boltzmann machines and deep belief networks. Neural Comput. **20**(6), 1631–1649 (2008)
8. Hinton, G., Osindero, I.Y.: A fast learning algorithm for deep belief nets. Neural Comput. **18**(7), 1527–1554 (2006)
9. Tieleman, T., Hinton, G.E.: Using fast weights to improve persistent contrastive divergence. In: Proceedings of the 26th International Conference on Machine Learning, Helsinki, Finland, pp. 1064–1071 (2008)
10. Deng, L.: A tutorial survey of architectures, algorithms, and applications for deep learning. APSIPA Trans. Signal Inf. Proces. **3**, 14–43 (2014)
11. Furundzic, D., Djordjevic, M., Bekic, A.J.: Neural networks approach to early breast cancer detection. Syst Architect **44**, 617–633 (1998)
12. Tieleman, T.: Training restricted Boltzmann machines using approximations to the likelihood gradient. In: Proceedings of 25th International Conference on Machine Learning, New York, pp, 1064–1071. ACM (2008)

A Knowledge-Based Health Question Answering System

Hongxia Liu$^{(\boxtimes)}$, Qingcheng Hu, Yong Zhang,
Chunxiao Xing, and Ming Sheng

Tsinghua National Laboratory for Information Science and Technology,
Department of Computer Science and Technology, Research Institute
of Information Technology, Institute of Internet Industry,
Tsinghua University, Beijing, China
panny_lhx@163.com, {huqingcheng, zhangyong05, xingcx,
shengming}@tsinghua.edu.cn

Abstract. With the quickly increasing of the Question Answering (QA) corpus, the health QA systems provide a convenient way for patients to provide instant service, and the effectiveness of the answer is a very important and challenging problem to be solved. Therefore, this paper proposes a solution based on medical knowledge base. In the process of generating answers, we utilize the entity set provided by medical knowledge base to calculate the correlation between answers and questions, at the same time we make use of the entities provided by relationships in the knowledge base but not appearing in the answers. Experiment conducted on a real data set in our HealthQA system shows that our method can effectively improve the relevance and accuracy of answer matching by using the medical knowledge base.

Keywords: Medical knowledge base · HealthQA · Entity relationship

1 Introduction

The question answering (QA) systems try to solve the shortcomings of the information retrieval system [1]. One of the main features is that people use natural language to express themselves and then QA system returns a more accurate and direct answer by Natural Language Processing and semantic analysis methods. This method not only saves people time to retrieve information, but also provides people with a more accurate and flexible interface. Therefore, QA systems have attracted many eyes.

Because of the limitation of the knowledge base, the early QA systems can only answer some field-specific questions, such as Baseball [2] and LUNAR [3]. In recent years, with the emergence of general domain knowledge base, such as DBpedia [4], Freebase [5], and Yago2 [6], a number of general domain QA systems arise. One of the most famous QA systems is the IBM's QA system Watson [7].

In this paper, we created one medical knowledge base with the help of medical professionals, and a question classification method aimed to capture the patient's intention.

© Springer International Publishing AG 2017
H. Chen et al. (Eds.): ICSH 2017, LNCS 10347, pp. 286–291, 2017.
https://doi.org/10.1007/978-3-319-67964-8_29

The remainder of the paper is organized as follows. Section 2 introduces the related work. Section 3 presents our research design. We report our experiments and results analysis in Sect. 4. The last section concludes this paper.

2   Related Work

There are two types of QA systems: domain-independent and domain-specific. Here we focus on the domain-specific QA systems. In the medical domain, there are two well-known QA systems - MedQA [8] and AskHERMES [9]. Few studies can be found for Chinese QA systems. Peng et al. [10] developed a domain-specific Chinese QA system based on an enterprise knowledge base. Zhang et al. [11] designed a document retrieval method for a Chinese QA system using professional documents.

A comprehensive and complete knowledge base is of great significance for constructing an intelligent QA system. Terol RM et al. [12] used two different knowledge: Unified Medical Language System (UMLS) to handle the medical terminology and WordNet to manage the open-domain terminology.

Although the research of healthQA system is quite universal, we rarely find the research work in Chinese. The main reason is the lack of Chinese medical or health knowledge base, which we can find is the Chinese version of DBpedia [4]. In our system, we have built a knowledge base in the medical field.

3   Research Design

Figure 1 is the framework of the HealthQA system, which consists of three parts: question analysis, medical knowledge base, and answer processing. This paper focuses on question classification and medical knowledge base construction.

3.1   Question Classification

Question classification can adopt classifier methods to deal with, such as SVM, Random Forest, Decision Trees, etc., but in this system we use a more simple and effective method: extracting interrogative sentences by using interrogative terms. By 1000 sampling statistics, the interrogatives and interrogative sentence patterns above can probably cover 90% of the interrogative sentences in the collection of questions.

When we extract the interrogatives, we explore the type of the questions. All the questions can be divided into two categories, closed questions and open questions.

For example:

Closed question: I would like to know whether diabetes will be inheritance to the next generation?

Open question: What should diabetes patients eat?

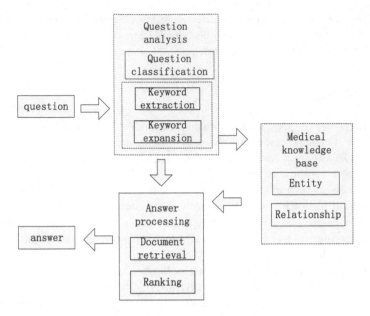

Fig. 1. HealthQA architecture

3.2   Medical Knowledge Base

It is of great significance to construct the knowledge base in medical field to understand the meaning of medical texts. Based on this, we construct a medical knowledge base by retrieving the professional dictionaries on the Internet and the medical authority books in the aid of medical professionals. The structure and content of our knowledge base is shown in Table 1.

Table 1. The structure and content of our knowledge base

Table name (Attributes)	#Records
Disease (name, subject, system, department, body part, alias)	512
Symptom (name)	2,162
Diagnosis (name, abbreviation)	1,080
Medicine (name, manufacturers, URL, alias)	3,200
Disease-Symptom (disease, symptom)	4,738
Disease-Diagnosis (disease, diagnosis)	3,049
Disease-Medicine (disease, medicine)	6,673

Based on the knowledge base, for the open questions, if the patient enters a symptom description, the system will be able to provide the corresponding disease, corresponding medicines and corresponding diagnoses, which could help the patient to obtain a more complete and more detailed answer.

3.3   Question and Answer Entity Expansion Based on Knowledge Base

Assuming a question q, and an answer is a, the entity set of q is Eq, and the entity set of a is Ea. By the relationship in the knowledge base, Eq is expanded to Eqk, $Eqk = Eq \cup$ {derived entities}, Ea is expanded to Eak, $Eak = Eq \cup$ {derived entities}.

Q: What does the diet of diabetes need to notice?

Eq = {diabetes}, according to searching knowledge base we know that "diabetes" belongs to the type of disease. What are related to disease are symptoms and medicines. Then Eqk = {diabetes, glycosuria, polydipsia, emaciation, Zhengtang Capsules, metformin, Pioglitazone}

> *A1: Eat less carbohydrate foods, such as sweet potatoes, lotus root and so on. Best not to drink. You can eat high-fiber foods to promote the body's sugar metabolism such as corn, wheat, and low sugar of vegetables such as pumpkin, vegetables, eggplant.*
>
> *A2: Diabetes is still not be cured and needs long-term medication control. Suggested that oral metformin and pioglitazone.*
>
> *A3: The typical symptoms of diabetes are three more, one less. That is, polyuria, polydipsia, polyphagia and emaciation. Diagnosis of diabetes need to measure blood glucose, glycosylated hemoglobin, etc. Patient should go to the hospital to identify.*
>
> $Eak1$ = {diabetes, potatoes, lotus root, corn, pumpkin, vegetables, eggplant}.
> $Eak2$ = {diabetes, metformin, pioglitazone}.
> $Eak3$ = {diabetes, polyuria, polydipsia, polyphagia, emaciation, blood glucose, glycosylated hemoglobin}.

3.4   Answer Ranking

There are several strategies for scoring one answer a in the candidate answer set A for a question q:

1. Similar to the scoring method of [13], which consider some indicators, including TFIDF, question keywords, statistics and question similarity.
2. Combine the knowledge base to extend the set of entities. When scoring, we utilize the existence of relationships between the answer entity set and the question entity set. If the relationship exists, the score of the answer will be higher.

4   Experiments

4.1   Data

We collected medical and health related QA data from three major Chinese QA websites: 39.net, xywy.com, and 120ask.com. On these websites, users can ask questions and get answers and/or advices from physicians and healthcare professionals. We extracted a data set consisting 135,709 QA pairs, each pair contains one question and at least one answer.

4.2   Experimental Method

In this paper, we consider not only the medical entities co-exist in the question and the answer, but also the similarity among the related entities that are retrieved from the knowledge base. For example, if the question contains disease a, the answer contains medicine b, there is a relationship in the knowledge base $a \rightarrow b$, then the question entity set is $\{a, b\}$, the answer entity set is $\{b\}$. With the knowledge base there is an overlap between question entities and answer entities although there is no intersection between them before.

We conducted a survey to evaluate the accuracy and richness of answers provided by our system. We carefully prepared 100 questions with the help of medical professionals, each of which has two answers. The first is produced by the original QA system without knowledge base, and the answer is related to the user query. The second answer is the result of combining the medical knowledge base, it not only contains the answers to user queries but also contains the extended answers from our medical knowledge base. The user needs to make a decision between the two answers: "answer 1 is better", "answer 2 is better", "equal" or "unknown". In the end, we evaluate the method by using the feedback from the users.

4.3   Experimental Result

We received a total of 42 users of the evaluation feedback. Table 2 shows the result of feedback to two kinds of answers. We can see from Table 2 that the Answer 2 won more than half of the votes because it contains more related information that the patients do not need to search again. Of course, there are some people who feel the same, because they can get the desired results in both answers. The data indicates that our HealthQA system based on medical knowledge base is accepted by the users.

Table 2. User's feedback to two kinds of answers

Selection	Answer 1 is better	Answer 2 is better	Equal	Unknown
Percentage	21%	57%	17%	5%

4.4   Result Analysis

In this optimized system, we highlight the role of the medical knowledge base in the process of searching for answers by improving the accuracy of the answer. For example: the question mentioned "diabetes", the answer includes "In this case, you should eat metformin". Only from the text itself, the answer is not relevant to the question. But through the medical knowledge base, we can see that "metformin" is a medication for treating diabetes, so the answer is relevant. Therefore, users can not only get the queried information but also can get relevant information, that's killing two birds with one stone.

5 Conclusion

It is important to build automatic health related QA systems to help people to get high-quality answers for their concerns. This paper proposes a solution based on medical knowledge base. In the process of generating answers, we utilize the entity set provided by medical knowledge base to calculate the correlation score between answers and questions. At the same time we make use of the entities provided by relationship in the knowledge base but not appearing in the answers.

Acknowledgments. This work was supported by NSFC(91646202), the National High-tech R&D Program of China(SS2015AA020102), Research/Project 2017YB142 supported by Ministry of Education of The People's Republic of China, the 1000-Talent program.

References

1. Xue, X., Jeon, J., Croft, W.B.: Retrieval models for question and answer archives. In: Proceedings of the 31st Annual International ACM SIGIR Conference on Research and Development in Information Retrieval, pp. 475–482. ACM (2008)
2. Green Jr., B.F., Wolf, A.K., Chomsky, C., Laughery, K.: Baseball: an automatic question-answerer. Papers presented at the 9–11 May 1961, Western Joint IRE-AIEE-ACM Computer Conference, pp. 219–224. ACM (1961)
3. Woods, W.A., Kaplan, R.M., Nash-Webber, B., et al.: The lunar sciences natural language information system: final report. Bolt Beranek and Newman (1972)
4. Auer, S., Bizer, C., Kobilarov, G., Lehmann, J., Cyganiak, R., Ives, Z.: DBpedia: a nucleus for a web of open data. In: Aberer, K., et al. (eds.) ASWC/ISWC -2007. LNCS, vol. 4825, pp. 722–735. Springer, Heidelberg (2007). doi:10.1007/978-3-540-76298-0_52
5. Bollacker, K., Evans, C., Paritosh, P., Sturge, T., Taylor, J.: Freebase: a collaboratively created graph database for structuring human knowledge. In: Proceedings of the 2008 ACM SIGMOD International Conference on Management of Data, pp. 1247–1250. ACM (2008)
6. Hoffart, J., Suchanek, F.M., Berberich, K., Weikum, G.: Yago2: a spatially and temporally enhanced knowledge base from wikipedia. Artif. Intell. **194**, 28–61 (2013)
7. https://en.wikipedia.org/wiki/Watson_(computer)
8. Lee, M., Cimino, J., Zhu, H.R., Sable, C., Shanker, V., Ely, J., Yu, H.: Beyond information retrieval—medical question answering. In: AMIA Annual Symposium Proceedings, vol. 2006, p. 469. American Medical Informatics Association (2006)
9. Cao, Y., Liu, F., Simpson, P., Antieau, L., Bennett, A., Cimino, J.J., Ely, J., Yu, H.: Askhermes: An online question answering system for complex clinical questions. J. Biomed. Inform. **44**(2), 277–288 (2011)
10. Peng, X.Y., Chen, Y., Huang, Z.W.: A Chinese question answering system using web service on restricted domain. In: 2010 International Conference on Artificial Intelligence and Computational Intelligence (AICI), vol. 1, pp. 350–353. IEEE (2010)
11. Zhang, H., Zhu, L., Xu, S., Li, W.: Xml-based document retrieval in Chinese diseases question answering system. In: Park, J., Adeli, H., Park, N., Woungang, I. (eds.) Mobile, Ubiquitous, and Intelligent Computing, vol. 274, pp. 211–217. Springer, Heidelberg (2014)
12. Terol, R.M., Martínez-Barco, P., Palomar, M.: A knowledge based method for the medical question answering problem. Comp. in Bio. and Med. **37**(10), 1511–1521 (2007)
13. Yin, Y., Zhang, Y., et al.: HealthQA: a Chinese QA summary system for smart health. In: ICSH, pp. 51–62 (2014)

Poster papers

Predictors for Switch from Unipolar Major Depressive Disorder to Bipolar Disorder: Applying Classification and Regression Trees Method to the Taiwan National Health Insurance Database

Cheng-Che Shen, Ya-Han Hu, and I-Chiu Chang[✉]

Department on Information Management,
National Chung Cheng University, Chiayi, Taiwan
misicc@mis.ccu.edu.tw

1 Induction

Unipolar major depressive disorder (MDD) and bipolar disorder are two common mood disorders in psychiatry. Both disorders are associated with chronicity, disability, and severe functional impairment, but they have different clinical courses, treatment strategies and prognoses. However, the course of bipolar disorder may begin with depression and could be diagnosed as MDD at the initial stage (Kawa et al. 2005). This kind of hidden bipolar disorder may contribute to the treatment resistance observed in unipolar depression (Correa et al. 2010). As previous studies shown (Akiskal et al. 1995; Angst 1985; Angst et al. 2005; Holma et al. 2008; Li et al. 2012), a significant proportion of patients who were diagnosed with MDD will over time develop bipolar disorder and the challenge is predicting the group of patients who are more likely to do this, as the change in diagnosis has important clinical consequences for both treatment and prognosis. However, the results of previous studies regarding the rate of MDD to bipolar conversion were inconsistent. In addition, there are several limitations of previous studies. First, most of these studies are based on small samples. Second, despite psychiatric comorbidity in MDD and bipolar disorder being very common (Mantere et al. 2006), the predictive value of comorbidity for bipolar switch has been examined surprisingly little in previous studies. In this population-based study, the rate of a bipolar switch was surveyed and a risk stratification model for bipolar conversion was developed for MDD patients using psychiatric comorbidities.

2 Methodology

The data source for our study was the Longitudinal Health Insurance Database 2000 (LHID 2000), which is a data set released by the National Health Research Institutes that contains all original claims data for 1 million randomly selected beneficiaries in the

© Springer International Publishing AG 2017
H. Chen et al. (Eds.): ICSH 2017, LNCS 10347, pp. 295–298, 2017.
https://doi.org/10.1007/978-3-319-67964-8

2005 Registry of Beneficiaries. Using the LHID2000, we conducted a retrospective cohort study involving patients who were newly diagnosed with major depressive disorder between January 1, 2000 and December 31, 2004. Major depressive disorder was defined based on ICD-9-CM Codes 296.2X and 296.3X. To ensure diagnostic validity and patient homogeneity, we included patients who were diagnosed only by psychiatrists. We excluded patients who were diagnosed with depressive disorder (ICD-9-CM Codes 296.2X, 296.3X, 300.4, and 311.X) in 1996 to 1999 and who were diagnosed with bipolar disorder (ICD-9-CM Codes 296.0, 296.1, 296.4, 296.5, 296.6, 296.7, 296.8, 296.80, 296.89) before enrolment. In addition, patients who were diagnosed with schizophrenia (ICD-9-CM code 295) were also excluded. The index date was defined as the date when an eligible depression patient was included in our cohort. All depression patients were observed until (1) diagnosed with a bipolar disorder (ICD-9-CM Codes 296.0, 296.1, 296.4, 296.5, 296.6, 296.7, 296.8, 296.80, 296.89) by a psychiatrist, (2) death, or (3) December 31, 2013.

Information on psychiatric comorbidities, which were diagnosed after enrollment, was also collected. In this study, psychiatric disorders including anxiety disorders (anxiety state, panic disorder, generalized anxiety disorder, social phobia, obsessive compulsive disorder, posttraumatic stress disorder), substance use disorder (e.g., alcohol use disorder, opioid use disorder, and amphetamine use disorder), personality disorder (affective personality disorder, schizoid personality disorder, histrionic personality disorder, dependent personality disorder, antisocial personality disorder, other personality disorder), sleep disorder, eating disorder (polyphagia, anorexia nervosa, bulimia nervosa, pica, rumination disorder), autistic spectrum disorder, mental retardation, and attention deficit hyperactivity disorder were categorized for the classification and regression trees (CART) analysis. To analyze personal characteristics, including age at enrollment and sex, and psychiatric comorbidities of interest in bipolar converters and non-bipolar converters, this study used Weka 3.6 open-source machine learning software (www.cs.waikato.ac.nz/ml/weka) to perform CART analysis. The simple CART module in Weka was adopted to generate a CART tree using a complete set of cohort data and variables. To simplify the generated CART tree, all internal and leaf nodes in the tree were constrained to have a minimum size of 20 samples. After the CART tree was built, the percentage of bipolar converter was calculated for each of the leaf nodes in the CART tree and used to generate the risk stratification model. Furthermore, the predictive value of this model was assessed by determining the bipolar odds ratio and 95% confidence intervals (CIs) between risk groups.

3   Results

There are 2820 MDD patients enrolled in our study, among whom 60.1% were women. The median age at enrollment was 38 years (interquartile range 26–52 years). During follow-up period, 536 patients was diagnosed with bipolar disorder (19.0%). The decision tree generated through CART analysis is shown in Fig. 1. Of the studied characteristics, the CART method identified other personality disorder (OPD) as the optimal discriminator between bipolar converters and non-bipolar converters.

For patients with other personality disorder, gender (female or male) provided additional prognostic value. This risk tree was able to stratify patients into high, intermediate, and low risk. The bipolar conversion odds ratio between the high- and low-risk groups was 8.84 (95% CI = 4.16–18.8).

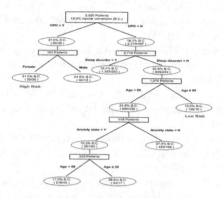

Fig. 1. The risk stratification model for the bipolar conversion in MDD patients.

4   Discussions and Conclusions

In our study, the CART method identified 4 variables as significant predictors of bipolar conversion. In a simple 2-*to 5-step process, these variables permit identification of patients with low, interme*diate, or high risk for bipolar conversion. Furthermore, this model can be easily applied in clinical practice. This model could help to identify patients with bipolar disorder early and to arrange appropriate treatment for these patients.

Our findings include some limitations. First, information regarding the family history of psychiatric disorders, lifestyle factors, and environmental factors are not included in the NHIRD, all of which might be associated with the risk of bipolar disorder. Second, in studies using NHIRD, it is unclear how the diagnostic classification was performed. Therefore, the diagnostic accuracy in our study could not be ascertained. Additional studies with patients diagnosed in structured interviews should be conducted to investigate the association between psychiatric comorbidities and the risk of BPD. Despite these potential limitations, the current CART-based analysis of the NHIRD has created a simple robust tool to predict the risk of bipolar conversion by using psychiatric comorbidities that is easy to use. Future population-based prospective studies are required to further validate our findings.

References

Akiskal, H.S., Maser, J.D., Zeller, P.J., Endicott, J., Coryell, W., Keller, M., Warshaw, M., Clayton, P., Goodwin, F.: Switching from 'unipolar' to bipolar II. An 11-year prospective study of clinical and temperamental predictors in 559 patients. Arch. Gen. Psychiatry **52**, 114–123 (1995)

Angst, J.: Switch from depression to mania–a record study over decades between 1920 and 1982. Psychopathology **18**, 140–154 (1985)

Angst, J., Sellaro, R., Stassen, H.H., Gamma, A.: Diagnostic conversion from depression to bipolar disorders: results of a long-term prospective study of hospital admissions. J. Affect. Disord. **84**, 149–157 (2005)

Correa, R., Akiskal, H., Gilmer, W., Nierenberg, A.A., Trivedi, M., Zisook, S.: Is unrecognized bipolar disorder a frequent contributor to apparent treatment resistant depression? J. Affect. Disord. **127**, 10–18 (2010)

Holma, K.M., Melartin, T.K., Holma, I.A., Isometsä, E.T.: Predictors for switch from unipolar major depressive disorder to bipolar disorder type I or II: a 5-year prospective study. J. Clin. Psychiatry **69**, 1267–1275 (2008)

Kawa, I., Carter, J.D., Joyce, P.R., Doughty, C.J., Frampton, C.M., Elisabeth Wells, J., Walsh, A.E., Olds, R.J.: Gender differences in bipolar disorder: age of onset, course, comorbidity, and symptom presentation. Bipolar Disord. **7**, 119–125 (2005)

Li, C.T., Bai, Y.M., Huang, Y.L., Chen, Y.S., Chen, T.J., Cheng, J.Y., Su, T.P.: Association between antidepressant resistance in unipolar depression and subsequent bipolar disorder: cohort study. Br. J. Psychiatry: J. Ment. Sci. **200**, 45–51 (2012)

Mantere, O., Melartin, T.K., Suominen, K., Rytsala, H.J., Valtonen, H.M., Arvilommi, P., Leppamaki, S., Isometsa, E.T.: Differences in axis I and II comorbidity between bipolar I and II disorders and major depressive disorder. J. Clin. Psychiatry **67**, 584–593 (2006)

A Cost-Sensitive Learning Framework
for Reducing 30-Day Readmission

Shaokun Fan[⊠] and Bin Zhu

College of Business, Oregon State University, Corvallis, OR 97331, USA

Background: Hospital readmissions are costly and have gained increasing attention from policy makers and healthcare providers. Recently, readmissions within 30 days of prior hospitalization are considered to be a focus for improvement of healthcare quality. In the United States, the 30-day readmission rate is estimated to be 18%. Readmissions are estimated to cost $17 billion annually for Medicare beneficiaries. Researchers believe that some of the readmissions can be avoidable if healthcare providers can improve healthcare processes via timely interventions. However, such interventions have not achieved the expected outcome yet in the healthcare industry. In 2016, the 30-day readmission rate has hit the historical high level and the US government will punish more than half of the nation's hospitals — a total of 2,597 — having more patients than expected return within a month.

Research Gap: Most of the existing studies on readmission rate mainly focus on whether readmissions can be predicted accurately. Various predictive models have been designed to accurately predict readmission risks of patients. It was hoped that patients with high risk of readmission will receive high attention from healthcare providers. For example, Amarasingham et al. (2015) proposed an automated model based on multivariable regression using only variables present on admission. Turgemen and May (2016) developed a hospital readmission predictive model, which enables controlling the tradeoff between reasoning transparency and predictive accuracy. They used a boosted C5.0 tree, as the base classifier, which was ensembled with a support vector machine (SVM), as a secondary classifier.

However, few approaches have taken the cost and effectiveness intervention into consideration. Without explicitly measuring the cost and benefit of certain intervention efforts, it is hard for healthcare provider optimally allocate their limited resources. For example, considering the following two confusion matrixes as the results from two prediction algorithms (Tables 1 and 2), it is obvious that Algorithm B outperforms Algorithm A in terms of accuracy. Assume an intervention program that helps prevent readmission cost about $500 each person and each readmission will cost $10,000. If a hospital provides such an intervention program to patients with predicted high readmission risk, Algorithm A would be able to cut the cost down 50%.

Table 1. Confusion Matrix for Algorithm A (Accuracy = 83% Cost = 350,000)

Actual	Predicted		
		Positive	Negative
	Positive	100 (Cost = 0)	25 (Cost = 10000)
	Negative	200 (Cost = 500)	1000 (Cost = 0)

© Springer International Publishing AG 2017
H. Chen et al. (Eds.): ICSH 2017, LNCS 10347, pp. 299–300, 2017.
https://doi.org/10.1007/978-3-319-67964-8

Table 2. Confusion Matrix for Algorithm B (Accuracy = 87% Cost = 800,000)

	Predicted		
Actual		Positive	Negative
	Positive	50 (Cost = 0)	75 (Cost = 10000)
	Negative	100 (Cost = 500)	1100 (Cost = 0)

To fill this gap, we propose a cost-sensitive learning framework to lower the cost of intervention to reduce readmission and improve patient outcome. The cost-sensitive learning is a type of learning that considers the different costs of different types of misclassifications, which is especially important for healthcare because prevention care are usually much cheaper than hospitalization. The goal is to minimize the total cost.

Data: We collected data about patient admission records that contain a diagnosis code for CHF from five hospitals located in Oregon State starting in the past 10 years. Our data records contains 72,164 patients without readmission and 7,794 patients with readmission. For each patient, we collected information about his or her demographics, hospital encounters, doctor diagnoses, social history, etc. Figure 1 shows the cost and benefit of using predictions results generated by three algorithms. The Neural networks model obtains the highest accuracy, but the CHAID tree model is the best in terms of cost savings (assume False positive cost is $500 and false negative cost is $10,000).

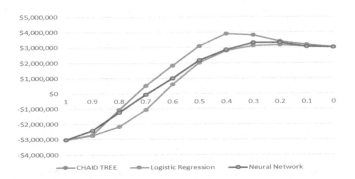

Fig. 1. Cost of three prediction algorithms in the dataset

Methods: Cost-sensitive learning can be categorized into two categories: direct method and wrapper method. The direct method is to design classifiers that are cost-sensitive in themselves (e.g., cost-sensitive decision tree (Ling et al. 2004)). The other category is to design a "wrapper" that converts any existing cost-insensitive classifiers into cost-sensitive ones (e.g., MetaCost (Domingos 1999)). In this research, we will apply different cost-sensitive learning methods to the data and compare the performance of different methods. We will also try to improve the existing cost-sensitive methods to help hospitals make optimal decision based on their available resources.

Author Index

Printed in the United States
By Bookmasters